Readings in
Community-
Based
Nursing

Roberta Hunt, RN, MSPH
Assistant Professor, Nursing
The College of Saint Catherine
St. Paul, Minnesota

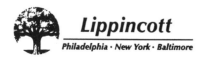

Lippincott
Philadelphia · New York · Baltimore

Acquisitions Editor: Susan M. Glover, RN, MSN
Editorial Assistant: Hilarie Surrena
Project Editor: Nicole Walz
Senior Production Manager: Helen Ewan
Production Coordinator: Mike Carcel
Design Coordinator: Brett MacNaughton
Manufacturing Manager: William Alberti
Indexer: Victoria Boyle
Compositor: PRD Group, Inc.
Printer: R. R. Donnelley

9 8 7 6 5 4 3 2 1

Library of Congress Cataloging-in-Publication Data

Hunt, Roberta.
  Readings in community-based nursing / Roberta Hunt.–1st ed.
    p. cm.
  Includes bibliographical references and index.
  ISBN 0-7817-2081-8 (alk. paper)
    1. Community health nursing. 2. Public health nursing. I. Title.

RT98 .H864 2000
610.73'43—dc21   99-058099

Care has been taken to confirm the accuracy of the information presented and to describe generally accepted practices. However, the authors, editors, and publisher are not responsible for errors or omissions or for any consequences from application of the information in this book and make no warranty, express or implied, with respect to the content of the publication.

The authors, editors, and publisher have exerted every effort to ensure that drug selection and dosage set forth in this text are in accordance with current recommendations and practice at the time of publication. However, in view of ongoing research, changes in government regulations, and the constant flow of information relating to drug therapy and drug reactions, the reader is urged to check the package insert for each drug for any change in indications and dosage and for added warnings and precautions. This is particularly important when the recommended agent is a new or infrequently employed drug.

Some drugs and medical devices presented in this publication have Food and Drug Administration (FDA) clearance for limited use in restricted research settings. It is the responsibility of the health care provider to ascertain the FDA status of each drug or device planned for use in his or her clinical practice.

To my mother, Ila Hunt Harris,
for her encouragement throughout the years.

Preface

The changing health care delivery system presents new challenges for contemporary nurses. Schools of nursing are struggling with the best way to restructure curriculum to meet current needs and give students experience in a variety of clinical settings that will prepare them for their careers in the diversified field of nursing. This textbook is designed to fill such a need. The foundational concepts in this text spring from the author's experience in more than 17 years of teaching community health, in both associate and baccalaureate nursing programs.

The idea for this textbook originated from a course developed by the author in 1983. The course, entitled "The Nurse in the Community," was designed in anticipation of the impact on nursing of the 1983 federal legislation, which implemented a prospective payment system for Medicare. Soon after, a course manual was developed which, along with the National League for Nursing 1993 recommendations in a "Vision for Nursing Education," became the basis for the first text by the author, *Introduction to Community Based Nursing*. Primarily intended for nursing curricula which offer community content in a distinct course, and secondarily for an integrated curriculum that threads community concepts throughout, *Introduction to Community Based Nursing* only partially met the need for textbooks in this area of nursing.

There was a need for a book primarily intended for those in nursing programs and majors where community content was integrated throughout the curriculum. An anthology addresses this glaring need, providing a variety of perspectives within a broad framework of community-based care. Further, *Readings in Community-Based Nursing* can be used in the very beginning of a nursing major or program to introduce students to community concepts, throughout a sequence of courses in an integrated curriculum or for a distinct course.

Delivery of health care in the community is changing with astounding speed, making it a challenging and exhilarating time to be a nurse. It is my hope that this anthology provides an inspiring introduction to the concepts, populations, and skills necessary for the nurse to find his or her niche in community-based nursing.

Acknowledgments

I am grateful to many individuals, especially family, friends, and colleagues, for their encouragement and assistance in the development of this textbook. Thanks to Kathleen Kalb for her exemplary editorial assistance, Marva Thurston for help choosing some of the articles, and Cyndi Winslow, for assisting with the photography. To all of my colleagues at the College of St. Catherine: Susan, Jean Marie, Linda, Marva, Suellen, Brenda, Barbara, Kathleen, JoAnne, Romana, Mary, Carol, Kaye, Cathy, Pam, Pat, Terri, Angela, Karen, Deb, Vicki and Alice, the most professional and supportive faculty group an educator could ever hope to work with, thanks for the daily sustenance. A special thanks to Susan Glover, Senior Editor at Lippincott Williams & Wilkins, for her ongoing encouragement.

Thanks to my family and friends who provide day-to-day support and encouragement. I especially would like to thank Meg Carolan and Sue Larson for their ongoing friendship and listening ear. Thanks to my family for encouragement, especially Becky Hunt Carmody, Ila and John Harris and Steve Hunt. To my terrific sons, Andy and Mark, who provide humor and balance in my life. Thanks to my wonderful daughters, Jackie and Megan, who are the light of my life and provide counsel and positive energy on a daily basis. Most of all, I am grateful to my loving husband, Tim Heaney, because without your committed attitude towards me and our children, I wouldn't be able to complete projects like this book.

Contents

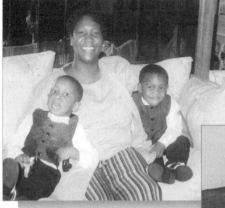

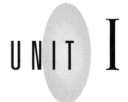

Basic Concepts of Community- Based Nursing

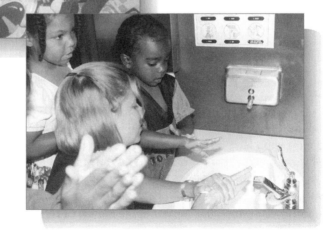

I n the last 15 years a major transformation in health care delivery has dictated that health care providers render care to not only ill but also well clients and families in a variety of diverse settings. These changes occurred as a result of cost containment efforts, which restructured the system for reimbursement of care. Increased participation from a better-informed consumer also created major reorganization in the delivery of health care. This evolution prescribed more emphasis on community-based care.

DEFINING THE ROLE OF THE NURSE

As health care delivery was transformed at an escalating pace, so to was nursing care. Care, which was once only provided in acute care settings, became routine in community settings. This dramatic paradigm shift created implications for all aspects of nursing. With this transformation, two significant questions arose about the practice of nursing in the future: who will provide care in community settings and what will be the focus of this care? In 1993, the National League for Nursing (NLN) addressed both of these questions in *A Vision for Nursing Education*.

In response to the questions who should practice in community settings, the NLN recommended that nurses at all educational levels be prepared to practice in community settings. This was a dramatic deviation from the traditional position that only nurses with a baccalaureate degree were qualified to practice in community settings. Before the early 1990s, distinctions between levels of practice were clear, but distinguishing roles and responsibilities became increasingly difficult. Confusion arose between community-based nursing and community health nursing, not only with definitions and philosophy, but also with goals and scope of practice. Numerous questions arose within the profession and the service community.

Secondly, the NLN addressed the question of the focus of care in community settings in the future. Their recommendations included:

1. The individual and the family have primary responsibility for health care decisions.
2. Health and social issues are acknowledged as interactive.
3. Treatment effectiveness, rather than the technologic imperative, drives decision-making.

Community-based nursing can be defined as nursing care directed toward specific individuals and families within a community. It is designed to meet needs of people as they move between and among health care settings. This level of care is possible only when health care providers are committed to collaboration and continuity. Thus, a new philosophy of care has emerged. In this textbook this new philosophy of practice will be defined as reflecting the components of:

- Self-care
- Preventive care within the context of the family, culture, and community

- Collaboration
- Continuity of care

SELF-CARE

An essential component of community-based nursing is self-care. Self-care charges the individual client and family with primary responsibility for making health care decisions and actions. Because clients are discharged earlier and sicker from the acute care setting, extended health care must be provided in the home. Often the costs associated with care provided by professionals is expensive, resulting in insurance and other reimbursement not covering care provided by health care providers in the home. Consequently, the client and family must assume responsibilities for self-care.

In discharge planning, for example, the role of the nurse in self-care includes teaching a diabetic client wound care based on the client's potential for performing his or her own care. This may involve assessing the client's knowledge base as well as evaluating the client's level of motivation regarding all aspects of self-care. A second example illustrating self-care is seen as the home care nurse assesses, plans, and evaluates the self-care abilities of the spouse of a client with cancer who is home with a central line. This nurse must determine how much care the spouse is reasonably able to provide. In all settings, nurses assess the client's ability to follow complex treatment regimens, intervening only as necessary. Promoting self-care requires that nurses be knowledgeable about outcome planning, intervention and evaluation, the teaching-learning process, and supportive techniques for ongoing care.

CARE WITHIN THE CONTEXT OF THE FAMILY AND CULTURE IN COMMUNITY-BASED NURSING

Another component of community-based nursing recognizes that health and social issues are interactive. The family is the basic social unit in American society. The client and family are closely interrelated in that the health of the client affects the family and the health of the family affects the client. Culture profoundly influences beliefs about health and family. The community where one resides affects health and access to health care. Nursing care is provided while considering the culture, values, and resources of the client, the family, and the community.

As the family is the basic social unit in American society, the family is also the most influential and dynamic unit. The family has been the primary focus of nursing care in the community since the establishment of public health nursing in the late 19th century. The family performs a variety of key functions and has a central role in promoting and maintaining the health of its members. If family members want to participate in the client's care but their skills restrict their ability to do so, the nurse will accommodate these requests within the constraints of time and safe care. Care within the context of the family is an essential component to community-based nursing care.

CULTURALLY SENSITIVE CARE IN COMMUNITY-BASED CARE

Just as the family is the basic social unit in American society, culture affects all areas of the client's life, including beliefs about health and illness. Culturally competent care that was once considered superfluous is today demanded by clients, families, and advocates as an essential component of health care. Consequently, nurses must consider cultural values in planning effective, individualized care.

For example, if the client requests a particular religious or social ceremony before a procedure, the nurse attempts, within the constraints of safety, to comply with this request. If the client lives in a community in which older individuals enjoy the social functions of religious services every week, the visiting nurse honors that community value by carefully scheduling visits. Nurses working in community-based care must consider cultural values, beliefs, and practices in planning effective and culturally competent nursing care.

Providing culturally sensitive care is complicated and challenging. Nurses must begin by identifying their own values and beliefs. Many times each of us may do things and not even know or think about why we do them the way we do. For example, consider the old story about a little girl watching her mother make a cake. As the little girl watches she asks her mother, "Mommy, why do you always put a pan of water on the bottom shelf of the oven when you make a cake?" The mother replies, "because that's the way Grandma made a cake." The little girl calls her Grandmother and asks, "Mommy says that she always puts a pan of water in the oven when she makes a cake because you always did that. Why do you put a pan of water in the oven when you bake a cake?" The grandmother responds, "I don't know why your mother does that, but I do it because my oven isn't level and the pan of water levels it out."

Many things we do and believe are based on what we learned and saw in our own families and communities. As we learn to understand our own values and beliefs, particularly as they relate to health, it becomes easier to understand and appreciate the cultural values and beliefs of others.

CONTINUITY OF CARE

Fragmentation of care has long been a concern of health care professionals. For instance, a client with a variety of problems may be seen by multiple health care providers, such as a family nurse practitioner, an internal medicine physician, a cardiologist, an endocrinologist, a social worker, an occupational therapist, and a surgeon. When health care providers do not communicate and collaborate with one another, fragmentation of care can result in conflicting directions for care, over- or undermedication, and a confused, frustrated client and family.

Further, there are tremendous external and internal pressures on the health care industry to control costs. Continuity of care saves money by reducing the number of visits to the emergency room and clinic, as well as hospital readmissions. Continuity of care creates a bridge to cost-effective, quality care; it is also the glue that holds community-based care together.

DISEASE PREVENTION AND HEALTH PROMOTION

Americans are moving from a narrow concept of health as the absence of disease to a broader definition that encompasses wellness and issues of quality of life. The consumer movement advocating increased participation in actively promoting wellness has resulted in the health promotion movement. Settings for practice have evolved as nurses focus on health rather than on disease and illness. Nursing has taken on a new look as it assumes the role of health promotion and illness prevention.

Health promotion has always been an essential component of the nurse's role. In the current environment emphasizing cost containment, reimbursement for health promotion activities by nurses has become increasingly difficult to procure. However, as a society we cannot afford not to continue to emphasize health promotion.

COLLABORATION

Collaboration between health care providers, whether disciplinary or interdisciplinary, is a foundation to the continuity of care. Although individual providers may be focused on a particular specialty, each provider must share information and evaluate the client's progress. Increased interaction among disciplines also generates more interdisciplinary referrals and encourages collaborative practice. If a single care provider in the chain of collaboration fails to communicate with the other providers, continuity is weakened and ultimately the quality of care is diminished. Interdisciplinary collaboration contains costs and maximizes effective interventions promoting the health of clients, families, and communities.

COMMUNITY-BASED NURSING CARE

The major paradigm shift from care in the acute care setting to community-based care dictates a major emphasis be placed on community-based care. For nurses this translates to a change in philosophy of practice. This philosophy requires that the nurse center care around the concepts of self-care and preventive care be directed toward specific individuals and families within the context of a culture and community. Continuity of care as well as collaboration are additional concepts essential to community-based care.

In 1993, the National League for Nursing (NLN) mandated inclusion of community content for all educational levels of nursing. Confusion arose between community-based nursing and community health nursing, not only with the definition and philosophy, but also with the goals and scope of nursing practice in the community. This article takes a giant leap in articulating the differences.

What is community-based nursing? What is community health nursing? What are the goals, clients, philosophical underpinnings, client characteristics, types of service, and service focus of each? What are the similarities and differences between community-based and community health nursing?

Zotti, M., Brown, P., & Stotts, R. (1996). Community-based nursing versus community health nursing: What does it all mean? Nursing Outlook, 44(5), 211–217.

Community-Based Nursing Versus Community Health Nursing: What Does It All Mean?

MARIANNE E. ZOTTI, PAUL BROWN, R. CRAIG STOTTS

With policy makers calling for the development of community-based, culturally appropriate, and comprehensive health care systems, it has become necessary for U.S. nursing schools to develop curricula and provide clinical experiences in community-based nursing. Articulating the differences between community-based and community health nursing practice is a necessary first step in improving any nurse's ability to care for individuals, families, and communities.

Today, perhaps more than at any other time, professional nursing is being challenged to actively participate in the development of cost-effective, high-quality, innovative systems of care that are accessible to all citizens. In this dynamic atmosphere of health care reform, policy makers are calling for the development of community-based, culturally appropriate, comprehensive health care delivery systems. Thus nurse educators need to prepare themselves and their students to practice in an increasingly community-oriented health care industry. The National League for Nursing, which accredits nursing schools, describes this phenomenon as ". . . realigning our [professional] allegiance and accountability away from institutions and toward populations."[1]

Marianne E. Zotti is an associate professor and chair of the Community, Psychiatric/Mental Health, and Gerontology Department of the College of Nursing at the University of Arkansas for Medical Sciences, Little Rock.

Paul Brown is an associate professor in the College of Nursing at the University of Arkansas for Medical Sciences, Little Rock.

R. Craig Stotts is an associate professor in the College of Nursing at the University of Arkansas for Medical Sciences, Little Rock.

Because of this realignment, the skills associated with community-based care need to be emphasized equally or to a greater extent than the more traditional tertiary care skills in nursing curricula.[2] In addition to the institutional-based primary, secondary, and tertiary skills usually taught in nursing schools, nursing students must master assessment skills that address the needs of individuals and families, their in-home and work environments, and the communities in which they live.

What does community-based care mean? What is entailed in community-based nursing (CBN)? Is CBN simply moving nursing as we have always known it to a new setting (i.e., the community)? How does CBN relate to community health nursing (CHN)? Does community-based care mean that we are expecting nurses in all specialties to become community health nurses?

We contend that CBN and CHN differ dramatically. Furthermore, we believe that CBN requires skills different from those previously required for institutionally based nursing. To demonstrate these differences, we have created two practice models, one illustrating CBN and one depicting CHN, for baccalaureate-prepared nurses. These models demonstrate a difference in overall goals, clients, underlying philosophies, autonomy, roles, service focus, types of service, and activities.

● DEFINITIONS

Community-based Nursing

In this article, the term "CBN" means a philosophy of nursing that guides nursing care provided for individuals, families, and groups wherever they are, including where they live, work, play, or go to school. CBN is characterized by an individual and family-centered orientation, the development of partnerships with clients, and an appreciation of the values of the community. According to this definition, CBN is not a specialty in nursing but a philosophy that guides care in all nursing specialties.

Community Health Nursing

In this article, the term "CHN" is synonymous with "public health nursing." Therefore, the definition incorporates writings from the Public Health Nurse Section of the American Public Health Association, 1980 and 1996, and the Council of Community Health Nurses of the American Nurses Association (1986).

CHN represents a systematic process of delivering nursing care to improve the health of an entire community. Although CHN may deliver care to individuals and groups, it is primarily responsible for the health of the population as a whole, with special emphasis on identification of high-risk aggregates. CHN practice synthesizes nursing theory and public health science and places priority on prevention, protection, and promotion.[3,4] CHN is a specialty in nursing.

● PRACTICE MODELS

Table 1-1 shows our conceptualization of the practice of CBN and CHN. A description of each section of the table follows.

Goals

Community-based nursing. The goal of CBN is to manage acute or chronic conditions while promoting self-care among individuals and families. In CBN the nurse may be

TABLE 1-1 ● Practice Models of CBN and CHN		
Model Component	*CBN*	*CHN*
Goals	Manage acute or chronic conditions Promote self-care	Preserve/protect health Promote self-care
Client	Individual and family	Community
Underlying philosophy	Human ecological model	Primary health care
Autonomy	Individual and family autonomy	Community autonomy Individual rights may be sacrificed for good of community
Client character	Across the lifespan	Across the lifespan with emphasis on high-risk aggregates
Cultural diversity	Culturally appropriate care of individual and families	Collaboration with and mobilization of diverse groups and communities
Type of service	Direct	Direct and indirect
Home visiting	Home visitor	Home visitor
Service focus	Local community	Local, state, federal, and international

meeting an acute need, but her/his goal is to enhance the individual or family's capacity for self-care. Because of its emphasis on enhancing self-care capabilities for individuals and families, this goal differs from past goals of episodic care in an acute care institution.

Community health nursing. The primary goal of CHN is to help a community protect and preserve the health of its members; the secondary goal is to promote self-care among individuals and families. In the health care reform environment, CHN will probably continue to include care for individuals and families, particularly for high-risk clients and those with communicable diseases.

Clients

Community-based nursing. Even though the individual is the client in CBN, nursing care must be family centered. The nursing of individuals within the context of the family (which is appropriate in an acute care institutional setting) is not the same as family-centered nursing. Within the institutional setting, nurses provide services and make priorities on the basis of client need, providers' schedules, and institutional practices. Families usually help in decision-making and teaching, but family-centered care is generally not the goal. "Family centered" means that the nurse believes in enhancing the competencies of families and designs her/his care in ways that are driven by families' needs and decisions.[5,6] The diversity among families and their values, beliefs, and coping styles are respected, accepted, and honored by nurses who provide family-centered care. Interventions, which are designed with the family, reflect agreed-upon strategies and support services. Family-centered care promotes family autonomy, enhancement of family competencies, and involvement of families in planning, implementation, and evaluation of services. Family-centered care is necessary in the community because most clients live and may be served in their homes, spend most of their time with their families, and depend on the family or other support members for most of their care and advocacy. Furthermore, because CBN services to families in the community may take a different form than institutionally based services of the past, family input is critical for the appropriate design and evaluation of services.

Community health nursing. In CHN the client is clearly the community, although the baccalaureate-prepared public health nurse may deliver care to individuals, families, and aggregates.[7–12] When community health nurses deliver care to these groups, they are evaluating the community to determine if conditions are signs of "immediate crises, enduring problems, or impending crises"[13] in the community. The responsibility of CHN extends beyond the individual client and family to the population as a whole for "preventive health services, health protection, and health promotion."[4]

Underlying Philosophy

Community-based nursing. The human ecological model, which underlies the CBN philosophy,[14–17] was first developed to describe effects on child development and now describes human development throughout the course of life.[17] This systems model consists of ecological units (social networks) that are represented by concentric circles, with each circle demonstrating social systems and units that affect or are affected by human development. The innermost circle, the "microsystem," contains the individual and the immediate family, who interact in a given setting. The second circle, the "mesosystem," consists of "interrelations among two or more settings in which the developing person actively participates."[14] Examples of the mesosystem include extended family and friends, human service programs, and neighborhoods or work groups. The "exosystem," the third circle, comprises one or more settings in which the developing person does not participate, but that affect or are affected by the developing person. Examples of the exosystem are local community values and policies. The outermost circle, the "macrosystem," consists of large social systems such as state and national government values and policies. The central tenet of the human ecological model is that "social units and their members do not act in isolation, but rather interact both within and between levels. . . ."[16]

The human ecological model underpins CBN because the nurse provides care wherever the client lives, works, and plays. The client will be interacting constantly with social networks in any of the human ecological model's concentric circles. Furthermore, what happens in each of these systems will affect the behavior of the client, directly or indirectly, and the client's behavior may affect any of these systems. The nurse needs to understand the client in terms of the many systems within which all individuals interact daily to provide holistic care to the individual and family in the community setting.

Community health nursing. The underlying philosophy for CHN is primary health care as defined by the World Health Organization.[18,19] Primary health care guarantees a minimum level of basic (essential) health care for all people. Four assumptions support the philosophy of primary health care:[18–24]

1. Health is a political and social right. Equity is fundamental and universal coverage is the norm, with care provided according to need.

2. The community as a whole, rather than the individual, is the client, and the community determines its greatest priority and resources allocation in health care. Thus the overall public good is promoted, but needs of individuals may go unmet.
3. Because conditions in many sectors of communities affect health, multisectoral cooperation is necessary to promote, maintain, or improve the health of the community.
4. The philosophy of primary health care can be applied to any country or community on the globe.

In CHN, primary health care services are essential, accessible, affordable, and acceptable to the people in the community. Furthermore, CHN emphasizes health promotion and disease prevention and promotes self-reliance. Essential elements of primary health care include health promotional activities, protective measures, and services to individuals and families. Health promotional activities include education about prevailing health problems and promotion of proper nutrition with an adequate and safe food supply. Basic sanitation and provision of adequate and safe water, immunizations against major infectious diseases, and control of endemic diseases are protective measures. Individual and family services include maternal and child health services, appropriate treatment of common diseases and injuries, and provision of essential basic household drugs.

Autonomy

Community-based nursing. The principles of family-centered care support individual and family autonomy in making decisions.[5,6] Nursing care provided in the community setting promotes this autonomy.

Community health nursing. CHN also promotes autonomy of the individual and family. However, CHN also adheres to the public health tenet that promotes the greatest good for the greatest number,[3] which may result in the sacrifice of individual and family rights for the common good. Examples include mandatory immunizations to control the spread of communicable diseases, restrictions on smoking to decrease effects of passive smoke on community members, and motorcycle helmet laws to protect individuals from injury and society from the costs associated with head injuries.

Client Character

Community-based nursing. In CBN the emphasis is limited to care of the individual and the family across the lifespan. In fact, if one uses a family-centered approach in CBN, the nurse would simultaneously be working with all members of the family, regardless of age. The community-based nurse might identify individuals and families who need care as they move from one ecological unit to another (e.g., the patient moving from hospital to home), or clients might be referred to the community-based nurse (e.g., a newly diagnosed client with a severe illness who comes to an ambulatory clinic). Community-based nurses may serve their clients in a variety of settings, such as specialty ambulatory clinics, home health agencies, and managed care organizations. Because CBN can enhance compliance with medical regimens and positively affect client outcomes, CBN may be supported by managed care systems or government programs.

Community health nursing. CHN has always involved care of individuals across the life-span and family-centered nursing. However, CHN also involves the identification of high-risk aggregates in the community and the development of appropriate policies and interventions to ensure accessible services for these groups.

Cultural Diversity

Both CBN and CHN emphasize sensitivity to cultural diversity issues. To be therapeutic, the nurse must acknowledge and value cultural differences and incorporate them into plans for care. In CBN, the nurse must be able to interact on a one-to-one basis with individuals and families of diverse ethnic or cultural backgrounds in a way that indicates respect for that culture and yields a mutually satisfactory exchange between nurse and client. In CHN, the nurse must have cross-cultural skills and be able to work with culturally diverse groups and organizations. Whether it is La Raza Unida, the National Association for the Advancement of Colored People (NAACP), or the Knights of Columbus, the nurse must involve each relevant community group in working on a particular community health problem and maintain their trust that each association's members will benefit from cooperation in joint community efforts.

Type of Service

BN and CHN involve direct service to individuals and families, but CHN also involves indirect services that can influence the health of clients. These indirect services include working with community leaders, being involved in relevant social action, promoting regulation or enforcement, and promoting health policy consistent with scientific knowledge.

Home Visiting

CHN has a longer nursing tradition in home environments than does CBN. CHN developed when nurses cared for the sick individual in his or her home. Thus, as the art and science of CHN evolved, it emphasized the home environment, the family, and client responsibility for health.

CBN, on the other hand, which is a product of recent times, has evolved from an acute care hospital orientation. Family involvement and client responsibility have been addressed by CBN but in a more peripheral manner than in CHN. However, both CBN and CHN involve visiting individuals and families in their homes and employ identical skills, such as environmental assessment. The primary change regarding home visiting lies in the education of nurses (i.e., all nurses, regardless of academic preparation, will need to develop home visiting skills). Furthermore, as educators develop community-based experiences across the curriculum, nursing students will need to learn home visiting skills early in their curriculum.

Service Focus

The primary focus of CBN is the client's immediate environment (the local community) and its impact on the health of individuals and families. In CHN, the nurse focuses on broader environmental and population-based factors that affect the health of communities. Therefore, the foci of CHN necessarily involve the local community, state, federal, and even international influences on health and health services.

Levels of Prevention

Figure 1-1 shows our estimation of the emphasis that each type of nursing places on the various levels of prevention. CBN places a much heavier emphasis on secondary and tertiary prevention, whereas primary prevention constitutes the largest proportion of CHN activities. Primary prevention, such as an immunization, means to prevent a problem before it occurs.[10] Secondary prevention involves early detection and treatment; examples include scoliosis screening and treatment. Tertiary prevention, such as cardiac rehabilitation, involves correction of a health problem or activities to prevent further deterioration.

Because CBN is primarily focused on the individual and the family, persons who have health problems receive the most CBN services. Persons with health problems want to feel better, learn to cope with their illness, or at least minimize the consequences of their illnesses. Thus the bulk of practice will focus on secondary and tertiary preventive services.

In CHN, however, the nurse works with people who are generally well, able to go to work, and may not have symptoms requiring them to see a health care provider. Thus the bulk of CHN practice falls within primary and secondary prevention. Using primary prevention, the nurse might work at a community level to improve the quality of life through safe food or at an individual and family level by conducting classes on individual-appropriate exercise regimens. Using secondary prevention, the nurse might engage in screening activities such as health fairs for the community or case finding for communicable diseases for an individual or family.

While Figure 1-1 represents a typical amount of emphasis placed by nurses in each type of practice, we do not mean that this is the amount of time each nurse should spend in each area. In fact, the amount of time nurses spend in each area can vary greatly week by week, depending on the needs of their clients and communities. The practice model described in this article results in different roles in CBN and CHN. Table 1-2 shows these roles, as described below.

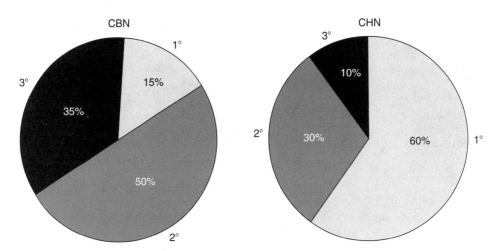

FIGURE 1-1. Levels of prevention used in CBN and CHN.

TABLE 1-2 ● Roles in CBN and CHN		
Roles	*CBN*	*CHN*
Client-delivery oriented		
Caregiver	X	X
Educator	X	X
Counselor	X	X
Advocator	X	X
Case manager	X	X
Group-oriented		
Leader	X	X
Change agent	X	X
Community advocate		X
Case finder		X
Community care agent		X

Roles

Roles may be divided into three groups: client oriented, delivery oriented, and group oriented.[25] Client-oriented roles involve direct service to clients, whereas delivery-oriented roles enhance service delivery to individuals and families. Nurses usually assume these two roles when providing services to individual or family clients. They assume group-oriented roles when working with community groups.

Client- and delivery-oriented roles. Client- and delivery-oriented roles, which include caregiver, educator, counselor, advocate, and case manager, may be similar in CBN and CHN. In CBN, the nurse is somewhat more likely to be a direct caregiver than in CHN, and the individual may need care for an acute or chronic condition. In both CBN and CHN, the nurse acts as an educator and counselor to promote enhanced self-care and serves as an advocate for the client and the family. The nurse assesses the client/family's needs and access to services and their effectiveness. Furthermore, the nurse determines the cause and solutions to problems while involving the client and the family. Traditionally, the nurse has served as case manager in CHN, but much of CBN also involves case management. In both CBN and CHN, the nurse may work in multidisciplinary and interdisciplinary teams in client- and delivery-oriented roles. These interdisciplinary teams could include a variety of partners, including physicians, social workers, nutritionists, pharmacists, and physical and occupational therapists.

Group-oriented. The primary difference between CBN and CHN involves the group-oriented roles. The roles of leader and change agent involve the same skills but different places and clients in CBN and CHN. For example, the community-based nurse might serve as a change agent in a managed care organization to change the package of services to clients with a specific diagnosis. The community health nurse might identify a group of people in the community who are at high risk for developing the same diagnosis, conduct screenings among the high risk group, and lobby for legislation to decrease exposures that predispose people to develop this diagnosis.

In CHN, however, the nurse has more group roles, that is, community advocate, case finder, and community care agent, which necessitate working in interdisciplinary teams. Community advocacy is practiced primarily in CHN. An advocate for the community knows what the community wants and needs and matches those needs with available resources.

The case-finder role is in the realm of CHN. Communicable disease control is primarily the responsibility of CHN. Although in CBN the nurse is responsible for reporting certain diseases to the health department (an important and essential element in disease control), this nurse typically has no other major responsibilities in this area. In CHN, the nurse is responsible not only for reporting diseases but also for helping to set up monitoring systems, educating providers about reporting, staying abreast of current epidemiological reports of disease outbreaks, and communicating this information to the public. The nurse in CHN also plans and implements programs to prevent disease outbreaks.

Another group-oriented role in CHN is that of community care agent.[25] The nurse may carry out this role through the core public health functions (i.e., assessment, policy development, and assurance).[13] In assessment, the nurse observes and records conditions in the community and participates in collecting and analyzing data about the community. The nurse also participates in the development of comprehensive health policies on the basis of scientific knowledge and uses the political process to actualize these policies. Two different types of activities are inherent in CHN.[3] "Engineering" means direct actions toward the management of risk by directly or indirectly managing variables in the environment. "Enforcement" involves more coercive measures that result in mandatory regulations to control risk. The nurse then participates in activities that assure that needed services are available. The assurance role can involve negotiations between agencies, development of regulations, or provision of services.

The proportion of time spent on any activity usually indicates the value the individual places on the activity. Nurses who spend significant periods of time on patient education, for example, can be implicitly imputed to have a high value for this activity. Both CBN and CHN have different valuing systems and patterns of service allocation. The following description and graphic of time allocation (Fig. 1-2) will illustrate the differences in these value systems.

Activities

Figure 1-2 depicts our estimation of the proportion of time spent on different categories of nursing service. As can be seen in Figure 2, substantial disparities in time allocations exist between CBN and CHN. In CBN, the largest time allotments are for case management, patient education, individual and family advocacy, and interdisciplinary practice. Together, these services account for 85% of the typical practice of CBN. In CHN, the services constituting the largest portions of time are case finding, patient education, and community development. Together, these services account for 45% of CHN practice. In CHN, the nurse also provides substantial services in program planning, implementation, and evaluation and community development. Thus, activities vary, depending on whether the nurse is practicing CBN or CHN.

● PRACTICE MODEL SUMMARY

We believe we have shown that CBN and CHN are different in practice, roles, and activities. Furthermore, we believe that CBN is different from institutionally based nursing as we have known it in the past. These differences require curricular changes in most schools of nursing. Our recommendations regarding curriculum follow.

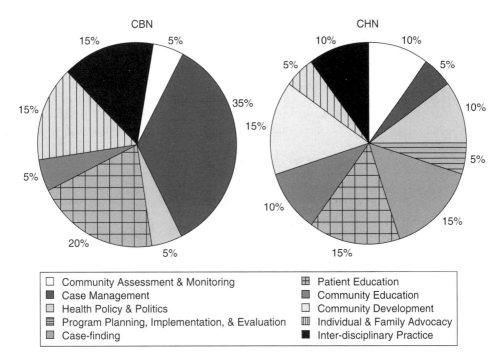

FIGURE 1-2. Proportion of time spent on category of nursing service.

Curriculum Recommendations

1. Include the philosophical base of the CBN human ecological model early in the curriculum. This philosophical base will enable students to view individuals, families, and environments together and understand nursing care of clients wherever they are. Educators can then easily teach the philosophy of primary health care in the CHN course.
2. Revise foundational courses to include content necessary for community-based experiences. Necessary content includes family theory, the tenets of family-centered care, community resources, principles of case management, roles and responsibilities in interdisciplinary teamwork, and principles of home visiting.
3. Expose students to community-based experiences early in the curriculum, with increasing responsibility and independence as the student progresses through the curriculum. Student progression should involve being an observer, participant, and team leader.
4. Have students conduct home visits throughout the curriculum, beginning early in the curriculum. Again, the student should progress through observational experiences, home visits with instructors, and visits made alone or with other students. Instructors would accompany students only in the event of complex cases or to perform an evaluation.
5. Develop case management skills throughout the curriculum, beginning early in the curriculum. The practice of case management should require development

throughout the student's program, with an increasing amount of responsibility and independence as the student progresses.

6. Encourage and promote interdisciplinary teamwork throughout the curriculum. Nursing has natural team partners, such as medicine and social work; students can develop relationships with colleagues in these disciplines. Students need opportunities to work in teams during clinical courses to enable them to understand their roles as team members. If possible, assign them to work as teams in the clinical area, composing teams of all three disciplines whenever possible. Didactic content on groups may also be helpful.

7. Retain an appropriate proportion of institutional experiences for efficiency of teaching to allow students to experience the gamut of acuity in medical conditions. Recognize that institutions such as hospitals offer experiences with sick clients who have a variety of conditions. Students need these experiences to enable them to truly understand health and threats to health.

8. Revise CHN after incorporating CBN into the curriculum. Students are exposed to much of the necessary content for CBN during their CHN rotation, usually late in the curriculum; examples include principles of home visiting and content related to community resources. Often, students never make home visits until they reach CHN. Therefore, if educators revise the curriculum to incorporate these experiences early, students will come to CHN with much more sophisticated skills. CHN faculty can then focus on content that relates to nursing a community and emphasize other content such as community development or participation in community assessment.

● SUMMARY

These are exciting times in nursing, with great possibilities for reforming nursing as we now know it. The desired outcome is to improve any nurse's ability to care for individuals, families, and communities wherever they are. We believe that articulating CBN and CHN practice is a necessary first step in achieving this outcome; however, it now becomes our challenge to advance this vision. We ask you to join us in this endeavor.

REFERENCES

1. National League for Nursing. *A Vision for Nursing Education*. New York: The League, 1993.
2. Edwards JB. Consultation at College of Nursing, University of Arkansas for Medical Sciences, May 19, 1994. Little Rock (AR): 1994.
3. Salmon White M. Construct for public health nursing. Nurs Outlook 1982;30:527–30.
4. Spradley BW. Community health nursing: concepts and practice. Glenview (IL): Scott, Foresman/Little, Brown Higher Education, 1990.
5. Northeastern Early Intervention Faculty Training Institute: a model for statewide faculty training. Presented at the Northeastern Early Intervention Faculty Training Institute, Philadelphia: 1993.
6. St Denis GC, Jaros KJ. Family centered health care: a public health social work perspective. Pittsburgh (PA): National Maternal & Child Health Clearinghouse, 1990.
7. American Public Health Association. The definition and role in public health nursing in the delivery of health care: a statement of the public health nursing section. Washington, DC: The Association, 1981.
8. American Public Health Association. The definition and role in public health nursing in the delivery of health care: a statement of the public health nursing section. Washington, DC: The Association, 1996.

9. Muecke MA. Community health diagnosis in nursing. Public Health Nurs 1984;1:23–5.
10. Albrecht M, Swanson JM. Health: a community view. In: Swanson JM, Albrecht M, editors. Community health nursing: promoting the health of aggregates. Philadelphia: WB Saunders, 1993:3–12.
11. Williams CA. Community health nursing-what is it? Nurs Outlook 1977; 25:250–4.
12. Williams CA. Community-based population-focused practice: the foundation of specialization in public health nursing. In: Stanhope M, Lancaster J, editors. Community health nursing: process and practice for promoting health. St. Louis (MO): Mosby-Year Book, 1992:244—52.
13. Institute of Medicine. The future of public health. Washington (DC): National Academy Press, 1988.
14. Bronfenbrenner U. The ecology of human development, experiments by nature and design. Cambridge: Harvard University Press, 1979.
15. Chamberlin RW. Beyond individual risk assessment: community wide approaches to promoting the health and development of families and children. Washington (DC): The National Center for Education in Maternal and Child Health 1988.
16. Dunst CJ. Rethinking early intervention. Analysis Intervention Dev Disabilities 1985;5: 165–201.
17. Vasta R. Annals of child development. Greenwich: JAI Press, 1989.
18. World Health Organization. Primary health care: Alma-Ata Conference. Geneva (Switzerland): The Organization, 1978.
19. World Health Organization. From Alma-Ata to the year 2000: reflections at the midpoint. Geneva (Switzerland): The Organization, 1988.
20. Flynn BC. Public health nursing education for primary health care. Public Health Nurs 1984; 1:36–44.
21. Maglacas AM. Health for all: nursing's role. Nurs Outlook 1995;43:66–71.
22. McElmurry BJ, Swider SM, Watanakij P. Primary health care. In: Stanhope M, Lancaster J, editors. Community health nursing: process and practice for promoting health care. St. Louis (MO): Mosby-Year Book, 1992: 34–44.
23. Salmon M, Talashek M, Tichy A. Health for all: a transnational model for nursing. Int Nurs Rev 1988;4:107–9.
24. Ulin PR. Global collaboration in primary health care. Nurs Outlook 1989;37:134–7.
25. Clark MJ. Nursing in the community. Norwalk (CT): Appleton & Lange, 1996.

This article discusses some common misconceptions about community care. Rather than considering community-based care as a setting for practice, the author suggests community-based care purports a particular philosophy of care. The basic tenets of community-based care apply to all practice settings.

When did community care evolve to be an important aspect of all nursing care? Why did this transformation occur? What are the principles of community care that apply to all practice settings?

Hunt, R. (1998). Community-based nursing: Philosophy or setting? *American Journal of Nursing*, 98(10), 44–48.

Community-Based Nursing

Philosophy or Setting?

ROBERTA HUNT

How you practice is no longer defined by where you practice.

It's difficult to be a nurse right now; change, often unwelcome, is everywhere. As the need for nursing in acute care settings wanes, there has been a lot of discussion about the increasing demand for "nursing in the community." When you hear about this trend, you may say, "If I had wanted to work in the community, I would have become a public health nurse."

But the shift to community care has already happened, and in some respects the role of the staff nurse has evolved to emulate this exemplar. In *A Vision for the Future of Nursing Education,* the NLN [National League for Nursing] defined essential components of community care. These include patient self-care; prevention; consideration of family, culture, and community; and continuity of care through collaboration.

Although you may not realize it, many of your everyday work activities are based on these principles.

- When you teach a patient about wound care—preparing him to be in charge of his care at home—you're enhancing his self-care abilities.
- When your patient teaching addresses avoiding repeat hospitalizations or clinic visits, you're providing preventive care.
- When you assess a patient's physical and psychological needs, determining how much support and assistance his family can provide, you're planning care within the context of the patient's family, culture, and community.
- When you coordinate discharge planning among a diverse team of professionals, you're using a collaborative approach.

Roberta Hunt is an assistant professor at the College of St. Catherine in St. Paul, MN, and author of Readings in Community-Based Nursing and coauthor of Introduction to Community Based Nursing.

As you can see, providing care with an emphasis on community and home is not a new concept for nursing. Until about 100 years ago, nurses usually practiced in homes and provided health education in rural areas and urban neighborhoods. From the late 1800s to the end of World War I, the rapid expansion of hospital-based schools of nursing began a shift in the care of the sick from the community and home to acute care facilities. And in the early 1950s, advances in health care technology and the introduction of third-party insurance payers prompted further growth of hospital care—a trend that continued into the 1960s with the expansion of ICUs. Escalating costs in the 1980s, however, returned nursing care to the home and community.

● MISCONCEPTIONS ABOUT COMMUNITY CARE

When nursing moved to inpatient care, how we practiced depended on where we were employed. This is no longer true. Now, the way we practice is changing, though for most of us, the way we *think* about care in the community is not. Let's consider some common misconceptions.

- *There are two "types" of nurses, those working in the community and those working in hospitals.* Numerous nursing positions don't strictly adhere to the traditional inpatient or community health roles. In fact, nurses in the community work in nursing homes, ambulatory facilities, community clinics, schools, and occupational and public health settings. The number of RNs working in health maintenance organizations and physician- or nurse-based group practices rose 15% between 1988 and 1992, while the number of those in public or community health grew by 38%, largely because of a near doubling of home health care jobs.
- *Community-based nursing describes a setting for practice.* Community-based nursing describes a philosophy of care applicable to all nurses in all settings, reflecting how nursing care is provided–not *where*. It's directed toward individuals and families within any community setting, and is designed to assist patients as they move between and among health care settings. Meg Jervis, for example, is a nurse working in an assisted-living facility. She is in frequent contact with a resident, Shirley Greenblatt, as well as her daughter. In order to assure continuity of care, Meg met with the nurse practitioner from the nursing home where Ms. Greenblatt lived before her admission to the assisted-living facility. Meg's primary nursing interventions emphasized strengthening Ms. Greenblatt's self-care in a culturally and socially sensitive manner, by acknowledging and working within her kosher diet. Meg knows that through collaboration she will improve the quality of Ms. Greenblatt's recovery.
- *Nursing in the community requires skills and knowledge different from those needed in the acute care setting.* There are certainly differences between the nursing responsibilities and skills in the acute care and the community-based settings. Some of these differences arise from the long-standing philosophies associated with each. Practice in the acute care setting, where the patient is defined by disease or condition, typically takes place in specialized units where family access and patient autonomy are regulated by facility policies. Health is viewed as the opposite of illness, and the focus of care is to eliminate illness. Nursing activities are geared toward short-term interventions.

In the community setting, the patient is seen within the context of his family and social network, and is treated in his own environment, where he is naturally more at ease. Illness is seen as a part of life, and the purpose of care is to limit patient disability and to improve functional capacity and quality of life. Nursing practice has greater autonomy with therapeutic interventions, mutually defined by clinician and patient, that hold the patient's values central to his care.

Although the traditional values and ways we think about each area of practice differ, nursing in each does not require widely different skills and knowledge. In both settings, nurses apply principles of interpersonal communication to interactions with client, family, and other caregivers. Similarly, in each setting nurses use leadership skills to plan, organize, coordinate, delegate, and evaluate care of patients. And in both, nurses provide effective physical care.

● THE PRINCIPLES OF COMMUNITY CARE

Advocating self-care. The self-care component of community care gives to patients and families the primary responsibility for health care decisions and actions. Nurses assist in the monitoring of health teaching and treatment. In all settings, nurses assess the patient's ability to follow complex medication regimens, and intervene only as needed. In the hospital, promoting self-care includes teaching based on the patient's motivation and ability to care for himself.

Consider Donald Watson, a patient with diabetes admitted to your unit for treatment of a leg ulcer. During assessment, you find that Mr. Watson is conscientious about taking his insulin, though he admits he doesn't pay close attention to skin care. You plan his discharge instruction, stressing the importance of good wound and skin care, and you refer him to a home care nurse. Once discharged, the home health nurse will continue to instruct Mr. Watson about wound care between scheduled hospital or clinic visits. Outpatient clinics provide another context for self-care promotion. Rickie James, for example, has been caring for her husband since he was discharged home from an acute care facility with a central line. During the past two months, the line site has evidenced transient signs of infection. Considering this, you assess Ms. James's skill and knowledge about caring for the central line, and you discover that she has been using cotton swabs dipped in a coffee cup full of tap water to clean the site. You devote your time to providing additional instruction, demonstrating proper care, and helping Ms. James look for signs of infection and perform the care. Such instruction strengthens her skills.

Focusing on prevention. Community-based nursing considers three levels of prevention: primary, in which the initial occurrence of disease or injury is avoided; secondary, in which early identification of disease or injury—with prompt intervention—prevents (or limits) disability; and tertiary, which helps minimize deterioration and improve quality of life. Preventive care is essential in all settings.

Assessing Ms. James's understanding of IV line care, and your instruction, reflects primary prevention of infection. And the referral you made for a home care nurse to follow Mr. Watson's ability to perform self-care with the diabetic regimen supports adherence to the treatment plan. Such tertiary prevention eliminates further progress of the disease, thus improving Mr. Watson's quality of life despite his illness.

Family, culture, and community. Community-based nursing recognizes that health and social issues are interactive, and when planning care, the patient's culture, values, and all external and internal resources including social support and family are considered.

RELATED RESEARCH
Feasibility and Effects of Nurse-Run Clinics

The purpose of this study, conducted in England, was to ascertain if patients with epilepsy would be willing to attend nurse-run clinics, whether there would be a difference between nurses and general practitioners in amount of advice given and monitoring of medications, and if documentation of advice would differ.

Of 127 patients offered a first-time appointment with a nurse, 83% (106) kept it. Ninety-two percent of these patients kept a second appointment with the clinic nurse. At the second visit, there was a significantly higher percentage of patient blood levels monitored, medication management advice given, and documentation of advice recorded by the nurse in the clinic compared to the physician in the traditional general practice. The nurse suggested improvements in drug management for one-fifth of the patients. The majority of recommendations were for re-evaluation of medications or modification of dosages. Patient satisfaction was assessed, but not reported. The researchers suggest that other outcome data should be collected.

COMMENTARY: Although limited, this study is important, as it documents the feasibility of such clinics, and raises questions about outcome measurement. One that comes to mind is: Of the nurse's medication management recommendations, what percentage was acted upon by the general practitioners?

This research addresses issues that also concern nurse-run community clinics in America. It points to the need for further examination of nursing practice's influence in nurse-run community clinics on both short- and long-term clinical outcomes. Ideally, outcome and satisfaction data could be collected by the nurse practitioner as part of point-of-service charting.

Other questions that warrant further study are: Is there a need for a minimum data set related to these practices that could guide nurses in determining what information should be included in case documentation, and is there a standard nomenclature appropriate for tracking outcomes (for example, the OMAHA system)? Both a minimum data set and standardized language would provide a benchmark against which nurse-run clinics could measure themselves. When nurses venture into new practice areas, they have to be aware of the need for assessing their impact upon patients and their families.—*Abstract/commentary by Judith A. DePalma, director of nursing research, AUH-Allegheny General, Pittsburgh, PA*

Source: Ridsdale, L., et al. *Br. Med. J.* (314)120–122, 1997

Marcus Morton, the son of a patient with Parkinson's disease who receives care at the local community clinic, wants to help care for his mother, but he has limited psychomotor skills. The nurse in the clinic accommodates his request by arranging for him to assist his mother with her evening meal. In another case, a visiting nurse honors a patient's cultural traditions by carefully scheduling appointments around the time of her weekly prayer group.

Continuity of care. Patients with a variety of health problems are often treated by several providers. Such fragmentation can result in conflicting directions of care, over- or undermedication, and a confused patient. Continuity of care is essential as a patient moves from one health care practitioner and setting to another.

When Wendy Smith, a school nurse, was advised that a student was undergoing chemotherapy treatments, she contacted the child's primary clinician. They discussed nutritional interventions that Ms. Smith could introduce during school hours to help maintain the child's dietary demands.

The concepts of continuity can be applied to almost all tasks. For example, completing all transfer information on a discharge form helps the next caregiver pick up where you left off. By emphasizing continuity, you can reduce the detrimental effect of multiple health care providers and decreased length of hospital stay.

Collaborative care. Though individual providers may be specialty focused, each must share information and evaluate the patient's progress. If one person in the chain of collaboration fails to communicate, continuity is weakened. And often, it's the nurse who coordinates the communication. Collaborative care is an integral part of nursing responsibility, and though it may be easier to coordinate joint planning with professionals working in the same facility than it is for the home-care nurse working in the field, the benefit to the patient and family is immeasurably satisfying.

● THE COMMUNITY-BASED NURSING PHILOSOPHY

Providing care with a community focus brings us back to our professional roots. When you emphasize patient self-care; prevention; care within the context of family, culture, and community; continuity; and collaboration, you're participating in community-based nursing. It's about *how* we practice—not *where* we work.

SELECTED REFERENCES

Clarke, P. N., and Cody, W. K. Nursing theory-based practice in the home and community: The crux of professional nursing education. *Adv. Nurs. Sci.* 17:41–53, Dec. 1994.

Craven, R. F., and Hirnle, C. J. *Fundamentals of Nursing: Human Health Function,* 2nd ed. Philadelphia, Lippincott-Raven, 1996.

De Tornyay, R. Reconsidering nursing education: The report of the Pew Health Professions Commission. *J. Nurs. Educ.* 31:296–301, Sept. 1992.

Hunt, R., and Zureck, E. L. Introduction to *Community Based Nursing.* Philadelphia, Lippincott-Raven, 1997.

National League for Nursing. *A Vision for Nursing Education.* New York, NLN Press, 1993.

Shindul-Rothschild, J., et al. Where have all the nurses gone? Final results of our Patient Care Survey. *Am. J. Nurs.* 96(11):25–32, Nov. 1996.

Self-care is a major theme in current health care policy, primarily because self-care has been associated with cost benefits. The emphasis on self-care shifts accountability and responsibility for care activities to clients and their families. This article discusses how to help clients and families achieve, maintain, or promote maximal health.

What themes in current health care policy have contributed to the increased value placed on self-care? What are the goals of the self-care movement? How is self-efficacy related to self-care? How does Pender's Health Promotion Model describe factors that influence readiness and motivation to learn?

Bonny, B. (1997). A time for self-care: Role of the home healthcare nurse. *Home Healthcare Nurse*, 15(4), 281–286.

A Time for Self-Care: Role of the Home Healthcare Nurse

BARBARA J. BOHNY

The concepts of self-efficacy and self-responsibility in personal health provide the framework for developing cost-effective nursing strategies that have positive outcomes for the consumer and the provider. Promoting self-care requires that nurses be knowledgeable about outcome planning, the teaching-learning process, and supportive techniques for ongoing care. The concepts outlined in this article can be used to provide care for those who require health promotion, health maintenance, and illness management.

The challenge of managing the care of growing numbers of clients within a constantly evolving healthcare delivery system while holding down costs requires highly competent and sophisticated nurses. The need to ensure appropriate outcomes in the context of this change challenges nurses to involve clients and their significant others in the management of their care.

Opportunity and change are the order of the day. The new healthcare system is influencing nursing as well as the consumer of nursing services. Cost-containment has become a cherished priority for those who pay for healthcare (Iglehart, 1992). This places constraints on the delivery of home healthcare services. Capitated reimbursement is at hand in home healthcare (Kientz, 1996). Capitation is the per capita payment for providing a specific menu of health services to a defined population over a determined pe-

Barbara J. Bohny, DNS, RN, CS, is Associate Professor and Graduate Program Coordinator, The William Paterson College of New Jersey, Wayne, New Jersey.

riod. This payment is the same regardless of the amount of service rendered by the care provider (Sperger-Nearpass, 1994). A reduction in the amount of time required to deliver direct care will result in increased revenue for home care agencies. The limitations imposed by capitation and other aggregated units of reimbursement on healthcare providers and consumers bear heavily on the need to change our strategy in delivering home healthcare.

The focus on cost-effective care compels us to implement nursing strategies that will reduce costs to the providers of home healthcare services. Responsibilities and expectations of the provider and the consumer are changing dramatically. Healthcare consumers are sharing more of the costs of healthcare, and as a result, are demanding active involvement in the decisions about and delivery of personal healthcare. Consumers are becoming more knowledgeable about their bodies and are demanding better outcomes. There is an increased interest in health and wellness as evidenced by the growing number of fitness programs that have become popular with the public and endorsed by the payers of healthcare. Self-responsibility and self-determination are becoming the norm. This change is prompted by inaccessibility to care that is related to rising costs, the diminishing availability of resources, and a rediscovery of the benefits of self-care.

Community-based home healthcare delivery involves taking healthcare to the consumer, in the home and through various community agencies. Increased and expanded healthcare services are being delivered by nurses in the workplace, schools, homes, ambulatory settings, assisted living and long-term care facilities, shelters, and community gathering places.

Changing needs of the consumer and the public require a partnership rather than a relationship characterized by professional dominance. Professional nurses in home healthcare must learn to use methods that foster the transition to self-determination in the various population groups that they serve. This requires that the nurse relinquish control in healthcare interactions and adapt styles of nursing intervention to meet the diverse needs of the population.

Home health nursing is well poised to develop systems of care that reflect strategies for health promotion, health maintenance, and management of illness in providing care for community-based clients. Home healthcare nurses have historically focused on the right and responsibility of the patient and family to be included in the plan of care.

In today's healthcare system, increasing responsibility is placed on clients and their families for self-care. Self-care has always been a part of family life and home care practices. However, there has been a rebirth of the self-care movement due to the economics of healthcare, consumer discontent with depersonalized care, and desire to control outcomes of care. J. Everett Koop, MD (1996), former Surgeon General, believes that self-care will eventually become the "other healthcare system in this country." The home care nurses' role in facilitating the self-care initiative should be grounded in an understanding of the concepts related to self-care and their application to practice.

● SELF-CARE

Self-responsibility and self-care are major themes in current healthcare policy. During the past decade, there has been an enormous increase in public and professional interest in the significance of self-care in health (Koop, 1996). During the past 5 years, we have seen a burgeoning growth in the self-care theme. Amid sweeping changes in the U.S. healthcare system. Americans are growing more aggressive about making their own medical decisions. Individuals spend most of their lives actively involved in caring for themselves. The clients in the community therefore are familiar with the self-care practice. According to Orem (1991), "Self-care is a universal requirement for sustaining and enhancing life and health." The competence with which this task is accomplished determines the quality of life experiences and has a significant impact on longevity and cost-effectiveness in health-care delivery.

Increasing client responsibility and competency for healthcare may be the most effective, safe, and economical way of meeting health needs and relieving the demand on limited resources. The client is a primary resource within the healthcare system. It has been estimated that informal self-care constitutes 85% of all healthcare within the United States (Spellbring, 1991).

The goal of the self-care movement is to empower the public for increased control over their own health. Self-care for health promotion requires that clients gain knowledge and competencies that can be used to maintain, enhance, and restore health. Self-care, a universal requirement for sustaining and enhancing life and health, is an ongoing activity for individuals and an area of competence to be developed. Self-care directed toward health protection, promotion, and restoration can be defined as "activities initiated or performed by the individual, caregiver and/or family to achieve, maintain or promote health" (Pender, 1996).

Effective health education informs, motivates, and encourages behavioral change in the client. Implementing this process, the nurse assists in the adoption and maintenance of health behaviors that result in the achievement of competence in self-care. Caporeal-Katz (1983) have identified the following components of self-care education:

1. Provision of a period for expression of feelings
2. Reinforcement of client self-esteem
3. Provision of open access to information related to health
4. Practice of self-care skills that can be applied immediately by the client
5. Presentation of alternative views on health-related issues
6. Critical evaluation of traditional and alternative therapies

Competence in implementing activities related to care is part of self-care; however, self-care also includes actions directed toward minimizing threats to personal health, self-nurturance, self-improvement, and personal growth.

● SELF-EFFICACY

Self-efficacy, according to Bandura (1986), refers to belief in one's own capacity to perform the behaviors needed to control events affecting one's welfare. In the realm of self-care, self-efficacy links knowledge and action because belief in one's ability to assume self-care must occur before self-care can be attempted (Damrosch, 1991). According to self-efficacy theory, self-care will be initiated if clients perceive that: (1) certain behaviors will lead to desirable results and (2) they possess the ability to successfully engage in the behavior.

For example, a client may believe not only that engaging in a smoking cessation program will produce good results (i.e., improve breathing capacity), but also that the client has whatever it takes to succeed in the program. This individual is likely to join the program. Another client may not be sure that a smoking cessation program will really help because he or she has been smoking for many years; therefore, the client does not participate. A third client might be convinced the program will work but does not feel equipped with the willpower to engage in it, and thus, is unlikely to join the program. To be effective in promoting self-care, the home healthcare nurse, using a theoretical base of self-efficacy must:

1. persuade the client that a particular action will work;
2. teach the client to implement that action;
3. get the client to believe that he or she can perform the necessary activities;
4. attribute the desired outcomes to the client's actions; and
5. prompt the client to value the outcomes sufficiently to maintain the behavior.

● CLIENT READINESS AND MOTIVATION FOR SELF-CARE

One of the advantages of self-efficacy is the direction it provides in modifying the client's health behavior. Clients who feel effective are empowered to exercise increased control over their own health. When clients perceive themselves as active participants of care, they will more effectively control delivery of care.

Perception is the key to self-care. Perception of a particular state creates reality for an individual more than the objective features of the circumstances themselves (Nolan, 1990). To successfully assist the client through self-care education, the nurse must develop a mutual understanding of the values, beliefs, and perceptions that affect the client's health. Because perception is a thought process, it can be affected by learning.

Individual perceptions identified in Pender's Health Promotion Model that may affect readiness and motivation to learn self-care include:

- Importance of health: The value placed on health influences the desire to achieve it. Individuals who have determined what is important in their lives tend to make responsible decisions regarding their lifestyle.
- Perception of health control: Clients who perceive themselves to be in control of their own health status are more likely to be receptive, motivated, and active in acquiring information about self-care.
- Perceived self-efficacy: The client's desire for efficacy or competence in self-care must be taken into consideration by the nurse. In many instances, the desire for competence has been frustrated by a healthcare system that makes people feel dependent and helpless. The nurse must assess the extent of self-care responsibility the client can manage.
- Personal definition of health: The client determines the importance and value of health education content based on what health means to him/her.
- Perceived health status: Individuals who view themselves as healthy possess a higher motivation to engage in health-promoting behaviors than do individuals who view themselves as only moderately healthy.
- Perceived benefits and barriers of health-promoting behavior: These beliefs are based on previous life experiences, contact with mass media, and interactions with health professionals. Assessing the confidence of clients in the benefits of specific health behaviors and their perceptions of barriers will provide the nurse with information important in understanding individual responsiveness to self-care interventions (Pender, 1987).

Individuals' responses to self-care education are multidimensional and thus extremely complex. The client brings to the learning situation a unique personality, established social interaction patterns, cultural norms and values, and environmental influences. Selection of appropriate teaching strategies and self-care content must take into consideration the chronological, intellectual, and emotional maturity of the client. Education in self-care must take into account physical, sensory, mobility, sexual, and psychosocial changes related to age. Older persons may require verbal persuasion, challenges, and support before they will try to perform new behaviors. Understanding clients' lifetime patterns of coping may facilitate teaching them self-care.

Demographic factors also influence the process of self-care education. In working with individuals or families of varying ethnic backgrounds, attempts must be made to incorporate traditional cultural beliefs into health education for self-care. The process of self-care education must be adapted to cultural beliefs and attitudes. Simply translating materials into the language of another culture is not effective. Educational materials to be used for specific cultures should be prepared by, or in consultation with, people within the target culture. Income affects the health priorities of families and accessibility of resources needed to follow through with recommended self-care behaviors. Lower-income groups experience limitations in their potential for acquiring the assistance needed to develop self-care skills.

The components of the health education process for self-care include:

● assessing self-care competencies;
● determining teaching priorities;
● identifying long-term and short-term objectives;
● facilitating self-paced learning;
● using positive reinforcement;
● decreasing barriers to learning;
● creating a supportive environment for learning; and
● evaluating client progress (Pender, 1987).

Focusing on the daily activities of the client's world and setting daily goals presents an opportunity for determining dimensions of the client's self-efficacy expectations and potential for self-care.

This case study illustrates the wonderful opportunity that nurses have in the home care setting. Clients come into the healthcare system with dated perceptions. They must be shown the benefits of assuming a responsible role in restoring, maintaining, and promoting their own health. Home health nurses have an obligation to update these perceptions. It's conceivable that Julie would have taken the same passive role she had on earlier admissions. However, the nurse provided the necessary information to empower Julie and once again let her take control.

Julie demonstrated a readiness to assume responsibility for herself. Her nurse Rosemary recognized her readiness and took advantage of the opportunity to teach Julie the important aspects of her care. She prepared Julie for the worst of the side effects of the transplant protocol.

This motivated Julie to take charge of her care. Julie did not perceive the potential side effects as a barrier; instead, she saw them as a challenge. Rosemary focused on maximizing Julie's independence, vigor, and life satisfaction and provided Julie with the information necessary to survive the transplant protocol at home. Julie knew that a successful outcome depended on her. She was no longer a victim. Rather, Julie had assumed an active role in her own healthcare. Julie had prevented major setbacks for herself by following all the recommended tasks of the client protocol.

Case Study

Julie is a 44-year-old divorced woman who worked as a waitress for 20 years, with an active social life, good health, high energy, and a bad habit of hopping the bus to Atlantic City at least once weekly. Three years ago, Julie found a lump in her left breast. She ignored the lump until the pain was unbearable: her first admission to the hospital was for a left radical mastectomy. She refused follow-up chemotherapy and within the year Julie had a right radical mastectomy for invasive carcinoma in the right breast. After the second surgery, Julie underwent follow-up chemotherapy. Julie remembered little about this treatment. She saw herself as a victim. Julie returned to work, but within the year was found to have lesions across her rib cage and in the axillary area bilaterally. She was unable to raise her arms over her head and felt "rocks" under her arms. Reluctantly, she returned to her physician, who gave her two choices: to have a stem cell transplant or die from the disease. Julie chose to have a stem cell transplant believing that it would buy her more time.

Julie was admitted to the outpatient hospital at a Medical Center near her apartment. She also had visiting nurses from the local home care agency for home care. Julie recalled that a nurse from this agency, Rosemary, helped her accomplish self-efficacy. Before her encounter with Rosemary, Julie did not view herself as an active participant in her own care. She did not perceive her ability to participate because of her being overwhelmed by the diagnosis. Rosemary took the time to be with and teach Julie the principles of self-efficacy. The goal of using self-efficacy to teach self-care is to shift the balance of power to the client. The nurse convinced Julie, through building her self-esteem, that she could do a better job of maintaining her health than could anyone in the medical community. Julie accepted the offer. Before this, she believed that her healthcare had to be managed solely by the caregivers.

Julie had a Hickman catheter inserted in preparation for her treatment. She was taught about all aspects of her care. Although she knew how to care for the catheter, Julie had to depend on the nurses to do it because of the limited range of motion in her arms. Julie monitored the nurses closely when they manipulated her catheter and demanded that sterile technique be implemented. Julie adhered to a low-fat diet, was meticulous in her oral hygiene, avoided all sources of infection, kept her regularly scheduled visits to the outpatient hospital, and kept her visitors to a minimum. She had come to realize that she was in charge of her health, and that her actions could impact the outcome of her treatment. After 3 months, Julie was ready to undergo the stem cell transplant. Her disease seemed to be out of control, but Julie wasn't. She had surmounted the barriers to self-care. She believed she had some power to affect what was going to happen to her.

Julie began to speak of what she planned to do when the treatment was over. She focused only on the positive. She was a beacon of hope and a tribute to the nurse who inspired her to take charge of herself. Despite a leukocyte count of $100/mm^3$ of peripheral venous blood, Julie remained infection-free, with no stomatitis and no temperature spikes. Julie sought Rosemary's input on methods of approaching self-care techniques. Together they evaluated the alternatives in treatment regimens. She followed every recommendation offered and elected precautions of her own. Within 3 weeks, Julie's blood count returned to normal, and she was released from the program for follow-up at her physician's office. She came into the protocol with a potentially complicated case, but she sailed through the treatment. She is a fine example of the influence of self-efficacy on self-care behavior.

● SUMMARY

The nurse-client relationship in the home care setting reflects the many changes in the healthcare system. The home care nurse serves as a facilitator in promoting, improving, or restoring health to the client, with the goal of teaching the client to take responsibility for self-care. This is not an easy task. It demands expert salesmanship. Many nurses are more comfortable in "doing" for the client. The transition from the client's passive to active role demands that nurses be informed, consistent, and supportive.

Promoting self-care requires developing a comprehensive plan, teaching, and being available to the client. When this is done well, the nurse spends less time with the client because the client assumes responsibility for care. The nurse, by serving as a resource for the client, then is able to be available to more clients. Consequently, the costs for direct care activity are reduced.

REFERENCES

Bandura, A. (1986). *Social foundations of thought and action: A social cognitive theory.* Englewood Cliffs, NJ: Prentice-Hall, Inc.

Caporael-Katz, B. (1983). Health, self-care and power: Shifting the balance. *Topics in Clinical Nursing, 5,* 31–41.

Damrosch, S. (1991). General strategies for motivating people to change their behavior. *Nursing Clinics of North America, 26,* 833–843.

Iglehart, J. K. (1992). Health policy report: The American health care system: Managed care. *New England Journal of Medicine, 327,* 742.

Kientz, C. (1996). A State Association's Executive Director speaks out about prospective pay. *The Remington Report, 4,* 22–23.

Koop, J. E. (1996). At time of diagnosis. *Time Life Medical Video Series.* New York: Patient Education Media, Inc.

Nolan, M. R., Grant, G., & Ellis, N. C. (1990). Stress is in the eye of the beholder: Reconceptualizing the measurement of carer burden. *Journal of Advanced Nursing, 15,* 544–555.

Orem, D. (1991). *Nursing concepts of practice* (4th ed.). Boston: Mosby-Year Book.

Pender, N. J., (1996). *Health promotion in nursing practice* (pp. 97–98). Stamford, CT: Appleton & Lange.

Pender, N. J. (1987). *Health promotion in nursing practice* (pp. 196–198). Norwalk, CT: Appleton & Lange.

Spellbring, A. M. (1991). Nursing's role in health promotion: An overview. *Nursing Clinics of North America, 26,* 805–813.

Sperger-Nearpass, M. (1994). Managed competition 101 [syllabus]. In M. D. Harris (Ed.), *Handbook of Home Health Care Administration.* Gaithersburg, MD: Aspen Publishers, Inc.

Steiger, N. J., & Lipson, J. G. (1985). *Self-care nursing and practice* (p. 12). Bowie, MD: Robert Brady.

SELF-CARE
....
This article demonstrates that a very simple intervention can promote self-care.

Lingerfelt, N. (1997). Would Connie ever take her medication? *Nursing*, 97(2), 32jjj–kkk.

4 Would Connie Ever Take Her Medication?

NANCY LINGERFELT

Working in the mountains of eastern Tennessee, I sometimes feel I've seen it all—like the woman whose venous ulcer was alive with wiggling maggots . . . or the man who promised to take his medications but dumped them in the creek behind his shack after I left (I found his walker there once too) . . . or the man who would shoot first and ask questions later if I didn't honk my car horn and wait for him to come out on the porch before getting out of my car.

Like these clients, Connie Jackson was memorable and challenging. At 80, Connie was thin, frail, and incredibly dirty. She wore layers of filthy clothing, even in the stifling summer heat, adding or subtracting layers as the weather dictated. Her bed was an iron cot with a woolen blanket. I'm not sure what color the blanket was originally, but whenever I brushed up against it, I would find a black stain on my white pants.

On one visit, I found a gun tucked under her pillow. I'd been visiting Connie for about 3 weeks, but I'd never noticed it before. Calmly, I asked her about it and, to my surprise, learned that she'd just used it. She gestured toward it and said, "You cain't be too careful. Did you see the dead snake out yonder? I shot hit this mornin', and now I'm waitin' for hit's mate to come so's I kin shoot hit too." I took Connie's advice and stepped carefully for the next few visits.

Connie lived in only two rooms of what had once been a fairly decent house. She had electricity (many mountain people don't), and a single bare lightbulb hung over her bed. Although she had an electric stove, circa 1950, she preferred the wood cookstove that dominated the kitchen. The legs of her little kitchen table were set in soup cans filled with water "to keep the ants away." She carefully tended a marijuana plant outside her back door; it was her means of supplementing her Social Security check.

● COMPLIANCE PROBLEMS

This was the backdrop for Connie's care. She had atrial fibrillation and heart failure, plus her mitral valve had been replaced years earlier. (Even from across the room, I could hear the ball valve "tick.") She was supposed to take digoxin (Lanoxin) and warfarin (Coumadin).

But compliance was a problem, and Connie's condition was deteriorating. Because she couldn't tolerate the 40-mile round-trip to her physician, I had to draw blood every week

Hospice Patient-Care Coordinator, Smoky Mountain Home Health and Hospice, Inc., Newport, TN to check her prothrombin time—a step the physician felt was necessary because we weren't sure how often she actually took her warfarin.

Ordinarily, my colleagues and I use the agency's standard teaching forms to help our clients understand their medications. But Connie couldn't read or write, so our written instructions were useless.

Explaining her medications and the importance of taking them according to schedule didn't work either—she was forgetful and would skip doses. So I tried dividing her medications in egg cartons, then pillboxes. But she couldn't remember where she'd put them. It would usually take an exhaustive search through, behind, and under piles of magazines, newspapers, clothes, and trash to locate them.

● FINALLY, A SOLUTION

In desperation, I went to the local office-supply store and bought 28 of the smallest manila envelopes I could find, about 4 × 6 inches. Next, I tacked four strips of cardboard to a door to represent morning, afternoon, evening, and bedtime. Connie took some of her medications four times a day; others, like digoxin and warfarin, less often.

I filled each of the 28 envelopes—a 1-week supply—with the appropriate medications for each time of day. Then I tacked the envelopes onto the cardboard strips.

Connie would remove an envelope, take the medication, and put the then-empty envelope in a special place in a kitchen drawer. She (and I) could tell whether she'd taken all her medications for the day by looking at how many envelopes had been removed.

Although this system sounds complicated, it really worked. Connie didn't have to search for her medications; they were right in front of her, ready for her to take. And I could stop worrying so much about her compliance and her prothrombin time.

● POSTSCRIPT

Two years and a lot of manila envelopes later, Connie developed chest pain and had to be hospitalized. She lingered for a couple of days, then her aged heart gave out.

Connie came home to be buried in her beloved mountains. She's fondly remembered by her neighbors, who refer to the dirt road leading to her shack as Connie Town Road.

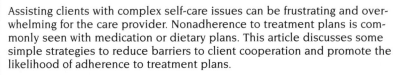

SELF-CARE

Assisting clients with complex self-care issues can be frustrating and over-whelming for the care provider. Nonadherence to treatment plans is com-monly seen with medication or dietary plans. This article discusses some simple strategies to reduce barriers to client cooperation and promote the likelihood of adherence to treatment plans.

What are the advantages to describing client behaviors rather than labeling them? How does culture influence client adherence to treatment? How does age influence adherence to treatment plans?

Ward-Collins, D. (1998). "Noncompliant" Isn't there a better way to say it? *American Journal of Nursing*, 98(5), 27–32.

"Noncompliant"

Isn't There a Better Way to Say It?

DIANA WARD-COLLINS

To influence a patient's behavior, we sometimes have to start by chang-ing our terminology.

Recently, a colleague contacted me because she needed to talk about a distressing professional experience. Nancy, a nursing care manager for the elderly, wanted to discuss an interdisciplinary care conference in which an elderly patient was referred to as noncompliant—in the presence of the patient and her family.

The incident involved a young student social worker who was discussing the patient, Ms. Miller. The student described the patient's behavior as "noncompliant" and "nonco-operative." Concerned about the impression the words might have on the patient and her family, Nancy said she diplomatically tried to divert the student from using that descrip-tion. While a social worker, two other nurses, and a physical therapist were also present at the conference, no one else seemed to react to the choice of words in the same way Nancy did.

Nancy gently but directly asked the student to use a term other than "noncompliant" to describe the patient's behavior. The purpose of the conference was to discuss a care plan involving the patient and family and to establish respectful therapeutic relationships. Nancy was concerned that Ms. Miller and her family might react negatively and be of-fended.

● WHAT'S COMMUNICATION, WHAT'S JARGON?

The word "noncompliant" has always troubled me. For a long time I wasn't sure why, but with experience, education, and curiosity nudging me, I embarked on a quest to better understand its meaning for myself and other providers.

Diana Ward-Collins is a nurse entrepreneur and president of the Legal Nurse Network and an adjunct faculty member at the University of Phoenix, Derwer, CO. The author dedicates this article to Nancy McCambridge, MS, RN, founder of Consultants for Aging Families, Fort Collins, CO.

This article will explore the meaning of the word as it relates to advocacy and transcultural, ethical, and transgenerational considerations. I hope to persuade you that we should eliminate the word from our professional vocabulary and consider better—more respectful and therapeutic, less negative, and more precise—words as alternatives.

First, let's consider some points about health care jargon and communication. Sometimes we get so used to a medical term that we don't think about the negative effect it might have. Our health care culture has developed a language of jargon, acronyms, and euphemisms. Some terms such as "STAT," "NPO," "DNR," and "Chem-12" have specific meanings to direct others to action or nonaction. Yet such terms might be inaccessible to those outside the health care profession. And in the world of our patients, the words might not be understood.

To health care consumers, some words are frightening or even demeaning. "Noncompliant" implies a negative judgment that patients, for whatever reason, won't do what we have advised them to do.

● IDENTIFYING CONTRIBUTING FACTORS

According to the *Nursing Diagnosis Reference Manual,* the definition of noncompliance is "unwillingness to practice prescribed health-related behaviors." In another text, Linda Carpenito describes noncompliance as "the state in which an individual or group desires to comply but is prevented from doing so by factors that deter adherence to health-related advice given by health professionals."

A diagnosis of noncompliance can be highly subjective. Consequently, it's important to identify causative and contributing factors that can help you intervene effectively. Keep in mind that the nursing model of autonomy allows patients to participate in planning their own care. It ensures that patients are made active participants in their care. This is supported by educating patients about their condition and related care without coercion based on practitioners' values.

Carpenito also addresses the importance of a person's right to self-determination through the process of informed consent. The principle of autonomy is related to and incorporated into the process of informed consent. When a patient refuses to comply with advice or instruction, it's important to ensure that the major elements of informed consent—information, voluntariness, and competence—are present. When you identify the reasons a patient chooses not to follow advice, you can then determine whether these factors can be decreased or eliminated.

Communication is a process consisting of a sender, the message—verbal and nonverbal—the channel, the receiver, and the response of the receiver. Verbal communication requires attention to the words chosen and the meanings that words have for the senders and receivers. Meanings and effects of words are influenced by receivers' and senders' values (see *How Values Influence Meanings and Effects of Words*).

As nurses, we need to consider ideas from all perspectives–including the exploration of conceptual meanings. We should raise questions, propose answers through critical thinking discussions, and research, and suggest implications for answers. The foundation of nursing science is its philosophical concepts and theories. Such philosophical questions are critical to the process of our scientific inquiry.

Thus we might ask, What is the meaning of the word "noncompliant"? Does this word project respect for patients and their right to direct their care? Will people who aren't nurses have the same interpretation as nurses? Will people working for insurance compa-

How Values Influence Meanings and Effects of Words

Values are action oriented and give direction and meaning to life. They don't exist separately and independently of people but are part of our conscious and unconscious processes as expressed in behavior.

Values are developed in a three-phase process of choosing, prizing, and acting. *Choosing* is a cognitive process that involves thinking and logic after receiving information. *Prizing* involves our affect—an emotional expression of values. Once received, accepted, and cherished, values become a source of positive self-esteem and willingness to affirm the choice. *Acting* is the behavioral component of valuing. After we choose our values, we prize them and choose to act on them. We repeat our choices consistently. Our values systems govern our conduct, shape our decision-making, and serve as filters for governing how we take in or exclude information.

nies understand that an individual identified as noncompliant has a legal right to make the decision that led to the diagnosis, or will they deny insurance benefits?

Seeing the phenomenon of noncompliant consumers only from the view of health care professionals limits our ability to see the patient's point of view. Perceptions vary for each of us even though we're in the same profession. Perceptions also vary among different health care providers as well as among our consumers. Perceptions are influenced by our culture, socialization, education, and experience. In short, the more we understand how beliefs arise and are sustained, the more we can understand why logical arguments are seldom effective in changing beliefs and faulty perceptions among providers as well as consumers. We need to understand that changes in perception have to occur before beliefs and prejudices can be altered.

RELATED RESEARCH
Reducing Barriers to Patient Cooperation

Nonadherence to either a medication or dietary plan to treat heart failure often results in negative patient outcomes such as hospital readmission. One approach to reducing barriers is implementing interventions that are individually designed for patients. In an attempt to understand patients' perceptions of the benefits and barriers to following a medication regimen and dietary sodium restriction, researchers at Indiana University developed the Beliefs About Medication Compliance Scale (BMCS) and the Beliefs About Dietary Compliance Scale (BDCS).

These instruments are based on the Health Belief Model, which defines benefits as positive aspects of performing a health behavior, and barriers as negative aspects of performing the behavior, which account for as much as 50% of nonadherence to medication and dietary changes required for some chronic illnesses, such as hypertension.

A convenience sample of 101 patients with heart failure participated in the study. Internal consistency reliability of the instruments was determined by Cronbach alpha. Subscales ranged from a reliability coefficient of 0.68 to 0.91. Construct validity was supported by a factor analysis, with the factors interpreted as benefits and barriers for each instrument.

The benefits of adhering to prescribed medications and suggestions for sodium restriction included decreasing the chance of being hospitalized, improving quality of life,

(continued)

RELATED RESEARCH
Reducing Barriers to Patient Cooperation (*Continued*)
•••

reducing symptoms, and decreasing worry. The barrier factor included unpleasantness, complicating everyday life, difficulty remembering to take pills or understanding the diet, and spending too much time and money following the regimens.

This initial test of the instruments has proven positive, but more needs to be done with other cardiac populations. The instruments appear to have potential for clinical application in attempting to understand why patients have difficulty following particular treatment plans. The next step is to determine the relationship between the measured benefits and barriers, and compliance of patients with heart failure. Then nursing and therapeutic interventions designed to decrease individual barriers can be planned and evaluated based upon findings from these instruments. This more individualized approach may yield improved patient cooperation with medications or dietary regimens.
—*Judith A. DePalma, MSN, RN, director of nursing research, Allegheny University Hospital-Allegheny General, Pittsburgh, PA*

Source: Bennett, S. J., et al. Beliefs about medication and dietary compliance in people with heart failure: An instrument development study. *Heart Lung* 26:273–279, July–Aug. 1997

● THE RISKS OF ADVOCACY

In the situation concerning Nancy and Ms. Miller, the presenter was offended by Nancy's suggestions and had a meeting with her faculty advisor to discuss the experience. The faculty member later contacted Nancy and expressed her dissatisfaction about the student being corrected in front of the patient and other members of the team.

Astounded by this response, Nancy reflected on the effects of the experience for the patient and student. Her dilemma: Should she speak up on behalf of Ms. Miller or remain silent? Whose feelings take precedence when there is such a difference of opinion? For whom is Nancy an advocate: the patient or the student? If a patient's self-esteem is determined to be at risk, should another's use of accepted but perhaps offensive vocabulary be curbed? Is the patient the pivotal person of concern? When professionals and students are present in a care conference, shouldn't a patient's right to be treated with respect and dignity take priority?

Prior to the care conference, Ms. Miller and her daughter told Nancy about their feelings that the staff had disregard for what they believed and valued. Nancy chose to act on behalf of the patient and family. She watched Ms. Miller's and her daughter's response to the care team's discussion and observed behavior that reflected controlled anger. Nancy's decision to be an advocate required introspection and reflection. Time spent in these activities helps us gain a clearer understanding of our roles and relationships with others.

Advocacy implies that we emphasize mutuality, facilitation, protection, and coordination. Two experts on concepts of professional nursing, Susan Leddy and Mae Pepper, describe patient advocacy as an appropriate role for nurses. It's an action that has evolved in harmony with a larger social movement characterized by self-care, human rights, consumer rights, and individual accountability for health. Nancy readily accepted the obligation to act as an advocate, knowing that two of the key activities for this role are providing informational support and helping patients make the wisest possible decisions in their pursuit of well-being.

Advocacy involves active support of autonomy, beneficence, and human dignity. It also incorporates understanding of and sensitivity to cultural and generational differences.

● CONSIDERING TRANSCULTURAL IMPLICATIONS

Nancy and the patient were from different generational and cultural backgrounds. Fortunately, Nancy was aware that transcultural nursing requires a sensitivity to our own and others' patterned ways of acting and thinking.

We have our own beliefs and values that influence our thinking as care providers and must work to understand how, when, and why our values come in conflict with others. We must also understand that sometimes conflict occurs simply because of our differences.

Another aspect of transcultural nursing is that professional nurses are from a health care subculture with a strong, traditional base. This subculture guides our thinking and acting about patients, illness, health-seeking behavior, and nursing care. We learn certain views early in our nursing careers and develop set patterns of actions, interactions, and expectations. But to be effective care agents, over the course of time we must be responsive to change and recognize the value and importance of culturally appropriate care.

A key component of successful interactions with culturally diverse patients is to avoid using stereotypical, judgmental words. Some transcultural experts suggest the term "nonadherence" as more appropriate than the term "noncompliance" because "nonadherence" more accurately reflects behavior resulting from differences in beliefs. It might also be less of a stigma to patients than the label "noncompliant." To advance this thought, perhaps we should consider other terms such as "difference in opinion," "different values," "knowledge deficit," or "financial constraint" as we attempt to describe why patients are reluctant or unable to do as we advise.

● WHY ETHICAL CONSIDERATIONS ARE IMPORTANT

When health care workers use the word "noncompliant," it can have the same effect as if they used the word "disobedient." We need to keep in mind that when we advise a patient to do something, that doesn't mean he must submit to our directions.

Another ethical consequence is that repeated attempts at rational persuasion might unduly influence a patient who is vulnerable and needs to be accepted by the caregiver. The effect can be the same as coercion.

So why don't some patients "follow advice?" A way to discover the reasons might be to simply say to a patient: "I see you haven't been following the advice of the doctor. I feel uncertain about that, and I'm wondering what information you can share to help me understand your situation." Then, if you hear the patient's answer without reacting to it, you are more likely to have a better understanding of the reasons influencing the patient's choice not to do what he was advised to do. You'll be better able to fill in knowledge gaps, clear up misunderstandings, and negotiate for actions that help to facilitate a positive outcome for the patient. However, there may be situations in which a patient consciously disagrees with your advice and chooses a course of action beyond your control.

● WHEN THERE'S A GENERATION GAP

Older adults are the major consumers of health care in our country. Although they experience loss in various aspects of their lives, they want the ability to make decisions regarding their care. When physical or mental limitations hinder their ability to manage daily activities, nurses can help them maintain their autonomy and control over choices.

Morris Massey, a values theorist, has proposed that core values are formed by the age of 10 and that we change our values only when confronted with significant emotional events. Massey also identifies Americans shaped by the events of the 1920s to 1940s as traditionalists. For many of these people, the traditional family, with assigned roles and recognition of authority granted to elders, was what they valued as they learned to master their world.

Included among the traditionalists are many individuals over age 65. By the year 2030, projections are that approximately 22% of the American population will be over age 65. Our nursing interventions must take into account the specific limitations and potential problems of this age group. We must support their right to self-directed care by recognizing that people who have demonstrated resiliency in tackling life's difficult issues during earlier stages of their lives will likely continue to do so as they age.

Ms. Miller's experience as an elder cared for by a younger generation of caregivers was a "battle of wills" during which she had to work hard to maintain self-control. Ms. Miller knew what her body could and couldn't do. She believed no one listened to her knowledge of what was important to her. Feeling frustrated, she became resistant and abrasive. Minor problems became major conflicts. Rather than using facilitation skills to determine Ms. Miller's reasons for nonadherence to the proposed therapeutic plan, her caregivers continued to press for what *they* wanted to occur.

● THREE MONTHS LATER

After Ms. Miller returned home, her behavior gradually changed as she developed trust and began to see the benefit of working with members of the care team—Nancy, her home health aide, and her family—toward mutually acceptable therapeutic goals. Soon she was taking full responsibility for activities such as bathing and walking.

Could Ms. Miller have become more independent sooner? Possibly. When individuals, especially the elderly, experience loss of control of valued aspects of their lives, they typically resist suggestions. When they believe that health care workers are pressuring them and not supporting their rights, the damage is often compounded.

Because use of the word "noncompliance" connotes judgment, it should be used cautiously—if at all, and nurse clinicians should avoid its use as a nursing diagnosis. And to document its negative implications, I believe nurse researchers should do linguistic analyses, in which the occasions, intentions, and practical sequences of using words relevant to the science are examined. When we understand more about how to help a patient decide which option is preferable, we might not need to attend to negative behavior so often.

Ensuring a patient's autonomy is a part of establishing a therapeutic regimen. For us to support a patient's autonomy, we should encourage that person to be self-directed and assume responsibility for his health and well-being. Judgmental terms such as "noncompliant" diminish the dignity of those we say we care for. Surely there's a better way to say it.

SELECTED REFERENCES

Beauchamp, T. L., and Childress, J. F. *Principles of Biomedical Ethics,* 3rd ed. New York, Oxford University Press, 1989.

Burns, N., and Grove, S. K. *The Practice of Nursing Research: Conduct, Critique, and Utilization,* 3rd ed. Philadelphia, Saunders, 1997.

Carpenito, L. J. *Nursing Diagnosis: Application to Clinical Practice,* 5th ed. Philadelphia, Lippincott, 1993.

Giger, J. N., and Davidhizar, R. E. [eds.]. *Transcultural Nursing: Assessment and Intervention,* 2nd ed. St. Louis, Mosby, 1995.

Leddy, S., and Pepper, J. *Conceptual Bases of Professional Nursing,* 3rd ed. Philadelphia, Lippincott, 1993.

Massey, M. *The People Puzzle.* Reston, VA, Prentice-Hall, 1979.

Sparks, S. M., and Taylor, C. M. *Nursing Diagnosis Reference Manual,* 3rd ed. Springhouse, PA, Springhouse, 1995.

Nurses are increasingly asked to include the whole family in the assessment and care of the client. Using a family systems approach, the nurse and the family can work together to promote the health, safety, and well-being of the client and family.

How can the nurse effectively maximize family strengths? How can the nurse effectively collaborate with the family to identify important family needs and match these needs with available resources?

MacPhee, M. (1995). The family systems approach and pediatric nursing care. *Pediatric Nursing*, 21(5), 417–423.

6

The Family Systems Approach and Pediatric Nursing Care

MAURA MACPHEE

The pediatric nurse is increasingly called upon to function as a family specialist, yet many nurses have assumed this role with little or no training in family systems theory. The family systems approach to pediatric nursing care maximizes family strengths. The nurse and family collaborate to identify important family needs and to match needs with resources. The primary goal is family empowerment. A basic understanding of the family systems approach to assessment and intervention can help pediatric nurses function more effectively in this role.

Pediatric nurses are often expected to function as family specialists. This role assignment has occurred with recognition that the child is a member of a family system. Pediatric health prevention/intervention outcomes depend on the functional status of the family system (Dunst, Trivette, & Deal, 1988).

Federal legislation and other factors have influenced this role shift. The *Education of Handicapped Act Amendments of 1986* (Public Law 99–457) (1986) requires that preschool intervention programs use a family systems model when designing early intervention plans for infants, toddlers, and their families. Health care professionals are frequently involved in the design and implementation of Individualized Family Service Plans (Newcomb, Stepanek, Beckman, Frank, & Brown, 1994). Technologic changes have resulted in medically complex children surviving and transitioning into the home and the community. Pediatric nurses often orchestrate the discharge preparations for these children and their families, and their knowledge of the family system affects the quality of their case coordination (Fleming et al., 1994). Recent health care reform activities, such as institutional downsizing, require pediatric nurses to assume multiple family-centered roles as budgets and positions are trimmed.

Maura MacPhee, MS, RN, is a Clinical Specialist at Children's Hospital of Denver in Denver, Co.

Many pediatric nurses have assumed expanded roles with little or no training in family systems theory. An overview of the purpose and function of the family systems approach in pediatric nursing care provides a starting point for pediatric nurses assuming these roles.

● THE FAMILY SYSTEMS APPROACH

"The family is a natural group which over time has evolved patterns of interacting" (Minuchin & Fishman, 1981, p. 11). These patterns reflect each family member's range of behavior and the rules that hold the family system together. A viable family system has clearly defined behavior patterns and rules that support the growth and development of individual family members while providing a sense of belonging and security.

The family systems approach is an amalgam of systems theory (von Bertalanffy, 1968) and family systems theory (Kerr & Bowen, 1988; Minuchin, 1974). This fusion characterizes a family as a system of interdependent, interacting individuals related to one another by blood or consent. Families are open, living systems, constantly exchanging information and energy with the environment. The environment is a series of other open, living systems, such as the neighborhood, the community, and society. Everything is interconnected and significant—from the relationships between individual family members to the health care reform policies of the society (Hymovich & Hagopian, 1992).

PRINCIPLES FOR PRACTICE

There are four major family systems principles to guide nurses working with children and their families (Dunst et al., 1988):

Principle 1. *Focus intervention/prevention on the family, not the child.* The family system nurtures the child, and by strengthening and supporting the family system, successful outcomes for the child are enhanced.

Principle 2. *Work with the family to create opportunities for ALL family members to acquire and employ competencies that strengthen the family.* Families are often passive recipients of professional "help." Rappaport (1981) stated:

> The pervasive belief that experts should solve all (the client's) problems in living has created a social and cultural iatrogenesis which extends the sense of alienation and loss of ability to control one's own life . . . This is the path that social as well as physical health experts have been on, and we need to reverse the trend (p. 17).

Noncontingent helping (Skinner, 1978) can be damaging and promote the sense of helplessness or lack of control. This occurs in situations when family members play little or no active part in meeting their needs.

Principle 3. *Respect the family's rightful role to decide what is important to them.* The nurse's role is to strengthen and support family decisions and actions. Many times the family's concerns and needs are very different from the nurse's. To forge a working relationship with the family, the nurse must respect the family's concerns and help them work through the issues they are expressing. With time, the nurse, as a facilitator, can help the family recognize and work through professionally identified concerns (Pilisuk & Parks, 1986).

Principle 4. *Acknowledge the positive aspects of the child and the family.* Too often professionals search for things that must be wrong, especially in families who have children with severe handicaps or significant chronic illness. "A family works when its members feel good about the family, when their needs are being met and the development of relationships flow smoothly" (Garbarino, 1982, p. 72).

EMPOWERMENT

The ultimate goal of the family systems approach is family empowerment. Empowered families can interact effectively (within their own system and with other systems) to obtain needed resources (Hobbs et al., 1984). The family systems approach acknowledges that the family is competent or capable of becoming competent. Families may appear dysfunctional or vulnerable. Rather than focusing on deficits within the family, family problems are viewed as our social system's failure to create opportunities for competence to be developed and displayed (Rappaport, 1987).

Traditional health caregiver models, such as the medical model, do not empower families (Brickman et al., 1982). These models focus on professional solutions; therefore, the client (family system) ascribes improvement to the professional. Any improvement in family function is temporary and only lasts as long as the professional is involved.

The family systems approach uses the compensatory model of helping: Clients are not responsible for their problems, but they are responsible for solutions. Head Start and CETA (Comprehensive Educational Training Association) are based on this model (Brickman et al., 1982). This model de-emphasizes past problems, which often are a source of guilt and low self-esteem, and focuses on helping the family obtain self-sustaining behaviors. Major professional empowering behaviors are summarized in Table 6-1.

Differences arising from intra- and extra-family influences are not viewed as deficits that have some pathologic origins requiring treatment. Rather, differences are seen as conditions that generate needs that can be met best by mobilizing resources that allow these needs to be met and thus stregthen families (Dunst, 1985).

● THE NURSE AS HELPER

The family systems approach empowers families through a collaboration process between the family and other systems, such as agencies. Certain skills enable the nurse to forge supportive, helping relationships with the family and with others. These skills include empathetic communication skills, honesty, and confidentiality (Dunst et al., 1988).

Active and reflective listening indicate the nurse's desire to learn about the family. Active listening involves listening with the whole body. Body posture is relaxed but alert

---

TABLE 6-1 ● **Points for Empowering Families**

1. Be positive.
2. Respond to *family*-identified needs.
3. Promote family success in mobilizing resources.
4. Promote the use of family/informal supports.
5. Promote an atmosphere of joint responsibility.

Note: Adapted from C. Dunst, C. Trivette, & A. Deal (1988). *Enabling and Empowering Families.* Cambridge, MA: Brookline Books.

and good eye contact is maintained. The nurse encourages conversation by providing simple reasons that let the speakers know she/he is listening ("Yes, that must be difficult for you."). Open-ended questions/responses can be used as prompts ("It sounds like you have a very hectic schedule. Tell me what a typical day is like for you."). Silence is another valuable communication skill; it allows time for the speakers to think, feel, and express themselves. Reflective listening rephrases what has been said to clarify what the family is saying. Paraphrasing provides a brief re-statement of the speaker's message ("I hear you saying that you are very concerned about your child's poor growth."). It is also important to mirror back the speaker's feelings in a brief, supportive way ("It seems that you are very concerned and worried about your child."). Major guidelines for effective listening are listed in Table 6-2 (Bolton, 1979; Dunst et al., 1988).

Honesty and confidentiality enhance communication and collaboration with the family. Every interaction with the family should include an explanation of the reason for meetings, what will be asked, and how the information will be used. The family needs to know if the information will be shared with other professionals and that the information is a professional confidence.

● FAMILY SYSTEMS ASSESSMENT

The family systems approach assesses three major areas: (a) family needs, (b) family functioning style (strengths), and (c) resources and supports.

The nurse explains the purpose and function of the assessment/interview: ("I would like to spend some time getting to know your family. This will help me provide the best possible assistance to you."). Each set of questions/questionnaires is prefaced with an explanation of its use and addresses the issue of confidentiality.

Family members are asked to introduce themselves and "tell their story," which helps the nurse clarify relationships and roles among family members. Using a recording sheet to document demographic information (age, sex, occupation, location) for each family member is helpful. One formal tool, the genogram (McGoldrick & Gerson, 1985), uses a family tree diagram covering multiple generations.

Symbols denote family member relationships (close, distant, divorced, deceased). Footnotes convey relevant information, such as brief medical and educational histories for members. Critical events, such as significant losses, can be highlighted. A similar tool, the ecomap (Hartman, 1978), diagrams the family's relationship with other systems, such as friends, church, social groups, and institutions. Symbols indicate the strength of helpful or not helpful associations.

Family needs. A need is defined as the family's perceptions of what is important for them to acquire. Family members will allot time, energy, and resources to meeting a need.

TABLE 6-2 ● Effective Listening Guidelines

1. Focus on feeling words.
2. Note the general content of the message.
3. Observe the speaker's body language.
4. *Do not* fake understanding.
5. *Do not* tell the speaker how he/she feels.

Note: Adapted from R. Bolton (1979). *People Skills.* Englewood, NJ: Prentice-Hall.

Unmet needs are hierarchically ordered from most to least important, and family heirarchies are highly unique. Often professionals describe families that fail to adhere to their child's prescribed treatment regimen as resistant and noncompliant. Actually, these families may be attending to other important needs and the professionally prescribed treatment regimen is a low priority.

Dunst and Leet (1987) asked parents of children with disabilities and developmentally at risk to assess their physical and emotional health and to indicate whether they had the time and energy to perform professionally prescribed child therapeutic interventions. They found significant correlations between parent needs assessments and personal well-being. The greater the number of unmet needs, the greater the emotional and physical problems reported. Significant correlations were found between need scores and commitment scores. The greater the number of unmet needs, the greater the probability that parents would not devote time or energy to performing therapeutic tasks for their children. These findings were significant regardless of parent age, education, or socioeconomic status.

Standardized, self-report tools can provide background information to assess family needs. These instruments are a springboard for discussion during the interview process to help the family clearly identify and specify their most important needs. Popular needs-based assessment scales include the *Family Needs Survey* (Goldfarb, Brotherson, Summers, & Turnbull, 1986), the *Parent Needs Inventory* (Fewell, Meyer, & Schell, 1981), the *Personal Projects Scale* (Little, 1983), the *Family Resource Scale* (Dunst & Leet, 1987), and the *Survey for Parents of Children with Handicaps* (Moore, Hammerlynck, Barsh, Spicker, & Jones, 1982). A text using a needs-based approach also provides assessment questions for the interview process (Hartman & Laird, 1983).

This assessment portion culminates with a prioritized list of the family's needs. A recording form, such as the *Needs by Sources of Support and Resources Matrix* (Dunst et al., 1988), can visually display each need with its subsequent sources of support.

Family functioning style (strengths). The family system is comprised of members with individual competencies. These competencies form a resource reservoir for the family to tap. Families sometimes have difficulty being objective about their intra-family resources. The nurse helps explore potential assets during the interview/assessment process.

Family strengths research (Curran, 1983; Stinnett & DeFrain, 1985) has identified 12 major qualities that characterize strong families (Table 6-3). Most families do not possess all of these qualities, but the presence of one or more of them is emphasized with the family systems approach. Each family's unique combination of strong qualities comprises the family's functioning style, which reflects how the family copes with life's challenges and how the family system grows (Folkman, Lazarus, Dunkel-Schetter, DeLorgis, & Gruen, 1986). Family functioning style can have a significant impact on life satisfaction (Sanders, Walters, & Montgomery, 1985) and dealing with stress (Folkman et al., 1986).

Examples of family strengths assessment tools include the *Family Strengths Inventory* (Stinnett & DeFrain, 1985), the *Family Strengths Scale* (Olson, Larsen, & McCubbin, 1983), the *Family Strength Questionnaire* (Otto, 1975), and the *Family Functioning Style Scale* (Deal, Trivette, & Dunst, 1987). Families are often asked to complete one of these questionnaires to use as a basis for discussion. For instance, one family member might identify communication as a family strength. The nurse might ask why the ability to communicate is a strength, how the family communicates, what family members usually talk about, how disputes are settled, et cetera. The nurse facilitates the family's efforts to operationalize their identified strengths so that these assets can be applied constructively.

TABLE 6-3 ● Qualities of Strong Families

1. *Commitment* toward promoting individual family members well-being
2. *Appreciation* for small and large things that family membes do well
3. Concentrated effort to spend *time* together
4. A sense of *purpose* for "going on" in good or bad times
5. A sense of *congruence* among family members when prioritizing needs
6. The ability to *communicate* positive feelings and support
7. A clear set of family *rules,* values, and beliefs
8. Coping *strategies* that promote positive functioning
9. *Problem-solving skills* for evaluating options
10. The ability to be *positive,* even in crisis situations
11. *Flexibility* and *adaptability*
12. A *balance* of internal and external resources for meeting needs.

Note: Adapted from C. Dunst, C. Trivette, & A. Deal (1988). *Enabling and Empowering Families.* Cambridge, MA: Brookline Books.

The *Family Strengths Profile* (Trivette, Dunst, & Deal, 1988) offers another creative assessment approach (see Fig. 6-1 for a portion of the profile). The family is asked to describe "a typical day–what each family member does during the day." Each member outlines his/her daily routine. The nurse lists key family member behaviors. The family and nurse review the list and decide how each behavior contributes to the family's strengths,

Family Behavior	Family Strengths														Type of Resource	
	Commitment	Appreciation	Time	Sense of Purpose	Congruence	Communication	Role Expectations	Coping Strategies	Problem Solving	Positivism	Flexibility	Balance			Intrafamily	Extrafamily

Note: From C. Trivette, C. Dunst, & A. Deal (1988). Family Strengths Profile. In *Enabling and Empowering Families* (pp. 202–203). Cambridge, MA: Brookline Books. Reprinted with permission.

FIGURE 6-1. Excerpt from Family Strengths Profile.

using a checklist of the 12 "strong family" qualities. The nurse reinforces how these strengths are important family resources.

The outcome of this assessment piece is a list of intrafamily resources. Families, especially families with many needs, may be unable to find positive things to say about themselves (Dunst et al., 1988). The nurse reframes concerns and problems in more positive ways, enabling the family to recognize alternative ways of viewing their situation and getting their needs met.

Extrafamily supports and resources. Social support from outside the family can be informal (neighbors, friends, church members) or formal (professionals and agencies). Dunst and colleagues (1988) report that the positive effects from informal supports are generally greater than those derived from formal support resources.

Dunst (1985) conducted a study to determine the importance of various kinds of resources on positive family outcomes. His subjects were parents of preschoolers who were retarded, disabled, or developmentally at risk. In this study, the significance of an intervention was defined as the percentage of variance. Intrafamily support accounted for a significant percentage of the variance for 5 of 10 outcome measures (parent well-being, management of child care demands, family integration, parent perceptions of child's abilities, and child–parent play opportunities). Informal support accounted for the major variance in 9 of 10 outcome measures (such as parent well-being, child care demands, management of child behavior difficulties, social acceptance). Formal support accounted for a significant percentage of the variance for only one outcome measure (family opportunities). Health care professionals often focus on the impact of their prevention/intervention programs. Studies such as Dunst's (1985) indicate that kinship and informal supports have a vital influence on family outcomes.

Other studies document significant relationships between extrafamily support (informal and formal) and personal health and well-being (Cohen & Syme, 1985), family well-being (Patterson & McCubbin, 1983), and satisfaction with parenting (Crnic, Greenberg, Ragozin, Robinson, & Basham, 1983). Successful outcomes were based on the match between family-identified needs and resources available.

Several scales that measure different components of the family's social support domain include questions about intrafamily and extrafamily (informal and formal) resources. The *Inventory of Social Support* (Trivette & Dunst, 1986) and the *Social Network Questionnaire* (Antonucci, 1986) have two parts: (a) a section to map out members' social support network, and (b) scales to indicate how each support source provides help or assistance with a variety of needs. The *Family Support Scale* (Dunst, Jenkins, & Trivette, 1984) is an 18-item questionnaire families use to assess the helpfulness of different support sources. Two other popular instruments include the *Perceived Support Network Inventory* (Oritt, Paul, & Behrman, 1985) and the *Personal Resource Questionnaire* (Weinert, 1987).

This assessment component allows the nurse to identify the family's social support network, which contains viable sources of support that family members are willing to ask for assistance. Some families include formal supports in their support network. More frequently, these supports are underused and may be introduced to the family in the next phase of the process.

● FAMILY SYSTEMS INTERVENTION

The nurse uses assessment information to help the family prioritize their needs and match them with family-identified resources. When gaps exist between identified needs and resources, the nurse queries the family about using formal support services, which are saved until last. The systems approach advocates for the family to identify their own needs and to meet these needs through their own competencies and/or through supports that they view as helpful. In this way the family is empowered.

During the matching process, the nurse pays attention to family members' verbal and nonverbal cues. Follow-up probes may indicate that the price of asking for help from a particular source outweighs the benefits. The nurse includes the pros and cons in the family discussion of exploring resource options. For instance, a family may recognize community health nurse visits as helpful, but the nurse detects the mother's hesitancy to have the nurse come into the home. The nurse could say, "You indicated that nurse visits could help you keep track of your baby's growth and development. I sense that there's a problem with this, though." The mother may reply, "She came out a couple of times after the baby was born. She was nice, but she came unannounced and I never felt prepared—kind of an invasion of privacy. We don't have a phone, so she can't call us." With this information, the nurse could mediate with the community nurse and the family to schedule regular visits with an agenda that directly addresses the family's needs.

The intervention phase consists of joint goal-setting between the family and the nurse and usually includes short- and long-term goals. Short-term goals often center around immediate family issues and help to stabilize the family system; long-term goals are usually concerned with helping the family adjust to long-lasting changes that have a major impact on family roles and interactional patterns (Captain, 1989; Kazak, 1989). When a child is newly diagnosed with a chronic illness, the family must deal with acute, short-term issues, such as finances, transportation, work releases to meet medical appointments, and child care for siblings. Long-term goals may entail sharing the diagnosis with family members and preparing the family to manage the responsibilities of a serious chronic illness.

The family systems approach provides tools to help the family establish realistic goals and manage them as competently as possible. The family must do the work, but the nurse helps bolster the family's functional skills and is sensitive to disruptive family interactional problems that affect outcomes. The nurse helps identify problems by observing the family's communication skills, problem-solving abilities, expression of feelings, and negotiation strategies. By reinforcing the use of "I" messages and positive statements and helping families develop these communication strategies, the nurse helps facilitate family interactions (Captain, 1989; Foster & Phillips, 1992).

Some families have unhealthy, entrenched patterns of behaving that require professional counseling or therapy. The family systems approach accentuates family strengths, even in instances where family discord is habitual and destructive. Therapists using the family systems approach employ the same systems principles to help the family establish healthy interactional patterns (Minuchin & Fishman, 1981). When counseling or therapy is indicated, the nurse helps the family make a working commitment with the therapist by encouraging and supporting their decisions and providing information (Whall, 1986).

● NURSING PROCESS AND THE FAMILY SYSTEMS APPROACH

Parallels exist between nursing process and the family systems approach. There is an assessment phase where needs and matching resources are identified. The planning and implementation stage consists of goal-setting and support for the family's chosen interventions.

There is also an evaluation phase. When the family system must change to accommodate new family tasks, established patterns need to be replaced with new ones. This change can take time and progress may be slow. The nurse helps the family recognize progress. The family is engaged in self-evaluation at regular intervals. Family conferences with invited staff recognize and reinforce identified gains as needs/goals are being achieved. Support is provided when families are discouraged. Change is continuous and so is the family systems process. Needs and resources are not static, and conferences can help reassess needs, resources, and strategies being employed (Captain, 1989).

The family system is composed of members who promote the health, safety and well-being of their members. To make the system work, nurses need to collaborate with the family to help the system seek out appropriate health care, monitor treatment, provide follow-up care, and encourage compliance with prescribed treatment regimens. Health care professionals have often assigned these duties to themselves where the family plays a passive role. The family systems approach works by acknowledging and strengthening the role of families in their own health care maintenance.

Case Study

This case study summarizes the major concepts of the family systems approach. It illustrates how a nurse collaborates with the family to create care strategies that enhance family competencies and offers professional help that the family acknowledges and solicits.

Alice is a 3-year-old girl with hemolytic uremic syndrome (HUS) resulting from an *E. coli* infection. She has a 6-year-old brother, Jason. Her mother, Wendy, is employed part-time (4 hours daily on weekdays) as a secretary. Wendy's contribution to the family income has been important. Her hours are arranged so that the family will not have to use day care or after-school care. The father, Robert, is a truck driver who is gone for a few days at a time. Wendy's mother, Abby, watches the children when Wendy is working. Other family members live nearby.

After the acute phase of her illness, Alice required peritoneal dialysis due to renal failure from HUS. Her laboratory values indicated that she was recovering and the physician estimated that she would be well-healed and ready for discharge within 2 weeks. The family anticipated a 2-week stay on the hospital's general ward. The parents arranged time off work for 2 weeks, and Abby helped Robert with household chores and Jason's care while Wendy stayed at the hospital with Alice.

By the end of the first week, it became apparent that Alice's kidneys were not becoming self-sufficient, and the renal staff informed the family that Alice's kidneys might not return to normal. The physician told the family that Alice would be on dialysis at the hospital for at least 2 more weeks, and, if no improvement occurred, he would help arrange home dialysis. This became a crisis event for the family.

The primary nurse helped the family and staff arrange a family conference. The nurse explained the purpose for the conference to the family: "Alice is going to be in the hospital for at least 2 more weeks, and she may need to go home with dialysis. You have coped so well with her time in the hospital and I want to help you identify what you'll need to get through the rest of Alice's hospitalization and her transition home. We can work on this together by having a conference with the rest of your family and a few of our staff who have been working with you. The conference will help us figure out what your major needs will be at the hospital and at home. We'll find out who can help with what and get a concrete plan together." The family's planning efforts helped them through a rough emotional time, and the staff reinforced all their positive work.

(continued)

The nurse and the hospital social worker helped the family generate a list of family members and close friends the family viewed as helpers. The social worker recommended inviting only the most significant supports to the conference. Four other people (Wendy's sister, Robert's parents, and Robert's sister) were invited to the conference, although the list of other potential helpers was kept on hand as a back-up. The child life specialist and a dialysis nurse were also invited to the conference. These professionals were well-known to the family and viewed by the family to be important in Alice's ongoing care.

At the beginning of the conference, the nurse explained that the conference was a brainstorming session to explore all the needs the family would have related to Alice's extended hospitalization and potential dialysis support at home. The nurse enlarged the *Family Support Plan* (FSP) (Dunst et al., 1988) to document participants' discussion (Fig. 6-2). The group agreed to use this format as a planning and tracking tool. Participants were given their own copies for jotting notes.

To help the family get started, the parents were asked to describe how their routine at home would be affected and what their major needs would be to normalize life as much as possible. Major needs for each immediate family member were raised and discussed. The mother stated that she needed to go back to work for financial reasons, but she did not want to leave Alice alone. The father stated that he wanted Wendy home more because he was having trouble with Jason. Both parents acknowledged that Jason was coping poorly with Alice's hospitalization and was acting out in school and having tantrums at home. Both parents were also worrying about Alice's regression. "The more she's in the hospital, the more baby-like she gets. She was going to be in preschool at home. She wouldn't be able to get along with other kids now." Finally,

Date	Need/Project	Source of support	Action
9/94	1) Coverage for Alice	Abby, Robert Sr., Doris, Margaret, Rachel, Sonia	See Alice's daily schedule for family coverage.
9/94	2) Wendy needs more time at home	Same as above	See Wendy's daily schedule for family coverage.
9/94	3) Normalizing Alice's routine	Play therapist Nursing staff	Special play times 2x daily. Meals with other preschoolers.
9/94	4) Information on home dialysis	Dialysis nurse	Home care protocol booklet. Staff numbers for questions.

Note: Form excerpted from C. Dunst, C. Trivette, & A. Deal, 1988. *Enabling and Empowering Families* (pp. 190–191). Cambridge, MA: Brookline Books.

FIGURE 6-2. Alice's Family Support Plan.

(continued)

the parents expressed concerns about how they would manage dialysis if Alice needed it at home. No one had talked with them about dialysis home care protocol.

These needs were listed and prioritized on the FSP as: (a) coverage for Alice during mom's absence; (b) more time for Jason, Wendy, and Robert to be together as a family; (c) age-appropriate activities for Alice to normalize her hospitalization; (d) clarity over family responsibility for home dialysis (see Fig. 2). The family felt that these were all short-term goals, and that long-term goals would involve home dialysis, if and when the physician said it was necessary. For now, the family just wanted information about home dialysis.

Each participant was asked to indicate how he/she could help support the family to get their needs met. Names and types of help were listed next to the needs. Due to time constraints, an assessment tool was not used to highlight family strengths. Instead, family strengths were noted by staff and reinforced as intrafamily sources of support were identified. This family system had many "strong family" qualities, including communication skills, commitment, and flexibility. Staff also discussed how they could help family members meet their needs. Care was taken to provide only solicited help. Verbal/nonverbal cues from the family were used to help staff determine whether they were offering needed services.

The final result was a contract from the family to provide coverage for Alice during the weekdays for the next 2 weeks. Wendy agreed to go back to work and to be home in the evening and overnight for 2 weekdays. On the weekend, the family would spend the majority of time together at the hospital with Alice. The family felt that this arrangement would be good for everybody. Wendy said, "I can work, spend important time with Jason and Robert, and also be with Alice. I feel that she will accept other family members being with her when I'm away." The staff assisted by devising a daily schedule plan for Alice's room with names of the family members staying with Alice. This schedule also identified procedure times, nap times, feeding times, and play times. This helped the family map out when it was important for certain family members to be with Alice. The child life specialist blocked out two daily therapeutic play sessions to work on Alice's developmental skills, and the nurse developed a care plan for feeding Alice out of her room with two other preschool-aged children. The family seemed very pleased with the normalization of Alice's hospital routine.

The final identified need, information about dialysis, was addressed by the dialysis nurse. She gave the family a home care booklet to peruse, and reassured them that if/when necessary, the dialysis staff would provide a thorough education program. The family indicated that their primary concern was how dialysis would disrupt their lives. The social worker suggested that the family talk with some families dealing with home dialysis, and the family liked the idea. The dialysis nurse and the social worker agreed to help the family make contacts with families in similar situations.

The staff commended the family for their ability to organize and to help each other in a demanding situation, and a date was set to meet again after the renal specialist decided whether or not home dialysis would be required. The nurse and social worker emphasized the importance of concentrating on short-term goals, and encouraged the family to call them with questions, concerns, or just to talk. At the end of this first family conference, the atmosphere between professionals and family was very positive and supportive.

REFERENCES

Antonucci, T. C. (1986, Summer). Social support networks: A hierarchical mapping technique. *Generations, 10*(4), 10–12.

Bolton, R. (1979). *People skills.* Englewood, NJ: Prentice-Hall.

Brickman, P., Rabinowitz, V., Karuza, J., Coates, D., Cohn, E., & Kidder, L. (1982). Models of helping and coping. *American Psychologist, 37*(4), 368–384.

Captain, C. (1989). Family recovery from alcoholism: Mediating family factors. *Nursing Clinics of North America, 24*(1), 55–67.

Cohen, S., & Syme, S. (1985). Issues in the study and application of social support. In S. Cohen & S. Syme (Eds.), *Social support and health* (p. 322). New York, NY: Academic Press.

Crnic, K., Greenberg, M., Ragozin, A., Robinson, N., & Basham, R. (1983). Effects of stress and social support on mothers of premature and full-term infants. *Child Development, 54*(1), 209–217.

Curran, D. (1983). *Traits of a healthy family.* Minneapolis, MN: Winston Press.

Deal, A., Trivette, C., & Dunst, C. (1987). *Styles of family functioning scale.* Morganton, NC: Family, Infant and Preschool Program, Western Carolina Center.

Dunst, C. (1985). Rethinking early intervention. *Analysis and Intervention in Developmental Disabilities, 5*(1-2), 165–201.

Dunst, C., Jenkins, V., & Trivette, C. (1984). Family support scale: Reliability and validity. *Journal of Individual, Family and Community Wellness, 1,* 45–52.

Dunst, C., & Leet, H. (1987). Measuring the adequacy of resources in households with young children. *Child: Health Care and Development, 13*(2), 111–125.

Dunst, C., Trivette, C., & Deal, A. (1988). *Enabling and empowering families.* Cambridge, MA: Brookline Books.

Education of Handicapped Act Amendments of 1986 (P.L. 99-457), 20 U.S.C. Secs. 1400–1485 (1986).

Fewell, R., Meyer, D., & Schell, G. (1981). *Parent needs inventory.* Seattle, WA: University of Washington.

Fleming, J., Challela, M., Eland, J., Hornick, R., Johnson, P., Martinson, I., Nativio, D., Nokes, K., Riddle, I., Steele, N., Sudela, K., Thomas, R., Turner, Q., Wheeler, B., & Young, A. (1994). Impact on the family of children who are technology dependent and cared for in the home. *Pediatric Nursing, 20*(4), 379–387.

Folkman, S., Lazarus, R., Dunkel-Schetter, C., DeLorgis, A., & Gruen, R. (1986). The dynamics of a stressful encounter: Cognitive appraisal, coping and encounter outcomes. *Journal of Personality and Social Psychology, 50*(5), 992–1003.

Foster, M., & Phillips, W. (1992). Family systems theory as a framework for problem solving in pediatric physical therapy. *Pediatric Physical Therapy, 4*(2) 70–73.

Garbarino, J. (1982). *Children and families in the social environment.* New York, NY: Aldine Publishing.

Goldfarb, L., Brotherson, M., Summers, J., & Turnbull, A. (1986). Family needs survey. In L. Goldfarb, M. Brotherson, J. Summers, & A. Turnbull (Eds.), Meeting the challenge of disability or chronic illness: *A family guide* (pp. 77–78). Baltimore, MD: Paul H. Brookes Publishing.

Hartman, A. (1978). Diagrammatic assessment of family relationships. *Social Casework, 59*(8), 465–476.

Hartman, A., & Laird, J. (1983). *Family-centered social work practice.* New York, NY: Free Press.

Hobbs, N., Dokecki, P., Hoover-Dempsey, K., Moroney, R., Shayne, M., & Weeks, K. (1984). *Strengthening families.* San Francisco, CA: Jossey Bass.

Hymovich, D., & Hagopian, G. (1992). *Chronic illness in children and adults.* Philadelphia, PA: W. B. Saunders Company.

Kazak, A. (1989). Families of chronically ill children: A systems and social-ecological model of adaptation and challenge. *Journal of Consulting and Clinical Psychology, 57*(1), 25–30.

Kerr, M., & Bowen, M. (1988). *Family evaluation: An approach based on the Bowen theory.* New York, NY: Norton Press.

Little, B. (1983). Personal projects: A rationale and method for investigation. *Environment and Behavior, 15*(3), 273–309.

McGoldrick, M., & Gerson, R. (1985). *Genograms in family assessment.* New York, NY: Norton Press.

Minuchin, S. (1974). *Families and family therapy.* Cambridge, MA: Harvard University Press.

Minuchin, S., & Fishman, H. (1981). *Family therapy techniques.* Cambridge, MA: Harvard University Press.

Moore, J., Hammerlynck, L., Barsh, E., Spicker, S., & Jones, R. (1982). *Extending family resources.* Seattle, WA: Children's Clinic & Preschool.

Newcomb, S., Stepanek, J., Beckman, P., Frank, N., & Brown, L. (1994). Providing family support services as part of a comprehensive early intervention system. *The ACCH Advocate, 1*(2), 21–24.

Olson, D., Larsen, A., & McCubbin, H. (1983). Family strengths. In D. Olson, H. McCubbin, H. Barnes, A. Larsen, M. Muxen, & M. Wilson (Eds.), *Families: What makes them work* (pp. 261–262). Beverly Hills, CA: Sage Publications.

Oritt, E., Paul, S., & Behrman, J. (1985). The perceived support network inventory. *American Journal of Community Psychology, 13*(5), 565–582.

Otto, H. (1975). *The use of family strength concepts and methods in family life education: A handbook.* Beverly Hills, CA: The Holistic Press.

Patterson, J., & McCubbin, H. (1983). Chronic illness: Family stress and coping. In C. Figley & H. McCubbin (Eds.), *Stress and the family: Vol. II. Coping with catastrophe* (pp. 21–36). New York, NY: Brunner-Mazel.

Pilisuk, M., & Parks, S. (1986). *The healing web: Social networks and human survival.* Hanover, NH: University Press of New England.

Rappaport, J. (1981). In praise of paradox: A social policy of empowerment over prevention. *American Journal of Community Psychology, 9*(1), 1–25.

Rappaport, J. (1987). Terms of empowerment / exemplars of prevention: Toward a theory of community psychology. *American Journal of Community Psychology, 15*(2), 121–148.

Sanders, G., Walters, J., & Montgomery, J. (1985). Family strengths of older couples and their adult children. In R. Williams, H. Lingren, G. Rowe, S. Van Zundt, P. Lee, & N. Stinnety (Eds.), *Family strengths VI: Enhancement of interaction* (pp. 85–97). Lincoln, NE: College of Home Economics, University of Lincoln.

Skinner, B. (1978). The ethics of helping people. In L. Wispe (Ed.), *Sympathy, altruism and helping behavior* (pp. 249–262). New York, NY: Academic Press.

Stinnett, N., & DeFrain, J. (1985). *Secrets of strong families.* New York, NY: Berkley Books.

Trivette, C., & Deal, A. (1986). *Inventory of social support: Reliability and validity.* Morganton, NC: Family, Infant and Preschool Program, Western Carolina Center.

Trivette, C., Dunst, C., & Deal, A. (1988). Family Strengths Profile. In C. Dunst, C. Trivette, & A. Deal (Eds.), *Enabling and empowering families.* Cambridge, MA: Brookline Books.

von Bertalanffy, L. V. (1968). *General systems theory.* New York, NY: George Barziller.

Weinert, C. (1987). A social support measure: PRQ85. *Nursing Research, 36,* 273–277.

Whall, A. (1986). *Family therapy for nursing: Four approaches.* New York, NY: Appleton-Century-Crofts.

Often when the family is involved in the care of a loved one, stress and tension can result. When families are assisted to mobilize their personal resources, they may experience some relief from these stresses and tensions. Nurses can assess families by using guidelines and a checklist designed to empower families to mobilize resources to ease the transition from hospital to home. Although this article describes caring for a child at home, the principles apply to clients across the life span.

What are some reasons that families may feel overwhelmed and consequently unable to ask for help when assuming the care of a family member at home? How can nurses encourage families to ask for help? What are some areas where families may benefit from help?

Dokken, D., & Sydnor-Greenberg, N. (1998). Helping families mobilize their personal resources. *Pediatric Nursing*, 24(1), 66–69.

Helping Families Mobilize Their Personal Resources

DEBORAH L. DOKKEN, NANCY SYDNOR-GREENBERG

With changes in delivery of and payment for health care, hospital stays may be shorter and children may be going home sooner and sicker. Therefore, more care may be required at home. Even with access to a variety of services and resources in the community, families of medically fragile or chronically ill children can be overwhelmed and stressed. Relief can be provided to some degree if families creatively mobilize their own *personal resources*. However, for a variety of reasons, families may find it difficult to do this. While nurses and other health care professionals are accustomed to helping families find professional services and resources in the community, they can also be invaluable *before discharge* by assisting families with their personal resources—from giving encouragement and motivation to outlining practical planning steps. Pediatric nurses can use guidelines and a checklist to assist families with mobilizing their resources to ease the transition from hospital to home for the whole family.

Deborah L. Dokken, MPA, and Nancy Sydnor-Greenberg, MA, were founding members of the Parent Partners Program at the George Washington University Hospital, in Washington, DC, and have been involved in NICU parent advocacy efforts. As family members and as parents, both have learned to use personal networks during times of medical need.

Families awaiting the discharge of a medically fragile or chronically ill child from the hospital face a broad range of practical and emotional life changes. The event may be anticipated with both excitement and trepidation. While these changes may be brief or long-lasting in duration, they place undue physical and psychic stress on families. Compounding this situation are the ever-evolving changes in the health care system. Nursing staff can help families with this transition by assisting them in the identification and organization of their own personal resources, specific to the needs of their children and the family as a whole. This should occur before the time of hospital discharge.

● TREND TOWARD CARE AT HOME

Nursing staff bear daily witness to the impact of shortened hospital stays and managed care. In recent decades, technological advances, reduced mortality rates, an increased focus on child development, and the movement toward deinstitutionalization have resulted in the social phenomenon of children with complex medical needs being cared for in the home. Children are discharged earlier and require more complex care at home, an approach generally more cost effective than institutional care (Weston & Keefe, 1993).

Recent nationwide surveys estimate that one fourth of all children have a chronic disease (Leyden, 1997). These situations may range from families with premature infants who are discharged with special equipment and medication, to families with terminally ill children having multiple needs. Families may have routine, intermittent, or no nursing care for support in the home.

As health care financing changes evolve, parents may find themselves performing care that used to be provided by hospital staff (Kuttner, 1996). The logical progression of these changes is that more families will be caring for medically fragile or chronically ill children in their own homes as we enter the 21st century. In a positive sense, the practice of families administering and managing care at home is a logical extension of the family-centered care model already adopted by pediatric hospitals and promoted by child and family-advocacy organizations (Johnson, Jeppson, & Redburn, 1992). Parents, after all, know the idiosyncrasies of their own child's nature and routine as well as those of the family best. Leora Kuttner, in her book on the management of childhood pain, refers to "the 21st-century philosophy of 'parents as partners-in-care'" and calls on parents to "learn more about pain and how to develop, flexible, nonfearful ways of coping with pain" (1996, p. 22).

Nurses and parents may extend the same philosophy to families readying for discharge of their children from the hospital. Part of planning for the inevitable changes in the health care system involves helping families mobilize a consistent array of resources adaptable to specific needs and to the medical, societal, and financial changes of that system over time. In more personal terms, helping parents mobilize their resources prior to discharge makes the unknown less frightening and more "do-able," while fostering high-quality, postdischarge care.

While families caring for medically fragile or chronically ill children at home may be a logical progression of the family-centered care model and may be beneficial to families and children, it is not without logistical and emotional consequences. Parents may, for example, have to incorporate providing medical care into the "normal" stresses of siblings, work, and maintaining continuing medical coverage. The "special" routine required by the newly discharged child adds to the existing demands and complicates logistics of daily family life, such as transportation, child care, and housekeeping.

● WHY IT MAY BE HARD TO ASK FOR HELP

A family whose child is medically fragile or chronically ill and being cared for at home desperately needs help—but may find it difficult to mobilize their own resources. They may be overwhelmed by the task for a variety of reasons including the following:

- Often, families are in a state of crisis and are feeling a host of emotions ranging from confusion and lack of control to actual clinical depression (Jarrett, Blinkoff, Dokken, & Freund, 1994). It is not uncommon that they also feel overwhelmed and stressed about their ability to care for their child (Ridgell, 1993). It may be simply too difficult for a family to begin the steps of planning and organizing.
- Families are also experiencing real physical challenges. They are exhausted from juggling many demands—their child, other family responsibilities, work, and financial issues. Any additional task to do—even if it would provide relief in the longer term—sounds daunting.
- Families may not recognize that people *other than professionals* could provide help that might relieve some of their stress and challenges. They may be focusing only on the child's care and medical help and forgetting the host of tasks that are needed to maintain "everyday life"—tasks that could be done by family, friends, and neighbors. It is not just the child, but indeed, the whole family who needs to be cared for.
- Some people are just not used to asking for help or delegating responsibility, whether at home or in the workplace. They are much more comfortable doing things themselves without relying on others. Other people may not be skilled at or experienced with planning and organizing. Faced with a seemingly overwhelming task, they may have trouble deciding how to begin.

Nurses and other health care professionals who are attuned to these factors can provide invaluable assistance in helping families to ask for help. Assistance can range from giving encouragement and motivation to suggesting specific areas in which personal resources might be useful. To help nurses in this role of "problem-solving coach," the discussion which follows includes: (a) general ideas to make families more comfortable with the process of asking for help and (b) specific areas in which families might mobilize their own resources. Asking for help may take on a new face when presented by involved nursing staff as a way of coping and caring.

● ENCOURAGEMENT FOR ASKING FOR HELP

- Encourage families to *ask for help* as a first step in the process. Assure them that asking for help is not a sign of poor coping but, rather, an important coping mechanism. Remind them that it is not a time to "go it alone." Reassure them that asking for help does not mean relinquishing control but rather gaining more control over their lives.
- Discuss with them the fact that family and friends may want to offer help but may not be sure what to do or may wonder if they are qualified to help. If they are asked directly to help with specific tasks, those same family and friends may actually be relieved and grateful.
- Suggest that they think about family members and friends and the tasks they are interested in and good at doing. Try to "match" those interests and skills appropriately with requests for help. Then people who are asked for help will feel especially selected and qualified. One family remembers the following examples of matching interests/skills and tasks: "My sister is a gourmet cook by avocation and, on a regular basis, brought meals for us. A friend who is a computer expert was delighted to select and install a personal computer so I could work at home. Another friend, a graphic artist, designed special and colorful posters for our child's room."
- Clarify that personal resources do not have to be used only for care of the medically fragile or chronically ill child; in fact, many people may not be comfortable providing hands-on care. With good discharge planning, families will hopefully have access to a variety of professional services and resources in the community. However, there are

many other nonmedical tasks which can help the family. The "Areas of Help" guideline and checklist provide a framework for beginning to identify tasks for which families could mobilize their personal resources (Table 7-1). Areas of help include overall coordination, communication, housekeeping, siblings, and information and resources.

● AREAS OF HELP GUIDELINE

The categories discussed and listed in the checklist represent areas in which families anticipating the discharge of a medically fragile or chronically ill child typically need help (see Table 7-1). They serve as a guide only. Categories and subcategories can be added or deleted depending on the needs of each family and child.

Overall coordination. Families may wish to designate one person to be "in charge" of assigning all the special tasks and coordinating individuals helping with the tasks. In this way, too much help in one area or too little in another can be avoided. Families also will not have to do all the asking themselves. The individual chosen will depend on the family's personal preferences and the interests and skills of their "resource pool." One parent may also want to assume the role.

Communication. Updating family and friends about the child's condition can be an overwhelming, repetitive, and sometimes emotionally painful task for exhausted parents. Two ways of streamlining the communication process are a telephone answering machine and a telephone tree.

Families can use their answering machine to give routine updates to callers. For example, "Things are fairly stable today. We appreciate your interest and concern but cannot talk now. Someone will call you as soon as possible. Please continue to check our answering machine for updates."

With a telephone tree, families first identify the people they would like to update on a regular basis. Then they select the one or two family members or friends whom they will call themselves with the information. Those individuals then pass the information along the phone tree. The system can be logically organized, for example, a work colleague calls others from work, and so on.

Housekeeping. Housekeeping, errands, laundry, and repairs are examples of everyday tasks that families may find difficult to fit into their schedules. It can be an enormous relief to have some of those jobs done by a volunteer. Tasks to consider include routine cleaning, special cleaning, errands, laundry, and home repair. Nurses can also assist families in determining what special housekeeping needs their situation requires. For example, an infant with asthma may require a particularly clean home environment.

Cooking, dietary needs, and grocery shopping. Families are often exhausted before the child comes home. Meal preparation and grocery shopping can certainly be done by other family members and friends; however, coordination is key so that too much food isn't given. With coordination, children's favorite foods can be prepared—a thoughtful way of maintaining their routines (see Siblings). In addition, the child or other family members may have special dietary needs. In either case, proper nutrition is important.

Siblings. Often it seems impossible to balance the care of a sick child with the other demands of life. The dilemma is particularly difficult when the family has other children. In addition to their standard needs, siblings may have new needs and feelings ranging from confusion and anxiety to rejection and anger. They may express these feelings through a variety of behaviors including withdrawal, regression, and acting out (Jarrett et al., 1994).

TABLE 7-1 ● **Areas of Help For Use by Parents and Nurses**

The following categories represent areas in which families preparing for discharge typically need help. They serve as a guide only. Adjust the list as needed depending on the needs of the family and child.

Overall Coordination
● Parent   Name/phone _____
● Family or friend   Name/phone _____

Communication
● Telephone answering machine updates
● Telephone tree

Housekeeping
● Routine cleaning   Name/phone _____
● Special cleaning   Name/phone _____

List needs: _____
● Errands   Name/phone _____
● Laundry   Name/phone _____
● Home repair   Name/phone _____

Cooking, Dietary Needs, and Grocery Shopping
Special dietary needs   _____
Grocery shopping   Name/phone _____
Cooking   Name/phone _____
                                            Time _____
                                            Name/phone _____
                                            Time _____

Siblings
● Extracurricular activities   Name/phone _____
● Playdates   Name/phone _____
● Weekend play/events   Name/phone _____
● Special homework projects   Name/phone _____
● Preschool coping   Name/phone _____
● Room parent responsibilities   Name/phone _____
● Errands (haircuts, new shoes)   Name/phone _____
● Carpooling   Name/phone _____

Transportation
● Medical appointments   Name/phone _____
● Emergency transportation   Name/phone _____
                                            Name/phone _____
                                            Name/phone _____
● Plan for the unexpected   Name/phone _____

Information and Resources
● Information and educational materials on diagnosis and related risks and conditions
                                            Source/phone _____
● Special support organizations   Source/phone _____
● Parent-to-parent support   Source/phone _____
● Respite care   Source/phone _____
● Insurance   Source/phone _____
● Other financial information   Source/phone _____

(continued)

TABLE 7-1 • **Areas of Help For Use by Parents and Nurses (*Continued*)**	
• Social services	Source/phone _____
• Other support services	Source/phone _____

Companionship

• Appointments	Name/phone _____ Date/time _____
• Errands	Name/phone _____ Date/time _____
• Shopping	Name/phone _____ Date/time _____
• Entertainment/break	Name/phone _____ Date/time _____
• Other	Name/phone _____ Date/time _____

Miscellaneous

Task/need	Name/company/organization/phone
_____	_____
_____	_____
_____	_____
_____	_____
_____	_____

Teachers and other school personnel can be asked to provide extra support to siblings. Additionally, by helping maintain the regular sibling routines, family, friends, and neighbors can help relieve both parental and child stress in several ways. Help with these tasks may free the parent to provide much needed emotional support. Tasks in this category include playdates, special homework projects, errands related to the sibling, and car-pooling.

Transportation. Families may have some special transportation concerns. Nurses can help by asking some very useful hypothetical questions. Does the child's condition warrant more than one adult on medical appointments? For example, does monitoring the child's respiratory status or managing the child and any accompanying equipment require two people? If so, families will want to prepare for these situations ahead of time by asking family members or friends for help. Do the parents know what their arrangements would be for emergency transportation? This includes a friend or neighbor who is willing to be called in an emergency, taxi services, and the local rescue squad. Most families who bring home a child with medical equipment are required to contact their local rescue squad in writing prior to discharge. Even if it is not required, a call or visit can be well worth the time later in case of an emergency. What have some of the family's transportation "crises" been before they faced this particular situation? Stranded in inclement weather? Out of needed cash for the cab or subway? Knowing that these "crisis" transportation situations are planned for can relieve everyday stress.

Information and resources. Even with good discharge planning, families may be faced with additional needs for information and resources, such as information about insurance coverage, the diagnosis, or treatment options. Once at home, families may find they need other community services and resources, including special support organizations. Remind families that these "research" tasks may be a perfect "match" with the interests or skills of friends or family. Other people can start the research process and present them with a summary of options.

When using the checklist, nurses may want to add categories or check off only specific categories within this area as the family's needs warrant, as well as refer the family to social workers or other appropriate resources for this information. Some of the categories listed include special support organizations, insurance, and parent-to-parent support.

Companionship. Remember that the entire family is affected (Baginski, 1994). Not only siblings but parents also need help and support as they face many emotional and physical challenges (Pokorni, 1996). Nurses can play an invaluable role by first giving parents "permission" to consider their own needs—by emphasizing that they will not be able to continue to help their child unless they take time out for themselves occasionally. Remind them that their partners might be reacting to the situation differently or have their own needs; and therefore, they cannot be relied on as a sole source of support.

Encourage parents to turn to close family members or friends as companions for themselves. These special companions could accompany the caregiving parent on follow-up hospital or physician visits–or even on errands. They could plan a weekly time away for the parent and take them shopping, for coffee, or to a movie. Above all, they would be available to the parent to listen, whether in person or on the telephone.

Miscellaneous. Urge families to consider the uniqueness of their situation and their own needs to determine what special "extra" help they need. For example, some parents have found the following information useful: pharmacies that deliver, pharmacies that carry special medical supplies, respiratory equipment supply companies, grocery stores that deliver, cleaning services, and companies that run errands and deliver.

● CONCLUSION

As changes take place in the delivery of health care, many more medically fragile and chronically ill children will be cared for at home. Families of these children, while overwhelmed and stressed, can find comfort from pediatric nurses who can provide assistance to the family before the child is discharged. By using the guidelines and checklist discussed, nurses can help families mobilize their resources so that the transition from hospital to home can be made as easily as possible.

REFERENCES

Baginski, Y. (1994). Roadblocks to home care. *Caring, XIII*(12), 18–24.
Jarrett, M. H., Blinkoff, R. I., Dokken, D. L., & Freund, M. B. (1994). *Parent partners listener training.* Washington, DC: The George Washington University.
Johnson, B. H., Jeppson, E. S., & Redburn, L. (1992). *Caring for children and families: Guidelines for hospitals.* Bethesda, MD: Association for the Care of Children's Health.
Kuttner, L. (1996). *A child in pain: How to help, what to do.* Point Roberts, WA: Hartley & Marks Publishers, Inc.
Leyden, C. (1997). Managed care fear not. *Pediatric Nursing, 23*(2), 176.
Pokorni, J. L. (1996). Promoting the overall development of infants and young children receiving home health services. *Pediatric Nursing, 23*(2), 187–190.
Ridgell, N. H. (1993). Home apnea monitoring: A systems approach to the family's home health care needs. *Caring, XII*(12), 34–37.
Weston, B., & Keefe, J. (1993). Pediatric home care and public policy. *Caring, XII*(12), 60–61.

Our culture influences what we believe about illness and health. Effective transcultural nursing requires self-awareness regarding our own cultural experiences as well as an ability to respect and understand cultures that are different from our own.

What have you learned from your own cultural heritage about rituals and symbols, language, dietary practices, style of communications, issues about time and personal space, and beliefs about health and illness? How do religious or spiritual practices influence your beliefs and values? Consider these questions as they relate to childbearing and childrearing as well as dietary practices, which are all aspects of family life that are expressed in a variety of ways in different cultural and religious backgrounds.

Spruhan, J. (1996). Beyond traditional nursing care: Cultural awareness and successful home healthcare nursing. *Home Healthcare Nurse*, 14(4), 445–449.

Beyond Traditional Nursing Care: Cultural Awareness and Successful Home Healthcare Nursing

JUDY BENNETT SPRUHAN

Culture affects all areas of clients' lives, including their beliefs about health and illness. Home care nurses must consider cultural values in planning effective and culturally competent nursing care. Getting in touch with one's own heritage helps nurses to understand and appreciate the cultures of others.

In recent years, nurses have become increasingly interested in the influence that culture and religion have on their clients' perceptions of illness and their willingness to cooperate with medical practitioners to achieve mutually satisfying goals of health and continued wellness. The pioneering work of nursing leaders such as Madeleine Leininger, founder of the Transcultural Nursing Society, has enhanced our knowledge of the tremendous importance of "culturally competent, congruent, safe, and beneficial care" (Leininger, 1991) (Fig. 8-1) and how that care is actualized in our nursing practice (Leininger, 1990). The American Academy of Nursing Expert Panel on Culturally Competent Nursing Care (1992) further emphasized the crucial significance of cultural competency in the delivery of effective nursing care.

Culture is defined as the communal life view of a particular group, including its beliefs, rituals and symbols, language, and dietary practices (Rempusheski, 1989). These be-

Judy Bennett Spruhan, RN, is the Clinical Specialist at Swedish Covenant Home Health Care, Chicago, IL

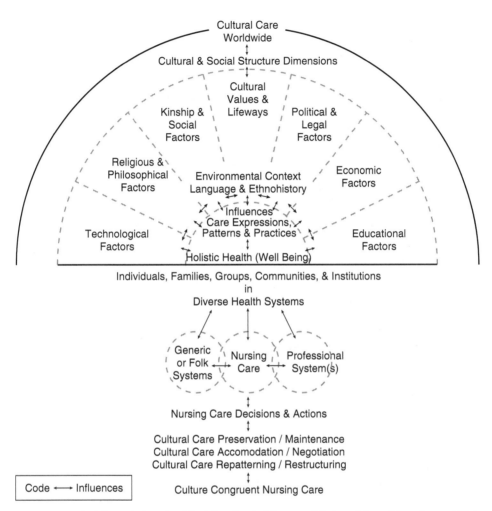

FIGURE 8-1. Leininger's Sunrise Model to Depict Theory of Cultural Care Diversity and Universality. Note. From Sunrise Model. 1991 In Cultural Care Diversity and Universality: A Theory of nursing. (p. 43), by M. Leininger, New York: New York National League for Nursing. Copyright 1991 by New York National League for Nursing. Reprinted with permission.

liefs are passed from grandparent, to parent, to child, "building a composite of prior experience" (Henkle & Kennerly, 1990). Other components of culture include education, communication style, time and personal space issues, family rituals, and beliefs about health and illness (Niederhauser, 1989). Religion and spirituality may be components of a particular culture, or they may be the primary identifiers defining a subcultural unit (such as the Amish or the Hare Krishna) (Morgan, 1992). The effect of subcultural identification within a dominant culture (such as Native American or rural Appalachian) (Hansen & Resick, 1990; Buehler, 1993) or racial identity such as African American is also important. These factors influence a client's receptiveness to teaching and willingness to engage in health-promoting behaviors, especially when these behaviors conflict with cultural or religious values. Only when a nurse recognizes and respects a client's cultural values can the basic rapport necessary for successful teaching occur.

● GENERAL CONSIDERATIONS

A common practice of many cultures is the use of home remedies (Hansen & Resick, 1990; Gonzalez-Swafford & Gutierrez, 1983). In addition to herbal teas, topical preparations such as rattlesnake oil, aloe vera, or alcohol with marijuana leaves, poultices, special prayers, and incantations are used. These preparations often are attempted first when illness occurs. They may be used exclusively or in conjunction with medications ordered by the physician. Because some of these remedies may interact adversely with prescription drugs, it is important that the nurse be familiar with them, or at least be willing to learn about them. It is un-

---

Case 1

M. was a 15-year-old Mexican girl who was recovering from meningitis. Some ataxia remained for which she was receiving physical therapy. The nurse was attempting to instruct the family on her anticonvulsant medications and basic safety issues. Although the nurse spoke some Spanish, it was obvious that something was wrong—the family was polite but did not follow through on any of the nurse's suggestions.

When the primary nurse became ill, another nurse visited the family. As with the previous nurse, the family was polite but appeared uneasy and somewhat defensive. During the visit, the mother set dinner on the table for the father, who was leaving for work. She invited the nurse to join them, who did so.

During the meal, the father suddenly turned to the nurse, and with tears in his eyes, asked, "What is wrong with us?" The nurse, confused, asked for clarification. The father replied, "The other nurse would not eat with us. I know we are poor, but we are clean people."

In this situation, the initial nurse did not recognize that her refusal to eat in the client's home was misinterpreted by the family. Within their culture, hospitality was imperative and food was meant to be shared, however meager the meal. The nurse's cultural values told her that eating at a client's home would make her gain weight. Her attempts to communicate to the family that she was on a diet confused them for two reasons. First, by their culture's standards, she was already too thin. Second, and most important, her refusal to share their meal was interpreted by the family as a statement that they were unclean and that their food was inadequate. Feeling that they were unacceptable, this family was unable to understand the importance of doing the things that the nurse was asking them to do.

Beliefs about health and illness can significantly affect a family's willingness to follow through on a plan of care. When considering these beliefs, it is important to determine what is thought to be the cause of illness and what is used to treat each illness.

For example, some Mexican American families believe in such traditional folk illnesses as mal de ojo (evil eye), empacho (surfeit), susto (fright), or caida de mollera (fallen fontanel) (Gomez & Gomez, 1985; Gonzalez-Swafford & Gutierrez, 1983). If a mother truly believes that one of these illnesses is the cause of her baby's symptoms, she will be much more likely to administer traditional folk remedies, such as oils, herbal teas, or charms obtained from a curandero (folk healer), than she would be likely to administer medications from a physician (Buehler, 1993; Reinert, 1986). Moreover, if a baby's treatment requires technology such as pulse oximetry or an apnea monitor, it may be difficult to assimilate these devices into the traditional treatment of infants with symptoms suggesting these folk illnesses.

Case 2

Baby A. was born at 34 weeks gestation, and apnea and bradycardia developed. She was discharged, given theophylline, and was using an apnea monitor. Her mother, who was Salvadoran, administered the theophylline every 6 hours as ordered. When the baby became irritable, the mother gave her chamomile tea (manzanilla). When she had difficulty sleeping, her mother gave her peppermint tea (hierba buena). Teaching regarding theophylline toxicity included recognizing irritability or sleeplessness that did not improve with the herbal teas. Although the mother had no problems with the medication, she refused to use the apnea monitor, despite persistent teaching regarding its importance. When asked about this refusal, the mother only would say that she was afraid of the monitor.

On a subsequent visit, the nurse arrived to find the mother smiling and the baby hooked up to the monitor. When the nurse asked what had changed her mind, the mother replied that her pastor had come to visit, had prayed over the monitor, and "anointed it with holy oil." In her opinion, it was now safe for her baby to use.

Family rituals that can affect nursing care may include shared holidays, religious practices, diet, or even furniture preferences. In one case, a client from India refused to lie anywhere but on the floor. The choice of his primary nurse was determined in part by her ability to provide nursing care while seated next to him on the floor. This same man's family brought water from the River Ganges to wash his body as he was dying.

Often, religious rituals overlap cultural preferences. The symbols, patterns and gestures, art forms, and prayer and meditation commonly associated with religion often make it difficult to separate religious from cultural factors (Gomez & Gomez, 1985; DiMeo, 1991).

---

likely that families will discontinue what has been used successfully for generations simply because their nurse is not familiar with them or doubts their efficacy.

Given these factors, how can home healthcare nurses effectively use the characteristics of their clients' cultures to increase health-promoting behaviors? First, cultural and spiritual assessment should be incorporated into the initial visit. Sev-

---

Case 3

Mrs. G. was a 52-year-old Mexican woman who had end-stage cervical cancer. She was taking morphine sulfate for pain when she began crying and shouting that there were demons in her television set. She eventually would fall asleep, only to awaken agitated, insisting that demons were in the room and were threatening her. Removing the television from her presence did not help. Her physician was notified. Assuming that these symptoms were hallucinations related to her morphine, the physician adjusted her medication, adding a mild tranquilizer. However, the agitation continued. The nurse discussed this with the patient's husband, who stated that he knew the solution. He brought the parish priest to visit. The priest sprinkled holy water throughout the apartment, especially in the client's room and on the television. After his visit, Mrs. G. rested comfortably. She did not see the demons again.

To provide healthcare interventions that "do not intimidate the spiritual integrity of a family" (Poma, 1983), it is often necessary to consider not only the country of origin, but the family's actual religion. Assuming without asking may lead to grossly incorrect presumptions.

Case 4

Mrs. S. was referred for home care after the birth of her first child, a healthy baby girl. Because healthy postpartum mothers and newborns usually were not referred for follow-up care, the primary nurse called the referral source for more information before the first visit. She was told that Mr. S. "went crazy in the labor room and attacked a doctor." He became angry again before discharge and informed the nurses on the unit that his wife would not return to the hospital, and he would not allow his baby to see a physician. The family was referred to home care to ensure follow-up care for postpartum and well-baby care.

On the first visit, the nurse found Mr. S. pleasant and cooperative. He allowed her to examine his wife and daughter, but repeated his insistence that they would never go back to the physician.

On a subsequent visit, the nurse discussed this with Mrs. S., discovering the root of the problem. The S. family were strict Moslems. During labor, a male physician not only approached Mrs. S. "boldly" when she was unveiled, but he proceeded to perform a vaginal examination without asking her husband's permission to touch her. (The boundaries of Moslem tradition do not allow unfamiliar men to touch another man's wife without permission.) After further questioning, Mrs. S. said that the hospital pediatrician also was a man.

On the next visit, the nurse informed Mr. and Mrs. S. that she had located a female gynecologist and a female pediatrician who were willing to see Mrs. S. and their daughter at a local department of a health clinic. Mr. S. agreed to this. Mrs. S. had her 6-week checkup, and Baby S. began her well-baby care on schedule.

When the nurse called the referral source and explained the problem, she asked if the hospital nurses had known the family's religion. The referral source replied, "We assumed they were Jewish. They were from Jerusalem."

In this case, the assessment of the S. family needed to include not only their country of origin, but, more importantly, their religion. By assuming that the S. family was Jewish, the hospital nurses missed the most important piece of the cultural puzzle. The husband's objection to male physicians was rooted deeply in the traditions of his Islamic faith. By suggesting female specialists for Mrs. S. and her daughter, the nurse showed her awareness and her acceptance of Mr. S's need to obey the proscriptions of his religion regarding touch.

---

eral useful tools are available for such assessment, from the comprehensive (such as those of Niederhauser and Leininger, which analyze culture from an anthropologic point of view) (Leininger, 1991; Niederhauser, 1989), to the less sophisticated (such as that of Rosenbaum) (Wald & Bailey, 1990). By learning a family's cultural and religious expectations, the nurse can plan interventions and patient teaching acceptable to individuals and their families (Peterson, 1985; Roberson, 1987).

Whenever possible, culture-specific teaching materials should be used (Henkle & Kennerly, 1990; Gorrie, 1989). For example, dietary guides developed by the American Dietetic Association (Henkle & Kennerly, 1990) and materials from the Office of Substance Abuse for prevention of alcoholism (Gorrie, 1989) are particularly effective because they present health-promoting behaviors within the context of Hispanic, Native American, and African American cultures.

In addition, community cultural associations are another valuable resource, not only for language assistance, but also for culturally acceptable assistance with psychosocial and socioeconomic needs.

No individual nurse can be expected to know the beliefs of all religious groups. However, referrals can be made to community religious centers regarding matters of spiritual guidance. Simple guides are available outlining basic beliefs of the major religious systems. Elizabeth DiMeo developed an easy-to-use reference chart for this purpose (Tripp-Reimer & Afifi, 1989).

Most important, we, as nurses must familiarize ourselves with our own cultural and religious values and expectations. As we learn to know and value our own heritage, we can understand and respect more fully the rich diversity of cultures represented by our clients.

REFERENCES

American Academy of Nursing Expert Panel on Culturally Competent Nursing Care. (1992). Culturally competent health care. *Nursing Outlook, 40,* 277–283.

American Dietetic Association. (1989). *Ethnic and regional food practices: A series.* Chicago: American Dietetic Association.

Buehler, J. (1993). Nursing in rural Native American communities. *Nursing Clinics of North America, 28,* 211—217.

DiMeo, E. (1991). Rx for spiritual distress. *RN, 54,* 22–25.

Gomez, G. E., & Gomez, E. A. (1985). Folk healing among Hispanic Americans. *Public Health Nursing, 2,* 245–249.

Gonzalez-Swafford, M., & Gutierrez, M. (1983, November/December). Ethno-medical beliefs and practices of Mexican-Americans. *Nurse Practitioner,* 29–34.

Gorrie, M. (1989). Reaching clients through cross cultural education. *Journal of Gerontological Nursing, 15,* 29–31.

Hansen, M., & Resick, L. (1990). Health beliefs, health care and rural Appalachian subcultures from an ethnographic perspective. *Family and Community Health, 7,* 145–149.

Henkle, J., & Kennerly, S. (1990). Cultural diversity: A resource in planning and implementing nursing care. *Nursing Science Quarterly, 7,* 145–149.

Leininger, M. (1990). The significance of cultural concepts in nursing. *Journal of Transcultural Nursing, 2,* 52—59.

Leininger, M. (1991). *Culture care diversity and universality: A theory of nursing.* New York: National League for Nursing.

Morgan, M. (1992). Pregnancy and childbirth beliefs and practices of American Hare Krishna devotees within transcultural nursing. *Journal of Transcultural Nursing, 4,* 5–10.

Niederhauser, V. (1989). Health care of immigrant children. *Pediatric Nursing, 15,* 569–574.

Office for Substance Abuse Prevention. *The discovery kit: Positive connections for kids.* Rockville, MD: Author.

Peterson, E. (1985). The physical . . . the spiritual . . . can you meet all of your patient's needs: *Journal of Gerontological Nursing, 11,* 23–27.

Poma, P. (1983). Hispanic cultural influences on medical practice. *Journal of the National Medical Association, 75,* 941–946.

Reinert, B. (1986). The health care beliefs and values of Mexican-Americans. *Home Healthcare Nurse, 4,* 23–31.

Rempusheski, V. (1989). The role of ethnicity in elder care. *Nursing Clinics of North America, 24,* 717–724.

Roberson, M. (1987). Home remedies: a cultural study. *Home Healthcare Nurse, 5,* 35–40.

Rosenbaum, J. (1991). A cultural assessment guide. *Canadian Nurse, 87,* 21–22.

Tripp-Reimer, T., & Afifi, L. (1989). Crosscultural perspective on patient teaching. *Nursing Clinics of North America, 24,* 613–619.

Wald, F., & Bailey, S. (1990). Nurturing the spiritual component in care for the terminally ill. *Caring, IX,* 64–68.

Since the early 20th century, health promotion has been considered the foundation of nursing practice. Gradually over time, less emphasis was placed on health promotion and more on the care of the acutely ill in the hospital setting. Recently, health promotion has enjoyed increasing attention as cost containment has dominated health care policy. Self-care is fundamental to health promotion.

How can nurses promote health within contemporary practice settings? What are the essential components of a health promotion assessment? What are effective strategies in health promotion practice?

Frenn, M., & Malin, S. (1998). Health promotion: Theoretical perspectives and clinical applications. Holistic Nursing Practice, 12(2), 1–7.

Health Promotion: Theoretical Perspectives and Clinical Applications

MARILYN FRENN, SHELLY MALIN

The article addresses the realities of health promotion practice in a managed care environment, synthesizing the most important findings from the midrange theories currently guiding wellness-oriented research. Factors that have been shown to predict engagement in a number of health behaviors are identified and are formulated into a guide for clinical assessment, intervention, and outcome evaluation for clients across the life span. Key words: *health behavior, health belief model, health promotion, health promotion model, nursing assessment, nursing intervention, nursing outcomes, self-efficacy, stages of change, theory of planned behavior.*

P romoting health has been fundamental to nursing practice since Nightingale. Various contemporary midrange theories guide health promotion activities in the current managed care environment. Additional areas require scrutiny, however. What conclusions can nurses draw from the theory-based research findings in promoting healthy behavior? How can health be promoted in the context of a 15-minute visit, a same-day surgery, or an acute hospitalization? Most crucial, how can health be promoted given the diminished resources and time available in public and community health settings? What are the essentials for health promotion assessment? Do differences in the way nurses intervene affect care? What sort of health promotion outcomes are acceptable and feasible to measure? Answers to these questions are essential to foster health in managed care environments.

Marilyn Frenn, PhD, RN, Assistant Professor and Shelly Malin, PhD, RN, Assistant Professor, College of Nursing, Marquette University, Milwaukee, WI

● PROMOTING HEALTHY BEHAVIOR: FINDINGS FROM MAJOR THEORIES

Most nursing and health promotion research has utilized midrange theories originating in cognitive or social psychology. Models include the health belief model,[1,2] the social cognitive model,[3–5] the theory of planned behavior,[6,7] and the transtheoretical model.[8–10] Elements of these models have been synthesized and extended for nursing purposes in Pender's revised health promotion model.[11–13] The findings of research based on these models consistently identify the importance of benefits of and barriers to behavior, self-efficacy, behavioral intention, and stage of change.

An individual's perception of barriers and benefits has consistently been most predictive of subsequent behavior.[14–17] When benefits outweigh barriers, behavioral change is likely to occur.[10] Research suggests that clinicians should develop interventions powerful enough to help individuals increase the benefits of a health behavior change and/or decrease the barriers to change.[18,19] Public health policies can also increase the benefits of health behavior changes; for example, laws can require reductions in health and life insurance premiums for seatbelt use or smoking cessation.

It is important to assess individuals' perceptions because what some experience as a barrier may be experienced as a benefit by others.[20] For example, family concerns over smoking can be perceived by some people as badgering, leading them to maintain their smoking behavior as a sign of personal freedom, whereas others perceive this concern as a benefit, fostering behavior change.

To overcome barriers to a desired action, self-efficacy, the belief in one's capacity to accomplish the desired action, is needed. Self-efficacy has been found to be predictive of a number of health behaviors,[21] such as breast self-examination,[22] safe sex,[23] exercise,[24] nutrition,[25] and smoking cessation.[26]

Self-efficacy is behavior specific. To evaluate self-efficacy in a clinical or research situation, a new instrument must be developed for each behavior.[3] Antecedents thought to enhance self-efficacy include verbal persuasion, modeling, emotional arousal, and enactment.[4] Verbal persuasion has been shown to promote development of confidence in one's ability to perform a desired behavior. Modeling, or observing others perform the desired action, also helps build self-efficacy. Emotional arousal is a factor to be considered, especially when phobias are encountered, because this may influence level of confidence. Overall, the optimal way to enhance self-efficacy is enactment. Nurses can encourage clients to try a healthy behavior. As the behavior is performed successfully, emotional arousal before performance decreases, and confidence increases.

Theorists suggest that, in addition to self-efficacy, subjective norms and affect influence behavioral intention, which then predicts actual behavior.[7,27] Across studies, behavioral intention is a significant predictor of actual behavior. Nurses can ask their clients about what they plan to do within a specific time frame. Research[28] suggests that nurses can set goals with clients to begin their intended health behaviors within a 2-month period.

Attitudes may influence behavioral intention. For example, women tend to favor seatbelt use and can be encouraged to share these attitudes with others.[29] Knowing the attitudes that influence specific behaviors in population subgroups also is important. Young men respond more favorably to teaching strategies suggesting that condom use may decrease their partner's worry and increase satisfaction. This is in contrast to attempts to try to change attitudes about risks of pregnancy or sexually transmitted diseases from lack of condom use.[30] Gay men also may be more influenced by peer-provided education and by perception of norms in the gay community than by health professionals' attempts to change attitudes toward condoms.[31] Subjective norms generally have been the least predictive construct in the theory of planned behavior, however.[32,33]

Pender's health promotion model incorporates predictive components of the aforementioned models with a unique perspective on promoting health, not just reducing health risks.[13] The health promotion model has been used with adolescents[34] through older adults[35–37] in various cultures.[38,39] Pender's model has evolved to incorporate variables consistent with nursing's holistic view. Major components of Pender's model include individual characteristics (prior related behavior and personal factors, such as biologic, sociocultural, and psychologic factors), behavior-specific cognitions and affect (perceived benefits and barriers, self-efficacy, and interpersonal influences, such as family, peers, providers, norms, support, and models as well as situational influences and options), and behavioral outcomes, mediated by commitment to a plan of action and immediate competing demands and preferences.[13]

Like Pender's model, the transtheoretical model[8–10] is integrative and comprehensive. Change processes for a wide range of behaviors (eg, smoking, delinquent behavior, exercise, and use of sunscreens[9,10]) have been studied using the transtheoretical model. People appear to move through a series of stages in their efforts to change or adopt a behavior.[40] These stages have been labeled as precontemplation, contemplation, preparation, action, and maintenance.

Precontemplation is a period in which the person is not thinking about changing or adopting a given behavior, at least not within the next 6 months. Contemplation is the period of time when the person ponders adopting a behavior in the next 6 months. Preparation is the time in which the person readies himself or herself to adopt a behavior in the next month. Action is a period ranging from the actual time of change to 6 months after the person has made the overt change. Maintenance is defined as the period beginning 6 months after action has started and continuing until the behavior is adopted or terminated. Only a small portion of a given population is ready to take action in changing behaviors,[41] so that nurses must assess the stage of change to focus interventions appropriately.

● HOW CAN NURSES PROMOTE HEALTH WITHIN CONTEMPORARY PRACTICE SETTINGS?

Given research outcomes and limited available time, how can nurses promote health in the context of office visits, same-day surgeries, acute hospitalizations, and, most important, public and community health settings? Major health promotion theories suggest critical factors that are of paramount importance when applied to nursing assessment, intervention, and outcome evaluation.

● HEALTH PROMOTION: ESSENTIALS OF ASSESSMENT

Research demonstrates that benefits and barriers to health are individually defined, necessitating individualized assessment. The relevance and critical nature of self-efficacy in major health promotion theories, as well as the usefulness of personal efficacy in overcoming barriers, make this construct another essential for assessment. Nurses need to assess when clients plan to make a change or the stage of change they are experiencing. Based on major research findings, four assessment questions are essential:

1. When did you begin [this behavior], or when do you plan to start? (This is a staging question.)

   • *Precontemplation:* No plans for 6 months or more
   • *Contemplation:* Plans within 6 months
   • *Planning:* Plans within 1 month or previous attempts
   • *Action:* 1 day to 6 months of new behavior
   • *Maintenance:* More than 6 months of new behavior

2. What benefits do you see in doing this behavior? (Ask the client to list as many as he or she can.)
3. What has been difficult for you about doing this behavior? (Then ask how the person has dealt with what has been experienced as difficult.)
4. How confident do you feel in being able to initiate and continue this behavior? (Prompt the person with example situations.)

Other assessment parameters that have received some research support include previous behavior and affect. Questions related to these areas may be added in subsequent interactions or if time allows.

Many times a client information sheet can be developed so that clients can review assessment questions while they are in the waiting room. Computerized systems may be used to highlight required immunizations or screenings and to identify goals set during a previous visit. Once particular health behaviors and concepts important to change have been assessed, appropriate individual or group interventions can be constructed. Nurses can then maximize their time with clients by focusing on areas most needed to promote their health.

● WHAT WORKS IN HEALTH PROMOTION PRACTICE?

Although many Americans need to change unhealthy behavior, most are not ready for action. Nurses can make the greatest impact if they match health promotion interventions with the client's stage of change. In addition, materials should be chosen carefully to reflect the needs of the population being served in terms of diversity, comprehension (reading level and language), and developmental level. In a weight reduction study in a health maintenance organization and community setting using this approach, 75% participation was achieved compared with 3% to 6% participation when materials were given to people regardless of their stage of change.[9]

After the client's stage of change has been determined, appropriate health promotion interventions can be chosen.

Precontemplation

Nurses can focus on developing relationships and establishing trust such that, when clients are ready to change, they will seek help as needed and know that user-friendly resources are available. Homework may be suggested to foster an enhanced list of benefits for the change. Provision of such homework assignments means that health care practitioners need to develop their own repertoire of benefits for given health behaviors. Provider preparation may include brainstorming with other providers to generate benefits identified by clients, reviewing research related to the behavior to identify additional benefits, and developing self-assessment cards for clients to check identified benefits. An alternative approach is to invite a group of precontemplators to brainstorm with a few members in action and maintenance stages to serve as role models. If such a strategy is used, however, "preaching" should be avoided because it may turn precontemplators away.

Contemplation

Many of the same strategies used with precontemplators are useful during contemplation. Additional strategies include affirming the movement into contemplation as an important step and assessing movement into preparation. A journal may be an important tool at this stage to provide clients with useful information about the designated behavior and how it is integrated into their lifestyle. Notations about benefits can be added to the journal.

Preparation

Clients have entered preparation when they have identified a start date within the next month or have made previous unsuccessful attempts. Nurses can provide preparatory guidance that "unsuccessful" attempts are often necessary to accomplish positive behavior change. Clients are more likely to believe that they are moving toward success rather than failing in their attempts. Nurses can commend any attempts and provide encouragement to those who have tried unsuccessfully that these actions are important, positive parts of the process of change. Contracting with clients is also important at this stage. The date of change, specific behaviors to be considered, responsibilities of client and provider, outcomes to be assessed, and target evaluation times should be included.

Action

Taking action is the most powerful way clients build their self-efficacy; it helps them sustain their efforts. Planned reinforcement and evaluation of progress are methods by which nurses can foster positive movement. Plans to deal with relapse need to be addressed so that clients feel comfortable discussing any encountered problems. Relapse discussions should include planning for the subsequent change attempts and strategies for overcoming barriers.

Maintenance

Providing leadership in groups may appeal to some clients in maintenance stages and acts as a further reinforcement of their continued maintenance. Involvement in providing testimony to change public policy relative to the societal influences on the health behavior may also be a relevant intervention in some cases. Continuing the journal and sharing excerpts with the nurse may be additional ways to reinforce expertise and contribute to the clinician's repertoire for future clients.

● HEALTH PROMOTION OUTCOMES: WHAT IS FEASIBLE TO MEASURE?

With a focus on matching stage of change and intervention, nurses' understanding of measurable outcomes must be reframed. Effective outcomes from visit to visit might mean simple movement from one stage to another. Given the evidence, most people attempting to stop an addictive behavior (eg, smoking) will have to try several times. A person who does not quit smoking the first time should be encouraged to try again and advised that there is an increased likelihood of success. Clinicians need to stay abreast of current research to integrate perceived benefits/barriers, self-efficacy, intentions, and parameters of behavioral change as expected outcomes.

Partnerships between clinicians and researchers may foster the most meaningful ongoing research needed to evaluate outcomes for clients within particular developmental and cultural groups. For example, use of a client information system that includes a rating on progress regarding specific behaviors would provide valuable outcome data for a given practice. Benchmarks for client progress can be set based on aggregated national or regional client data if a standardized system is used. These data can inform further intervention research to help clients reach benchmarks with the most efficient use of health care resources.

Time constraints on clinical practice within managed care make effective use of the time nurses have with clients a priority. Accurate assessment regarding factors that precede behavior change helps nurses focus their action-oriented interventions on clients who will best profit from them. Clients who are not ready for change can be helped to move in that direction by assistance with identifying benefits to healthy behavior change and the potential hazards in the status quo.

Nurses can organize health promotion systems so that assessments are completed by clients before visits. Time with clients can be efficiently planned through the use of expert system technology, groups, and media-assisted interventions that address readiness to change, reading level, and cultural issues. Computerized information systems can enhance clinical efficiency as well as contribute useful data in the refinement of interventions to foster clients' health most effectively and economically. Technology cannot replace nurses' clinical judgment and the relationship needed with clients for interventions based on their readiness to change. Nurses' knowledge of the key factors involved in successfully maintaining health promotion changes is essential to successful client outcomes.

REFERENCES

1. Becker MH, Haefner DP, Kasl SV, Kirscht JP, Maiman LA, Rosenstock IM. Selected psychosocial models and correlates of individual health-related behaviors. *Med Care.* 1977;15:27–46.
2. Rosenstock IM, Strecher VJ, Becker MH. Social learning theory and the Health Belief Model. *Health Educ Q.* 1988;15:175–183.
3. Bandura A. *Social Foundations of Thought and Action: A Social Cognitive Theory.* Englewood Cliffs, NJ: Prentice-Hall; 1986.
4. Bandura A. Self-efficacy mechanism in psychobiologic functioning. In Schwarzer R, ed. *Self-Efficacy: Thought Control of Action.* Washington, DC: Hemisphere; 1992.
5. Bandura A. *Self Efficacy: The Exercise of Control.* New York: Freeman; 1997.
6. Azjen I, Fishbein M. *Understanding Attitudes and Predicting Social Behavior.* Englewood Cliffs, NJ; Prentice Hall; 1977.
7. Azjen I. *Attitudes, Personality, and Behavior.* Chicago: Dorsey; 1985.
8. Prochaska JO, DiClemente CC. Stages and processes of self change of smoking. Toward an integrative model of change. *J Consult Clin Psychol.* 1983;5:390–395.
9. Prochaska JO, Norcross JC, Fowler JL, Follick MJ, Abrams DB. Attendance and outcome in a work site weight control program: Processes and stages of change as process and predictor variables. *Addict Behav.* 1992;17:35–45.

10. Prochaska JO, Velicer WF, Rossi JS, et al. Stages of change and decisional balance for 12 problem behaviors. *Health Psychol.* 1994;13:39–46.

11. Pender NJ. *Health Promotion in Nursing Practice.* Norwalk, CT: Appleton-Century-Crofts; 1982.

12. Pender NJ. *Health Promotion in Nursing Practice.* 2nd ed. Norwalk, CT: Appleton & Lange; 1987.

13. Pender NJ. *Health Promotion in Nursing Practice.* 3rd ed. Norwalk, CT: Appleton & Lange; 1996.

14. Fischera SD, Frank DI. The health belief model as a predictor of mammography screening. *Health Values.* 1994;18:3–9.

15. Hahn EJ. Predicting Head Start parent involvement in an alcohol and other drug prevention program. *Nurs Res.* 1995;44:45–51.

16. McInyk KAM. Barriers: A critical review of recent literature. *Nurse Res.* 1988;37:196–201.

17. Watts RJ. Beliefs about prostate disease in African American men: A pilot study. *ABNF J.* July/August 1994;102–105.

18. Champion VL. Beliefs about breast cancer and mammography by behavioral stage. *Oncol Nurs Forum.* 1994;21:1009–1114.

19. Champion VL. Results of a nurse-delivered intervention on proficiency and nodule detection with breast self-examination. *Oncol Nurs Forum.* 1995;22:819–824.

20. Frenn M. Older adults' experience of health promotion: A theory for nursing practice. *Public Health Nurs.* 1996;13:65–71.

21. Schwarzer R, ed. *Self-Efficacy: Thought Control of Action.* Washington, DC: Hemisphere; 1992.

22. Lu ZJ. Variables associated with breast self-examination among Chinese women. *Cancer Nurs.* 1995;18:29–34.

23. McKusick L, Coates TJ, Morin SF. Longitudinal predictors of reductions in unprotected anal intercourse among Gay men in San Francisco: The AIDS behavioral research project. *Am J Public Health.* 1990;80:978–983.

24. Duncan TE, McAuley E. Social support and efficacy cognitions in exercise adherence: A latent growth curve analysis. *J Behav Med.* 1993;16:199–218.

25. Shannon B, Bagby R, Wang MQ, Trenker L. Self-efficacy: A contributor to the explanation of eating behavior. *Health Educ Res.* 1990;5:395–407.

26. Velicer WF, DiClemente CC, Rossi JS, Prochaska JO. Relapse situations and self-efficacy: An intergrative model. *Addict Behav.* 1990;15:271–283.

27. Burns AC. The expanded health belief model as the basis for enlightened preventive health care practice and research. *J Health Care Market.* 1992;12:332–45.

28. Sharpe PA, McConnell CM. Exercise beliefs and behaviors among older adult employees: A health promotion trial. *Gerontologist.* 1992;32:444–449.

29. Martin GL, Newman IM. Women as motivators in the use of safety belts. *Health Values.* 1990; 14:37–47.

30. Lavole M, Godin G. Correlates of intention to use condoms among auto mechanic students. *Health Educ Res.* 1991;6:313–316.

31. Ross MW, McLaws MI. Subjective norms about condoms are better predictors of use and intention to use than attitudes. *Health Educ Res.* 1992;7:335–339.

32. Jemmott LS, Jemmott JB. Applying the theory of reasoned action to AIDS risk behavior: Condom use among Black women. *Nurs Res.* 1991;40:228–234.

33. Kimiecik J. Predicting vigorous physical activity of corporate employees: Comparing the theories of reasoned action and planned behavior. *J Sport Exerc Psychol.* 1992;14:192–206.

34. Garcia A, Broda MA, Frenn M, Coviak C, Pender NJ, Roans DL. Gender and development differences in exercise beliefs among youth and prediction of their exercise behavior. *J School Health.* 1995;65:213–219.

35. Duffy ME. Determinants of health promotion in mid-life women. *Nurs Res.* 1988;37:358–362.

36. Duffy ME. Determinants of health promoting life styles in older persons. *Image.* 1993; 25:23–28.

37. Walker SN, Volkan K, Sechrist KR, Pender NJ. Health promoting lifestyles of older adults: Comparisons with young and middle-aged adults, correlates and patterns. *Adv Nurs Sci.* 1988;11:76–90.
38. Ahijevych K, Bernhard L. Health-promoting behaviors of African American women. *Nurs Res.* 1994;43:86–89.
39. Duffy ME, Rossow R, Hernandez M. Correlates of health-promotion activities in employed Mexican American women. *Nurs Res.* 1996;45:18–24.
40. Marcus BH, Simkin LR. The transtheoretical model: Applications to exercise behavior. *Med Sports Exerc.* 1994;26:1400–1404.
41. DiClemente CC, Prochaska JO, Fairhurst S, Velicer WF, Velasquez MM, Rossi JS. The process of smoking cessation: An analysis of precontemplation, contemplation and preparation stages of change. *J Consult Clin Psychol.* 1991;59:295–304.

Facilitating continuity means facilitating a client's progression from a clinical environment to home. Identifying environmental, medical, psychosocial, financial, and functional issues that may cause setbacks after discharge is an essential nursing strategy to ensure that continuity of care is managed across health care settings. This article discusses how this can be accomplished.

What are some of the strategies that enable staff nurses to coordinate a safe discharge? How can visualizing the client at home enhance discharge planning? What are some issues to consider before referring a client to home care?

Green, K., & Lydon, S. (1998). The continuum of patient care. *American Journal of Nursing*, 98(10), 16BBB–16DDD.

The Continuum of Patient Care

KAY GREEN, SUSAN LYDON

You can ease a patient's progression from a clinical environment to his home.

*H*ospital supervisor: *"This is Jack Sorenson's second admission to the hospital in a week! Can't the home health nurses figure something out to keep him home?"* Home health nurse: *"I wish the hospital nurses had seen that Mr. Sorenson's discharge plan couldn't work. We're not miracle workers!"*

Jack Sorenson, a 69-year-old patient with a diagnosis of diabetes and two recent below-the-knee amputations, was readmitted to the hospital just four days after his discharge with a high fever, signs of infection at the surgical site, and hypoglycemia. The discharge planner had developed a plan based on the information he gleaned from interviews with the patient and his wife. However, the Sorensons had high expectations of their ability to manage his recovery at home, and the hospital staff had overestimated the assistance the home health agency would be able to provide. Unfortunately, this scenario of unsuccessful transition from hospital to home is a common one.

Home health care has grown tremendously in the past 10 years in an effort to treat patients in less costly settings. Many patients leave the hospital with ongoing medical needs, and they need a health care continuum that works. According to authors Pamela Bean and Kathryn Waldron, seeing care as a continuum is a return to the basic principles of health care: treat the whole person from wellness to illness to recovery, within the community.

Home health care and other community resources help to meet patient needs and prevent rehospitalizations. Nurses in acute care settings must view the inpatient experience

Kay Green is the vice president of ambulatory services at Desert Regional Medical Center in Palm Springs, CA. Susan Lydon is the director of case management at Desert Regional Medical Center in Palm Springs, CA.

as a relatively small component of treatment for a critical illness or injury. Nurses are evolving rapidly to also function as patient advocates—key participants in bridging the continuum, and managers of patients' transitions between levels of care.

● CHANGES IN HEALTH CARE

There's tremendous pressure on the health care industry to control costs: Congress is currently struggling to prevent the looming bankruptcy of Medicare, and businesses are demanding affordable health plans to offer employees. Managed care is a direct result of these pressures.

Length of hospital stay has shortened from the standard of 10 to 15 years ago. For example, a patient admitted in the 1980s for a coronary artery bypass graft surgery stayed seven to 10 days. Today, these patients are typically discharged after three or four days of acute hospitalization. A study completed by the Rand Corporation, a health care and social policy research company, confirmed what many of us have personally observed—that since the advent of Medicare's prospective payment system, patients are being discharged in less recovered states. Discharged patients may still be receiving ongoing intravenous infusions such as TPN, antibiotics, chemotherapy, or a variety of other medical treatments that previously had been administered exclusively in hospitals. Now more than ever, nurses in acute settings have a responsibility to recognize patients with ongoing needs and to secure appropriate follow-up care for them. Health care continuity is also increasingly important as the "baby boomer" generation ages and receives more frequent diagnoses of disease and disability.

● ASSURING SAFE DISCHARGES

Often in inpatient settings, discharge planners don't have the opportunity to observe a patient's functional abilities, making it difficult to identify pertinent issues that may affect the patient's release. That's why it's so important that nurses who provide a patient's primary care also become involved in his discharge.

As patient advocates, nurses can "build the bridge" that allows patients a smooth transition from one care setting to another. Many hospitals and health systems have made significant improvements in the delivery of ongoing care. Some hospitals have introduced new staff positions to help improve the continuum of care for their patients, including home health liaisons, who identify home care needs and coordinate appropriate referrals, and resource managers, who monitor quality of hospital services and identify interdisciplinary discharge needs. Although these specialized roles have improved the transition process, the primary care nurse remains critical.

We're often so busy trying to meet the immediate needs of patients that it's difficult to imagine how to anticipate their future needs. But this can be incorporated into patient care. You may, for example, observe visual impairment in a newly diagnosed patient with diabetes who lives alone. By anticipating his need to independently prepare an insulin injection, you may realize that he'll require adaptive equipment or the assistance of a community agency. You can then inform him and the discharge planner what you recommend upon the patient's release.

Most nursing programs focus on developing the knowledge and skills necessary for acute care. Unfortunately, this lack of educational preparation and experience in identifying continuing care needs makes it difficult for nurses to visualize patients in other settings and contribute to a smooth transition. You might need a better understanding of the services other care settings provide and how they could affect the success of the discharge plan. It's also crucial that all caregivers share the information that each has gathered.

● HOME HEALTH CARE

Nurses aren't always able to help patients understand their ongoing health care needs before they are released. But even if you do manage to instruct the patient, he is often so ill or anxious about his pending discharge that he may not fully comprehend. And patients and their families are now expected to learn complex medical procedures that have historically been performed exclusively by licensed professionals. For example, patients now manage sterile dressing changes, intravenous infusions, intramuscular injections, and site care of central venous catheters.

When patients are in their own homes, they are less anxious and more inclined to learn. Under these circumstances, home health care can be highly effective in providing education in complex technical procedures and disease management concepts.

Home health care professionals provide clinical assessment, education, and specific health maintenance skills such as wound care and intravenous infusions. Visits typically last 45 minutes to an hour and may occur two to three times a week. The scope of home care is limited to intermittent and medically necessary services such as those provided by licensed nurses, physical therapists, occupational therapists, speech therapists, and social workers. Although home care prepares patients to function independently, the home care discharge plan may depend on the capabilities of family members who are helping the patient recuperate and their communication with the home health agency.

When a patient's needs have not been adequately addressed in the hospital before discharge, the consequences can be serious. Because the first home health care visit may not occur until 24 to 48 hours after a patient is discharged home, it's important that nurses help patients identify their needs during that time, to ensure that they can function independently. If a patient can't successfully function without home health intervention within the first 24 hours, the acute care nurse should alert the discharge planner so that she can revise the discharge plan and possibly arrange for a home health agency nurse to visit the patient on the day of discharge (see *Home Health Interventions*).

● VISUALIZING THE PATIENT AT HOME

It's important to a successful discharge that nurses gain insight into the patient's home environment. If you identify problem areas before the patient goes home, you may find that he needs an alternate plan. For example, Olivia Simpson, diagnosed with end-stage pancreatic cancer, was scheduled to be discharged into her husband's care, with the support of a hospice home care program. The primary clinician found that Ms. Simpson's husband was seriously depressed and had been unable to care for himself. The nurse contacted the hospice program to inform them of this. Instead of continuing with her original discharge plan, Ms. Simpson was released to a nursing facility for a week while the hospice program coordinated additional family support to assist her husband in caring for her at home.

Environmental factors can also affect the success of a patient's discharge. Someone who requires a walker or wheelchair, for example, would be quite limited in a home with narrow doorways or stairs, or in an apartment building with no elevator, and would clearly require assistance. A patient who might otherwise be active and mobile could literally be confined to one room in a home with inadequate adaptations for this support equipment. The nurse can proactively identify some of these concerns before the patient is discharged.

Home Health Interventions
· ·

Here are the various steps that a home health nurse takes to treat a homebound patient.

ASSESS: Evaluate a patient's physical, environmental, psychosocial, and functional status.

TEACH: Explain disease progression, medication administration, possible side effects, signs of exacerbation, safety measures, wound care, bowel and bladder management, and how to perform activities of daily living.

PERFORM: Carry out nursing procedures such as intravenous infusions and maintenance of sites, wound care, or venipunctures for laboratory specimen collection; administer injectable medication; or insert urinary catheter.

COUNSEL: Assist patients in long-term planning to identify future health needs.

COORDINATE: Supervise care plans implemented by other professionals, such as physical therapists or social service representatives.

REFER: Contact community resources, such as durable medical equipment companies, meal delivery services, private duty nurses, and other programs. Act as the patient's advocate.

Sometimes the most basic concerns are the most critical. Consider these questions: How will the patient get food? How will he get his medications? How will he get to the bathroom?

To understand a patient's future care needs as he's returning home, you might ask several more questions: Will the patient and caregiver be able to perform a dressing change? Does the patient have a memory deficit that may alter his compliance with an exercise or medication regime? Does he have the financial resources to purchase medication or foods for a special diet? Does he require special supplies, and can he access them? (see *Identifying Issues for Hospital Discharge*)

● THE RIGHT HOME CARE

Psychosocial factors can largely influence a patient's recovery. You have the opportunity to observe interactions between the patient and the person who will be providing his care at home. Notice whether the caregiver assists the patient in the hospital. Does he provide support as needed? Are interactions between them congenial and caring? Are there signs of resentment or apathy? Does the patient act differently when the caregiver isn't present? Does the caregiver have functional deficits or health problems that may impede his ability to assist the patient? Answers to these questions can provide important clues to the quality of care the patient will receive at home.

Often, a patient's physical strength decreases during the course of his illness. Or the patient may have a long-term functional deficit—like paralysis—which would significantly limit performance of ADLs [activities of daily living]. How will he adapt to such deficiencies? To assistive devices? To a caregiver's assistance? Will the patient's home environment support these adaptations?

Wendell Anderson, for instance, a man who was rendered paraplegic from an automobile accident six years ago, was discharged after a six-day hospitalization for pneumonia. Mr. Anderson had lived alone for years, and his home accommodated his disability.

Identifying Issues for Hospital Discharge

This chart lists points to consider before referring a patient to home care.

MEDICAL CONCERNS
- Instruct the patient on the purpose and schedule of medications.
- Discuss whether the patient will be able to fill necessary prescriptions.
- Evaluate whether the patient will need medical intervention within the first 24 hours—for example, for wound care or IV infusions.
- Make arrangements for the immediate delivery of durable medical equipment.
- Ask the discharge planner the need to make arrangements with the home health agency to visit the patient on the day of discharge.
- Instruct the patient and caregiver on early symptoms of exacerbation and on most probable side effects to medications.
- Provide instructions on how and when to report changes in his condition or how to ask questions about his medical treatment plan.
- Give the patient the phone number of a 24-hour home health agency nurse if available.

FUNCTIONAL CONCERNS
- Determine whether the patient will need a support device, such as a bedside commode, an oxygen unit, or a walker, for activities he'll have to perform before the first home care nursing visit.
- Evaluate the patient's ability to independently perform ADLs as well as the caregivers' capacity to provide assistance.

ENVIRONMENTAL CONCERNS
- Address the patient's mobility limitations.
- Determine whether special arrangements should be made, such as providing a refrigerator for IV solutions, ensuring cleanliness for sterile procedures, or taking dust control measures for respiratory conditions.
- Assess whether there are physical barriers, such as stairs or narrow doorways, in the patient's home.
- Educate him about assistive devices such as a walker.
- Evaluate the patient's access to transportation for doctor appointments, or grocery shopping.

PSYCHOSOCIAL CONCERNS
- Find out if the patient has support systems, such as friends, family, church volunteers, and community social groups available to him.
- Determine the willingness and competency of the caregiver to provide support to the patient.
- Note whether there are difficult interactions between the patient and caregiver.

FINANCIAL CONCERNS
- Address the patient's ability to pay for basic needs such as groceries, transportation, electricity, and prescription medications.
- Discuss the patient's concerns about insurance coverage.

However, his upper body strength had deteriorated during his hospitalization, hindering his ability to get into and out of his wheelchair by himself. The nurse informed the discharge planner, who made appropriate changes to the release plan.

● CLOSING THE GAP

Identifying environmental, medical, psychosocial, financial, and functional issues that can potentially cause setbacks after a patient's discharge is one of the most significant contributions you can make, bridging these gaps of care through education and communication.

Patient education is often an appropriate intervention for many discharge issues, but effective teaching can become very difficult. Patients may be upset about the transition from the hospital to their homes. They may worry about being able to care for themselves properly, think that they're a burden to loved ones, have financial concerns or anxiety about body changes, or they may fear injury or recurrence of their illness.

Focus on information that will help him in the first 24 to 48 hours at home. This may include how to empty a drainage bag; when to take medications; symptoms that would prompt a call to the physician; circumstances in which he would contact emergency medical assistance; and the name and phone number of the home health agency that will be providing services. Teach only the most critical issues and make sure that your patient understands them. Remember that providing too much information at this point can make him more anxious.

Carefully record pertinent information on the patient's discharge summary or home health referral form. This information is used to determine the day and time of the first home visit, assign a nurse with appropriate skills, and ensure that appropriate supplies and equipment are available for the first home visit. Failure to carefully document pertinent information can delay medical services.

Through bridging the continuum, nurses can truly serve as advocates for the patients who depend on them.

SELECTED REFERENCES

Proctor, E. K., et al. Implementation of discharge plans for chronically ill elders discharged home. *Health Soc. Work.* 21(1):30–40, Feb. 1996.

Anderson, M. Interorganizational Communication: Home Care Referral of Elderly Following Hospital Discharge. Unpublished doctoral dissertation, University of Iowa, Iowa City, 1991.

Bean, P., and Waldron, K. Readmission study leads to continuum of care. *Nurs. Manage.* 26(9): 65–68, Sept. 1995.

To facilitate continuity of care, the nurse must have knowledge of community resources as well as the ability to access and coordinate these resources. Such knowledge and skill are requisite to select resources that are available in your community and to determine which of these resources is appropriate for your client's specific needs. The following article discusses how to identify and use community resources to plan care.

What community resources are available in your community? Which resources are available for clients with chronic illness . . . for clients with financial needs . . . for children . . . for pregnant teens . . . for the underinsured and uninsured?

(1998). Using community resources effectively to plan care. *Home Healthcare Nurse*, 16(5), 309.

Using Community Resources Effectively to Plan Care

The changes in home care reimbursement, Medicare coverage criteria, and the pressures of managed care have left field staff, especially nurses, finding new ways to plan patient care. Home care nurses are used to planning for discharge and for assuring that abandonment of the patient doesn't occur. However, in these times all home care staff must become creative in working with community resources.

As agencies more efficiently prepare patients for discharge, providers may feel as though they are leaving the patients without the assistance necessary for them to remain safely in their homes. Since the majority of the patients affected are considered chronic and can barely manage to remain in their homes with the assistance of the home care agency, these fears may be well founded. Where will these patients and their families turn when the home health agency is no longer able to provide needed oversight and personal care services for them?

Home Healthcare Nurse discussed these concerns with Michelle Alvarez, MSW. Michelle has used her extensive networking experiences to develop a strong support system for the elderly in a previously underserved rural area. She suggests home health providers seeking assistance for the elderly use one or more of the following information sources:

- Regional United Way offices have a referral line that can be called to determine what resources they are offered for the elderly. In addition to providing a list of available community resources, they also publish a resource guide with names and phone numbers of groups that may offer elderly assistance.
- Contact any organization in the area that has the words "aging" or "senior" in their name. Many times such groups will provide services such as transportation or grocery shopping for the elderly.
- Call local government agencies. Ask which departments may provide assistance for elderly citizens. Some assistance with financial difficulties may even be available at

the county or township level. While there may be nothing available in your area, you won't know unless you call.

- Contact your state Board of Health. They may be aware of assistance available for the elderly through state level providers.
- Access the state information line; their phone number is listed under state governmental agencies in the phone book. A toll-free number is usually available.
- Contact churches, particularly if the client is a member of the church or of a certain denomination. Many times churches provide transportation, cleaning, and other assistance as service opportunities for members. Some even have "fix-it" men who make minor repairs that are difficult for the elderly to perform.
- Some churches have parish nurses who provide services such as dressing changes, blood pressure checks, etc., for members of their parochial district. Contact the church or synagogue for information.
- Contact schools of nursing. Occasionally, universities sponsor screening clinics for blood pressure, cholesterol, and blood sugar monitoring.
- Call the American Association of Retired Persons (AARP) at (202) 434-2277. Ask what is available through their organization to help elderly clients' transition through this difficult period.
- Connect the patient with a prescription assistance program. Several of the larger pharmaceutical companies offer assistance in obtaining medications to elderly clients who have limited resources. Income restrictions and other guidelines exist, but it is well worth the time invested to determine eligibility for the program.
- Some independent laboratories will make visits to perform venipunctures. This service would be very beneficial for the elderly client who doesn't have transportation to the hospital or physician's office.

Although the above list is not all-inclusive, it provides for identifying ways to develop an assistance plan for elderly patients. All members of the home health agency should be familiar with the role and functions of the social work staff in the office and in community agencies. By working together to clarify the specific problems encountered by the patient and family, the most appropriate avenues can be pursued.

Collaboration is an essential component of community-based care. Believed to contain costs and maximize effective interventions, successful collaboration is a challenge worth the effort. This article outlines a collaborative effort between nursing and occupational therapy.

What are the principal domains of the occupational therapist? How do these areas translate to the activities involved in self-administration of medication? What are the areas of overlap between the role of the nurse and the role of an occupational therapist?

Touchard, B., & Berthelot, K. (1999). Collaborative home practice: Nursing and occupations therapy ensures appropriate medication administration. Home Healthcare Nurse, 17(1), 45–51.

Collaborative Home Practice: Nursing and Occupational Therapy Ensure Appropriate Medication Administration

BARBARA MOLLERE TOUCHARD, KIM BERTHELOT

In rehabilitation, interdisciplinary collaboration is frequently recommended to contain costs and maximize effective intervention and outcomes (Oriol, 1997). Skillful communication practices along with strong interpersonal skills are behaviors exhibited by effective interdisciplinary teams (Robertson, 1996). Cohesive rehabilitation teams composed of nurses, physical therapists, occupational therapists, speech pathologists, rehabilitation counselors, and physicians have the potential to generate holistic and comprehensive care.

Interdisciplinary collaboration may be even more important in home healthcare. Current communication technologies offer independent clinicians a variety of means by which to contact and discuss patient care with other team members (e.g., e-mail, voice mail, paging, fax, etc.). However, team members may not have frequent opportunities as a group to review the patient's treatment or discuss interventions at a common time and place with all team members present. Continuity and consistency of services may suffer, and several logistical obstacles exist that make comprehensive patient care challenging.

Barbara Mollere Touchard, MHS, LOTR, BCN, is an Assistant Professor in the Department of Occupational Therapy, School of Allied Health, Louisiana State University Medical Center, New Orleans, and an occupational therapist for St. Charles Parish Hospital Home Health, Luling, LA. Kim Berthelot, RN, is a nurse at St. Charles Parish Hospital Home Health, Luling, LA.

● ISSUES AFFECTING CARE CONTINUITY

1. Clinicians assigned to patients are required to collaborate with other disciplines involved and document evidence of the collaboration.
2. Team members often provide direct patient care independently of each other and may possess different levels of experience, employ varying treatment methods, and have diverse communication styles.
3. Patients usually are scheduled at varying times of the day, by individual disciplines, so interaction between team members may be limited.
4. Most important, team members may be unaware of the skills and services offered by their coworkers.

Wheelan and Hochberger (1996) noted additional problems inherent to rehabilitation teams composed of interdisciplinary members, including organizational issues, delineation of territory, and role ambiguity. Ensuring that home healthcare teams thoroughly understand the roles of their team members is vital to maximizing patient outcomes.

● SOLUTIONS TO THE PROBLEM

Education

Home healthcare organizations are mandated by regulatory agencies to provide educational opportunities for their employees. Through continuing professional education, team members can be encouraged to engage in collaborative home practice. This education can occur during team meetings, organized in-service sessions, or patient case conferences. Many health professions are currently experiencing technological advances or evolutions in practice due to healthcare changes. Therefore, the necessity to update and inform team members of new information related to individual disciplines becomes essential for interdisciplinary understanding of the comprehensive rehabilitation process.

Although the scope of practice in allied health professions remains relatively constant, home health rehabilitation has undergone its own changes to clarify services and ensure reimbursement in response to managed care (Schulman, 1994). These changes can have an effect on treatment duration, interventions used, elements of documentation, the way disciplines collaborate, and even which disciplines are involved in provision of services.

Uniform Technology

The American Occupational Therapy Association (AOTA, 1996) now encourages use of uniform terminology for occupational therapy not only to establish a consistent language in documentation, but to provide an "outline of the domain of concern of occupational therapy . . . and to capture the essence of occupational therapy succinctly for others" (p. 273). Clinicians readily use jargon specific to their discipline that may be unfamiliar to coworkers. Unless team members are educated in the language, miscommunications or misunderstandings may result. This type of information can be shared between the members of the home healthcare team to foster a thorough understanding of each discipline.

The Domain of Occupational Therapy

1. performance areas
   "broad categories of human activity that are typically part of daily life" (AOTA, 1996, p. 273), including ADL, work/productive activities, and play/leisure activities.

2. performance components
   "fundamental human abilities that, to varying degrees and in differing combinations, are required for successful engagement in performance areas" (AOTA, 1996, p. 273), including sensorimotor, cognitive, and psychosocial areas.

3. performance contexts
   "situations or factors that influence an individual's engagement in desired and/or required performance areas. . . [including] temporal and environmental aspects." (AOTA, 1996, p. 273–274)

Collaboration

Education of team members regarding other disciplines has the potential to create true multidisciplinary, patient-centered care (Coles, 1995). Increased interaction between disciplines can generate more interdisciplinary referrals and encourage collaborative practice.

The case study presented later illustrates the successful outcomes that occurred as a result of education and communication among the home healthcare team. The successful collaboration between nursing and occupational therapy enabled the patient to live independently in her home environment and maintained her ability to engage in productive activities of daily living (ADL).

● EVOLUTION OF ONE AGENCY'S TEAM

The rehabilitation home healthcare team from a local rural hospital previously consisted of only a nurse and physical therapist. To develop the team further and expand services, an occupational therapist and a speech pathologist were hired. For the new employees, the home health director suggested that each discipline conduct an in-service session to educate other team members about its role in home healthcare service delivery. This was scheduled during a regular staff meeting so all staff members could attend.

● OCCUPATIONAL THERAPY SERVICES DEFINED

The occupational therapist presented an in-service session defining the scope of occupational therapy and implications for referral. A copy of *Uniform Terminology for Occupational Therapy*, 3rd ed. (American Occupational Therapy Association [AOTA], 1996) was distributed to participants as a guide for the presentation. *Uniform Terminology* is organized in an outline format, enabling the person unfamiliar with the scope of occupational therapy services to view the information in a concise, understandable fashion (Table 12-1). The document, although developed to increase consistency in clinical documentation language for the occupational therapy profession, also serves as a comprehensive listing of areas for intervention that may concern the occupational therapist.

TABLE 12-1 ● **Uniform Terminology for Occupational Therapy, Third Edition Outline**

I. Performance Areas

A. Activities of Daily Living
  1. Grooming
  2. Oral Hygiene
  3. Bathing/Showering
  4. Toilet Hygiene
  5. Personal Device Care
  6. Dressing
  7. Feeding and Eating
  8. Medication Routine
  9. Health Maintenance
  10. Socialization
  11. Functional Communication
  12. Functional Mobility
  13. Community Mobility
  14. Emergency Response
  15. Sexual Expression

B. Work and Productive Activities
  1. Home Management
    a. Clothing Care
    b. Cleaning
    c. Meal Preparation/Clean-up
    d. Shopping
    e. Money Management
    f. Household Management
    g. Safety Procedures
  2. Care of Other
  3. Educational Activities
  4. Vocational Activities
    a. Vocational Exploration
    b. Job Acquisition
    c. Work or Job Performance
    d. Retirement Planning
    e. Volunteer Participation

C. Play or Leisure Activities
  1. Play/Leisure Exploration
  2. Play/Leisure Performance

II. Performance Components

A. Sensorimotor Component
  1. Sensory
    a. Sensory Awareness
    b. Sensory Processing
      (1) Tactile
      (2) Proprioceptive
      (3) Vestibular
      (4) Visual
      (5) Auditory
      (6) Gustatory
      (7) Olfactory
    c. Perceptual Processing
      (1) Stereognosis
      (2) Kinesthesia
      (3) Pain Response
      (4) Body Scheme
      (5) Auditory
      (6) Form Constancy
      (7) Position in Space
      (8) Visual-Closure
      (9) Figure Ground
      (10) Depth Perception
      (11) Spatial Relations
      (12) Topographical Orientation
  2. Neuromusculoskeletal
    a. Reflex
    b. Range of Motion
    c. Muscle Tone
    d. Strength
    e. Endurance
    f. Postural Control
    g. Postural Alignment
    h. Soft Tissue Integrity
  3. Motor
    a. Gross Coordination
    b. Crossing the Midline
    c. Laterality
    d. Bilateral Integration
    e. Motor Control
    f. Praxis
    g. Fine Coordination/Dexterity
    h. Visual-Motor Integration
    i. Oral-Motor Control

B. Cognitive Integration and Cognitive Components
  1. Level of Arousal
  2. Orientation
  3. Recognition
  4. Attention Span
  5. Initiation of Activity
  6. Termination of Activity
  7. Memory
  8. Sequencing
  9. Categorization
  10. Concept Formation
  11. Spatial Operations
  12. Problem Solving
  13. Learning
  14. Generalization

C. Psychosocial Skills and Psychosocial Components
  1. Psychological
    a. Values
    b. Interests
    c. Self-Concept
  2. Social
    a. Role Performance
    b. Social Conduct
    c. Interpersonal Skills
    d. Self-Expression
  3. Self-Management
    a. Coping Skills
    b. Time Management
    c. Self-Control

(continued)

TABLE 12-1 ● Uniform Terminology for Occupational Therapy, Third Edition Outline (*Continued*)	

III. Performance Contents

A. Temporal Aspects	B. Environmental Aspects
1. Chronological	1. Physical
2. Developmental	2. Social
3. Life Cycle	3. Cultural
4. Disability Status	

From *Reference Manual of the Official Documents of the American Occupational Therapy Association*, 6th Ed., (p. 278), by the American Occupational Therapy Association, 1996, Bethesda, MD: Author. Copyright © 1996 by the American Occupational Therapy Association, Inc. Reprinted with permission.

The occupational therapist can use the performance areas as a guide for assessing a patient's functional ability to perform specific tasks that fall under the heading of ADL, work, or play/leisure. The performance components such as sensorimotor, cognitive, or psychosocial allow the therapist to analyze impairment areas that may be affecting performance of ADL, work, or play/leisure. The performance contexts of temporal and environmental aspects give occupational therapists still other factors to consider, such as a person's developmental stage or physical environment, that also will affect ADL, work, or play/leisure performance.

As a guide for occupational therapy assessment and intervention, *Uniform Terminology* emphasizes the holistic nature of occupational therapy and cues the clinician to consider the many factors that contribute to independent living. For example, an elderly homemaker who sustained a stroke with resulting hemiplegia may be unable to transfer to her commode and toilet independently, resulting in frustration and anger. In this instance, the homemaker would require assistance in the performance area of ADLs, specifically toileting/hygiene.

The performance components affecting her ability to perform the task could include sensory-perception deficits, neuromusculoskeletal impairments, or motor deficits. The psychosocial aspects of her frustration and anger will possibly inhibit independence in the task. In consideration of performance contexts, the homemaker's age (temporal context) may indicate previous functional deficits or disabilities that should be taken into account, and modification of the physical environment may be necessary. In this manner, *Uniform Terminology* can assist occupational therapists in treatment planning and in educating other team members and the patient about the scope of services and supports offered by occupational therapy.

This information was presented to the other team members at the in-service session. Most staff were unfamiliar with the document, and appreciated the clarification of services. Furthermore, members of the home healthcare team responded positively to the information, reporting they were unaware of the many areas in which occupational therapy intervention may be warranted.

● OCCUPATIONAL THERAPY AND MEDICATION ROUTINE

The nursing members of the team requested clarification about the Medication Routine heading under Activities of Daily Living in the Performance Areas section. This area of intervention for occupational therapy is defined as follows:

Medication Routine—[describes patient's ability to . . .] obtain medication, open and close containers, follow prescribed schedules, take correct quantities, report problems and adverse effects, and administer correct quantities by using prescribed methods." (AOTA, 1996, p. 280)

Further information was provided to the nurses regarding the occupational therapist's ability to assess the cognitive, perceptual, and motoric aspects of patients' ability to administer their medications correctly. Whereas the nurse has expertise related to specific medication and administration, the occupational therapist is able to interface with nurs-

---

Case Study

Mrs. E was a 79-year-old female with an extensive history of numerous medical problems, most notably, congestive heart failure, hypertension, chronic edema of the lower extremities, and a right cerebral vascular accident (CVA) that occurred in 1991. The CVA had left her with partial use of her left (nondominant) upper and lower extremities, and asymmetry in her trunk. She underwent comprehensive inpatient rehabilitation for approximately 6 weeks, followed by home health services that included nursing and physical and occupational therapy.

Mrs. E. previously lived in her own home, where two of her sons, who worked during the day, resided with her. After her CVA, two daughters lived with her and provided constant care during her recovery. Mrs. E had continual family support, but she displayed a remarkable determination and motivation to return to living independently and alone. An accomplished cook and homemaker, she often told stories of growing up in rural Louisiana and helping her mother to care for her large family. She had been performing household chores since the age of 12 years, and homemaking was an important part of her daily routine.

Mrs. E was discharged from all home health services approximately 3 months after her CVA. At that time, she continued to exhibit motor deficits in the left upper and lower extremities, but could ambulate short distances in her home and use her left upper extremity for simple household tasks, primarily those requiring gross grasp. Isolated finger movement was limited, and flexor patterns dominated her left upper extremity resting posture. Her daughters were still needed to assist her with dressing, grooming, and hygiene tasks. Mrs. E was not yet able to resume homemaking tasks.

During the subsequent year, Mrs. E continued a home program of exercises and activities learned in rehabilitation to attain a level of function that allowed her daughters to return to their homes. Her determination and drive compelled her to attempt various homemaking skills gradually. Over time, with dedication and persistence, she resumed an independent level of function in her home.

Mrs. E was referred to home health services in October of 1997. After a short medical stay, she was fully independent in all areas of home management, which included making homemade bread from her mother's recipe. She had regained functional use of her left upper extremity, including isolated finger return and a fair to good level of strength.

However, due to a recent medical exacerbation, Mrs. E was required to take five different medications daily. She exhibited intermittent lapses of memory, and occasionally became confused when trying to administer her own medications. Because research showed that elderly individuals with cognitive impairment may benefit from home healthcare, occupational therapy services were initiated with Mrs. E to maximize her independence and ensure continued independent living (Dellasega, Dansky, King, & Stricklin, 1994).

ing by assessing the specific performance components (sensorimotor, cognitive, psychosocial, etc.) that may be preventing successful performance of this daily task. The occupational therapist can then address the impairment area through *remedial, compensatory,* or *adaptive* methods. Together, the two disciplines can offer unique skills that complement each other and help in providing true comprehensive interdisciplinary coordinated care.

The team nurses began to report a specific case of a current patient who would benefit from training in administering her medications independently. Nursing services had recommended discharging this patient due to her high level of independence in other self-care and home management activities, but she remained unable to administer a large number of medications accurately. A physician's order for occupational therapy services was obtained, and an evaluation was scheduled.

● NURSING AND OCCUPATIONAL THERAPY COLLABORATION

The occupational therapy evaluation revealed that Mrs. E was cognitively able to process written language and graphic information. She wore reading glasses and exhibited no field cuts or hemianopsias. Sensory processing throughout the left side generally appeared intact, and no attentional deficits were noted.

First, the occupational therapist contacted the nurse for practical information regarding the schedule and specifics of Mrs. E's medications. Questions were asked to discover whether grouping medications for simplification could be done or whether the medications had restrictions (e.g., to be taken only at bedtime because of drowsiness effects, or with meals, etc.). The home health nurse served as a great source for information and practical experience with the medications and was instrumental in establishing a simpler method of grouping pills to ease the administration process. Attempts were successfully made to have each day's medication routine exactly alike, except for medications to be taken as needed. This would potentially ease the process for Mrs. E and possibly reduce errors in administration.

Second, Mrs. E's current pillbox required modification. She used a device divided into smaller compartments representing each day of the week and four times of the day. Across the horizontal top edge of the box were abbreviations for the days of the week: M, T, W, Th, F. Down the left vertical edge of the box, times of the day were listed: Morning, Noon, Afternoon, Evening. Through constant use, many of the words had become worn, and most of the ink had faded. Mrs. E was familiar with this pillbox, and preferred to modify her current equipment rather than purchase a new device. To simplify and clarify the compartments, new bold labels were attached to each compartment separately so she could easily discern the specific compartments rather than rely on column headers only. Employing this process reflected occupational therapy's ability to *adapt* equipment so as to maximize Mrs. E's independence in identifying and use the correct compartments of her pillbox.

Third, Mrs. E required a cueing device, primarily for loading the pill compartments for the week. Although she understood and could verbalize when her medications were to be taken, she showed difficulty translating this information into a spatial arrangement (loading the separate compartments to correspond to appropriate date and times for her medications). When the pills were appropriately loaded into the compartments, a particular visual pattern emerged for each day. All the pills were different colors, sizes, and shapes, but the formation of pills for each day was consistent. If Mrs. E could use a guide to load the pills for 1 day, she could successfully load the entire box, thus becoming independent in this task.

Fourth, a visual guide was constructed for Mrs. E. This drawing depicted a column of compartments corresponding to the exact size of her pill compartments for 1 day. Her specific medications were traced and color coded to correspond exactly with the shape, size, and color of the actual pill. These pictures were then drawn in the appropriate compartments according to the time of day each medication was to be taken. (If Mrs. E. would have had difficulty generalizing the drawn pill to the actual pill, then the actual pills could have been glued to the visual guide.) The guide was laminated to prevent deterioration that possibly could be caused by daily handling. Due to Mrs. E's deficits in memory, the occupational therapist used this compensatory method to help her remember which pills were to be inserted in the individual compartments.

Finally, the visual guide was presented to Mrs. E. She was trained in using the guide to load the compartments of the pillbox with close supervision over the course of two sessions. By the third session, Mrs. E was loading the pillbox independently before the therapists' arrival, and only a check for errors was necessary. Nursing also used the guide to reinforce correct administration of medications. Through collaborative nursing and occupational therapy practice, Mrs. E's dependence in medication administration was *remediated*.

● CONCLUSION

Through a combination of interdisciplinary education, collaboration, and creative problem solving, one home healthcare patient was able to resume an independent level of function in her home that included administering her medications regularly and accurately. It is believed that structured team education, effective use of clinicians' expertise, and interdisciplinary collaboration were related to the successful outcomes in this scenario.

Structured education between home healthcare team members regarding the scope of the disciplines' services provided new information, opened a line of communication, and generated an interdisciplinary referral. Team members (primarily nursing and occupational therapy personnel), after learning to identify roles more clearly, were able to understand scope of services more readily.

Team member expertise was used effectively. Occupational therapy was able to enlist the expertise of nursing to plan an effective medication routine for the patient. Nursing identified areas of intervention that could warrant an occupational therapy referral.

Interdisciplinary collaboration was ongoing through the course of rehabilitation and helped to integrate treatment planning. Nursing and occupational therapy identified the problem area and practiced open communication, team problem solving, and collaborative resolution. By having both team members working toward similar goals, patient care was focused and consistent.

Collaborative home healthcare practice can potentially improve outcomes for patients. With thorough understanding of each discipline, true knowledge of roles, and a willingness to share expertise and collaborate, home healthcare team members can have a positive and profound effect on the quality of their patients' lives.

● ACKNOWLEDGMENT

The author thanks Dr. Patricia Snyder for her expert editing and continual support.

REFERENCES

American Occupational Therapy Association. (1996). Uniform terminology for occupational therapy (3rd ed.). In *Reference Manual of the Official Documents of The American Occupational Therapy Association*. (6th ed.). Rockville, MD: Author.

Coles, C. (1995). Educating the health care team. *Patient Education and Counseling, 26,* 239–244.

Dellasega, C., Dansky, K., King, L. & Stricklin, M. (1994). Use of home health services by elderly persons with cognitive impairment. *Journal of Nursing Administration, 24*(6), 20–25.

Oriol, M. (1997). Specialty team development: One agency's formula. *Home Healthcare Nurse, 15*(7), 505–508.

Robertson, S. (1996). Team building and leadership. In *The Occupational Therapy Manager* (rev. ed.). Rockville, MD: American Occupational Therapy Association.

Schulman, C. (1994). The impact of managed care on rehabilitation in home health care. *Journal of Home Health Care Practice, 6*(2), 24–29.

Wheelan, S., & Hochberger, J. (1996). Assessing the functional level of rehabilitation teams and facilitating team development. *Rehabilitation Nursing, 21*(2), 75–81.

Technologic advances in neonatal care have resulted in increased survival rates of low-birth weight infants, many who have complex medical needs. This article discusses a collaborative consultation project among physical therapy, occupational therapy, and nursing to serve infants and children with sensorimotor impairments.

What are the principal areas of expertise of the occupational therapist? What are the principal areas of expertise of the physical therapist? How do these scopes of practice translate to the activities involved in promoting the motor development of a young child? What are the areas of overlap between the role of the nurse and the roles of an occupational therapist and a physical therapist?

Pokorni, J., & Sippel, K. M. (1997). Consultation with physical and occupational therapists to promote the motor development of young children. *Home Healthcare Nurse,* 15(5), 331–339.

Consultation With Physical and Occupational Therapists to Promote the Motor Development of Young Children

JUDITH L. POKORNI, KIRSTEN M. SIPPEL

Increased survival of infants with complex medical needs combined with fiscal constraints have resulted in more young children receiving home care nursing. Home care nurses can enhance their role by understanding how physical and occupational therapists provide consultation to the family and nursing staff.

Technologic advances have increased the survival rates of very-low-birth-weight infants and other neonates with complex medical needs (Goldson, 1996; Ventura, Martin, Taffel, Mathews, & Clarke, 1994). Although the overall percentage of the survivors who sustain significant motor impairments has not changed, the number of children requiring long-term care has increased as more children survive early neonatal problems (Hack,

Judith L. Pokorni, PhD, is from the Georgetown University Child Development Center, Department of Pediatrics, Georgetown University Medical Center, Washington, DC.

Kirsten M. Sippel, MPP, PT, is physical therapist at the Westchester County Early Intervention Program and the Westchester School for Special Children.

This article describes work that was funded in part by a grant from the U.S. Department of Education, Office of Special Education Projects (Grant No. HO29K20012) but does not necessarily reflect the views of this agency.

Friedman, & Fanaroff, 1996). These increases and the concomitant financial constraints of healthcare systems have resulted in a greater number of infants receiving home health services (Singer, 1996). Infants receiving home nursing services who have sensorimotor impairments may have physical or occupational therapy prescribed to address their motor needs. The purposes of this article are to review the consultative role of physical and occupational therapists in providing services to young children receiving home nursing and to provide an overview of basic motor concepts that can be incorporated into home nursing care plans.

● THE THERAPIST AS CONSULTANT

Consultation by professionals working with children has been described in the literature for almost 20 years (Bailey, 1996). With the advent of early intervention, the fields of physical and occupational therapies have been involved actively in developing service-delivery models including consultation (Brown, Wyne, Blackburn, & Powell, 1979; Hanft & Place, 1996; Rainforth & Roberts, 1996). Direct services, monitoring, and consultation are three models that have been used by motor specialists in recent years (Dunn, 1996). Direct services include immediate and ongoing contact with a child either alone or in a small group. The monitoring model is used when a therapist develops an intervention plan and then supervises the individuals who implement the plan. The consultation model uses collaboration of the physical and occupational therapists with family members and other professionals in the development of the intervention plan. This model is particularly appropriate for use with a young child receiving home nursing because the fragile health of the child and the nurse's caregiving role should be taken into consideration as the motor intervention plan is designed. The consultation model also facilitates the development of comprehensive, interdisciplinary nursing care plans.

Therapeutic models have evolved along with contemporary thought regarding the nature of developmentally appropriate services for infants and young children. Although physical and occupational therapy traditionally were limited to direct, therapeutic handling of patients, the younger and sicker clientele requires services that are designed to minimize the number of adults who handle a child. Because all young children, including those with special health needs, thrive when their overall development is nurtured by their primary caregivers during everyday care, an important job of the therapist is to assist the family in learning appropriate handling and positioning techniques. In the case of a child who receives home nursing, the primary caregivers also include members of the nursing team. Although a child may need specialized treatment provided by the occupational or physical therapist, the ideal treatment plan emphasizes the primary caregivers in implementing strategies for achieving a child's therapeutic goals.

Physical and occupational therapists along with specialists from the disciplines of early intervention, speech and language, and psychology are trained to address various developmental areas of need. Figure 13-1 outlines the areas of primary concern of each discipline. In the case of young children, physical and occupational therapists may address similar areas, although physical therapists typically address gross motor areas of concern and occupational therapists focus on fine motor concerns. Assessment, direct intervention, and consultative services concerning motor development may be addressed by either or both occupational and physical therapists. Young children with special health needs who may need occupational or physical therapy include children with multiple physical disabilities or genetic disorders. In addition, infants and young children born preterm and who experience prolonged early hospitalization may have atyp-

Factors Influencing Motor Development	Areas of Expertise		
	Occupational Therapy	Physical Therapy	Nursing
Sensorimotor Development	Sensorimotor processing	Sensorimotor processing	Impact of sensory impairments on child's daily functioning during routines
	Specialty: influence of sensory input on adaptive behavior & functional movement	Specialty: posture, balance, & quality of movement	
Neuromuscular function	Evaluates muscle tone, reflexes, and range of motion of legs/arms/head & how they influence self-care, play & motor skills	Evaluates muscle tone, reflexes and range of motion of legs/arms/ head, & how they influence self-care, play, & motor skills	Impact of medical status on movement, self-care, & play in home
	Specialty: arm and hand function	Specialty: mobility & stability of back, hips, legs	
Motor development	Gross & fine motor skills and impact of neurologic status on motor development	Gross & fine motor skills and impact of neurologic status on motor development	Use of gross & fine motor skills during daily routines at home
	Specialty: fine motor, eye–hand coordination, visual–motor	Specialty: gross motor, balance & equilibrium, coordination	
Adaptive equipment	Evaluates & recommends positioning equipment, i.e., corner chairs, wheelchairs, prone stander, based on functional need	Evaluates and recommends positioning equipment, i.e., corner chairs, wheelchairs, prone stander, to prevent structural deformity	Use of positioning equipment in home and play environment
	Specialty: making hand splints; adapting feeding utensils, toys & environment	Specialty: training to use leg braces, orthotics	
Functional movement	Use of body for play, communication and self-care	Mobility & walking	Impact of medical issues on movement at home.
	Specialty: feeding; play; toileting; dressing	Specialty: locomotion, especially walking; body mechanics, energy conservation	

FIGURE 13-1. A chart of the types of specialists working with young children. *Note.* From B. Hanft, K. Sippel, & Judith Pokorni, 1994. Originally presented at the Case Management for Children with Disabilities Course of the Office of the Surgeon General, U.S. Army Medical Department, Atlanta, Georgia, May 17–19, 1994.

ical muscle tone that would benefit from consultation by a physical or occupational therapist (see Figure 13-1).

There is a growing recognition that therapeutic strategies and techniques should be embedded into daily routines to facilitate improvement in a child's functional level (McEwen & Shelden, 1996). A child's sensorimotor needs should be addressed within the child's daily activities, such as bathing, feeding, dressing, and playing. Specialized treatment techniques implemented by a therapist may be indicated for some young children to assist them in adapting their movement patterns so that they become more efficient and more effective. Because a child needs to practice these evolving patterns daily, the therapist consults with the family and nursing team on the integration of these techniques into daily routines to maximize the opportunities to practice evolving skills. Although a young child's motor needs may necessitate an exercise regime, most goals can be accomplished through a combination of direct services and implementation of strategies within a young child's regular activities. It is through continual opportunities to practice skills that young children learn and develop their abilities.

Through consultation with family members and a child's nursing team, the physical or occupational therapist provides information about the motor goals for a child. In turn, family and nurses share information about the child's physical needs, daily routines, and other pertinent information needed to develop a plan that can be used throughout the day. Through this collaborative consultation, an effective plan to meet the individual child's goals can be developed. Therefore, implementing developmentally appropriate therapeutic services for young children requires a conceptual shift from the medical model of the therapist working in isolation to "treat" the child to a model in which the therapist facilitates the child's motor development by collaborative consultation with the primary caregivers to assure that therapeutic recommendations are integrated into the child's daily care plan.

The use of collaborative consultation is consistent with the principles of care for children with special healthcare needs, which were mandated through an amendment to Title V of the Social Security Act, supporting the Maternal and Child Health Services Block Grant (Maternal and Child Health Bureau, 1994). These standards of care were highlighted at the 1987 Surgeon General's workshop focusing on children with disabilities and their families. These same standards also were articulated for nurses as "guiding principles" in the Standards of Nursing Practice for the Care of Children and Adolescents with Special Health and Developmental Needs (Maternal and Child Health Bureau, 1994). Both sets of standards mandate that care for children with special health needs should be family-centered, developmentally appropriate, culturally competent, collaborative, comprehensive, community-based, and coordinated. The consultative model of therapeutic services is responsive to these standards by promoting services that are family-centered, developmentally appropriate, coordinated, and collaborative.

This shift in emphasis from direct services to consultation is unique to pediatric therapy and has arisen, in part, because of the requirements of federal legislation regarding services to young children with disabilities (Brown et al., 1979). Therefore, therapists new to the pediatric arena may be unfamiliar with the change. As consultation becomes more firmly established in policy and practice, more therapists will embrace a consultative role as a means to encouraging a holistic approach to promoting the development of a young child with special health needs.

Successful consultation is collaborative and requires specific skills of the therapist and members of the nursing team. Along with their disciplinary expertise, therapists, nurses, and family members must develop communication skills that enable them to articulate informa-

TABLE 13-1 • **Strategies for Optimal Communication Among Team Members**	
Method of Communication	*Purpose*
Communication book	To provide ongoing communication for therapists, nursing team, and family members
Charts and photos	To display positioning and handling techniques, exercise routines and schedules
Video tapes	To demonstrate exercises, use of adaptive equipment and assistive devices, handling techniques, feeding

tion, to listen to other members, and to integrate information from various perspectives. On the one hand, therapists need to know about a child's respiratory and cardiac functioning, about concerns regarding feeding and sleeping, and about the child's daily routines that are most conducive for achieving the motor goals. They also need to be informed of the family's priorities and the child's functioning within the family. Nurses, conversely, need demonstrations of recommended handling and positioning techniques. They also need suggestions for incorporating activities into a child's care plan and periodic updates on the child's progress. Because it is sometimes difficult for members of a child's team to meet regularly, alternative strategies for ensuring communication are needed. Table 13-1 lists some suggestions for ensuring ongoing communication between therapists and members of a child's nursing team. By working closely with therapists, home care nurses gain a better understanding of a child's therapeutic plan and are better equipped to develop care plans that integrate a child's motor needs (see Table 13-1).

● BASIC MOTOR GUIDELINES AND ACTIVITIES FOR INTEGRATION INTO CARE PLANS

There are a few basic motor guidelines that can be incorporated into care plans of many infants and young children receiving home nursing. Nurses who are aware of these guidelines will be able to work more effectively with therapists. The four important guidelines listed in Table 13-2 are each described here.

Positioning a Child in the Most Stable and Normal Positions

The midline position is an important element of normal positioning and contributes to the optimal functioning of a child by providing maximum stability and by allowing a child to use both sides of the body. Infants who tend to move out of alignment need supports

TABLE 13-2 • Guidelines for Home Nurses Regarding Motor Activities for Young Children
Providing a variety of environments
Positioning a young child in the most stable and normal positions
Providing a variety of positions each day
Promoting many opportunities to use hands and fingers
Incorporating functional movements into routine caregiving

to assist them in remaining in the midline position. Consultation may be needed to demonstrate the use of blanket rolls, wedges, or other objects to prop a child in the correct position in the bed, highchair, or other piece of furniture. Demonstrations to caregivers of the use of their own hands to improve a child's stability and alignment also may be helpful. In some cases, special equipment may be needed to position a child effectively. The midline and upright positions help a child maintain good respiratory function, an important goal for children with special health needs. Appropriate positioning also allows greater opportunities for developmentally appropriate play.

Providing a Variety of Positions

Unfortunately, caregivers of a young child with reduced mobility may be unaware of the importance of providing a variety of positions during the day. Varying a child's position throughout the day promotes the development of a wide range of important muscles. The schedule for changing positions depends on the specific needs of the individual child with reduced mobility. Schedules may change often as the young child develops and changes. The physical or occupational therapist can provide guidelines for use of various positions for each child. The use of various positions to further a child's motor development is described here.

Supine. This position is used by almost all nursing staff in acute care and home settings. Unfortunately, an infant or young child with reduced mobility may be placed in this position for long periods. Although a mobile hanging above the crib (if placed in midline and at chest level) may be useful visual stimulation, there are additional ways to promote a child's development while in the supine position. For example, blanket roles placed under the child's shoulders will encourage reaching or grasping for toys that are hung on a crib gym within the child's reach. Placing weighted toys with sound at an infant's feet may encourage a kicking motion that activates the sound.

Prone. In contrast to the supine position, this position is less often used with young children with complex medical needs. Because the prone position may be somewhat aversive to an infant who has experienced limited time in this position early in development, family members and nursing staff members may tend to avoid placing a child in a prone position. Placing an awake child in a prone position, if medically appropriate, encourages the development of trunk muscles. Because a child who has experienced prolonged hospitalization may tolerate only short periods in a prone position, it may be necessary to help the child gradually tolerate longer periods by talking to the child, singing, or using toys. It is important for a nursing team to understand the importance of using the prone position during playtime for a young child's overall motor development and to identify specific opportunities for incorporating this position throughout the child's day.

Sidelying. A child with minimal mobility should be repositioned from side to side during the day. Blanket rolls or other props placed along a child's back will help a child maintain the sidelying position. Once again, when the sidelying position is used, interesting toys can be placed in front of a child and within reach to encourage play. Placing a mirror or busy box on the side of the crib can be a good source of stimulation for the child in the sidelying position.

Upright or supported sitting. The upright or supported sitting position allows a child to engage in experiences that are unavailable to a child who is lying down. Exercises that support head control are important precursors and an ongoing part of independent sitting activities. When a young child is positioned on the lap, varying levels of support can be given. By gradually withdrawing some support for short periods, nurses can promote the development of the muscle tone and strength needed to maintain independent sitting. Demonstrations of the use of blanket rolls and other aids to enable a child to remain upright in an infant seat, swing, high chair, or, when necessary, adaptive equipment such as a corner chair, may be useful.

Each of the positions described above may be appropriate at different times and for different reasons. Table 13-3, using positions to encourage gross motor development, can be discussed with therapists and family members during consultation. These activities are designed to promote a young child's overall motor development in each position. Table 13-4 lists a variety of toys that can be used to encourage motor development while a child is in various positions (see Tables 13-3 and 13-4).

Providing a Variety of Environments

In addition to facilitating the use of a variety of positions each day, home care nurses can encourage the positioning of a child in a variety of environments. Caregivers of a child who has spent prolonged periods in a hospital should vary the child's environment as soon as the child is medically stable and able to tolerate such movement. Repositioning a child from a crib to a blanket on the floor and taking the child from inside the house to a deck, the park, or even a restaurant promotes a child's overall development. The family and nursing team has important information to share as they participate in making decisions about where the child will be taken.

TABLE 13-3 ● Using Positions to Encourage Gross Motor Development

Supine

Hold toys above child and within reach to promote reaching and grasping.
Use crib gym with toys that can be changed to maintain the child's interest.
Alternate frequently with other positions.
Use small rolls under the shoulders to bring the child's arms forward.

Prone

Use to promote development of trunk muscles.
Gradually increase the time the child tolerates this position by using toys or your voice to distract the child.
Place busy boxes or other bright objects directly in front of the child for play.

Sidelying

Use rolls along the child's backside to maintain the position.
Position the child to enjoy visual stimulation of the environment.
Position the child to promote touching and batting at toys.
Place toys within reach so the child can play.

Upright or Supported Sitting

Use hands to provide support as needed when holding a child upright on the lap.
Gradually reduce the support to encourage muscle development.
Use rolls next to each hip to support the trunk when sitting in a chair.
Use rolls behind each shoulder to bring the child's shoulders forward in a high chair or infant seat.

TABLE 13-4 ● Toys for Young Children to Foster Motor Development	
Toys	*Possible Use*
Brightly colored rattles dangling from crib gym	Swiping, batting, or kicking of rattles
Small lightweight rattles	Grasping, waving, shaking, mouthing
Wrist or leg rattles	Waving arms, kicking legs
Busy boxes	Poking, batting, pushing parts with hands, fingers, feet
Containers	Putting small objects in, taking objects out, dumping contents out
Durable picture books with bright colors	Practice turning pages, looking at pictures, listening to single words and short stories
Blocks	Banging together, stacking
Simple shape sorters	Matching similar shapes
Dolls and stuffed animals	Patting, hugging, pretend feeding and bathing

Providing Many Opportunities to Use Hands and Fingers

A young child who has been hospitalized for a long period may not have had the full range of experiences that promote the ability to use hands and fingers. Home care nurses can play an important role in helping a young child to develop fine motor skills. Nurses can encourage a young child to finger and manipulate toys, equipment, and other objects to develop fine motor and cognitive skills. Equipment must be handled under the direct supervision of the caregiver to ensure that objects are safe. The

TABLE 13-5 ● Activities to Encourage Fine Motor Development

Grasps Object Placed in Hand

Place small rattle into the child's hand before, during, and after diapering.
Hold small rattle in the child's field of vision and shake it, encouraging the child to reach and grasp it.
Pause often during play with a rattle, providing verbal praise as the child attends to the object.
Encourage the child to bat at toys hanging from a crib gym.

Reaches, Grasps, and Holds Object in Hand

Encourage the child to reach and hold a variety of objects.
Encourage the child to explore objects with one and then two hands.
Encourage the child to feel toys and objects of many different textures—rough, smooth, hard, soft.

Uses Individual Fingers to Explore Objects

Encourage the child to poke and move small parts of complex toys.
Allow the child to touch caregiver's face and clothing when the child is being held.

Grasps Small Object with Fingers

Encourage the child to finger feed cereal and other small foods.
Encourage the child to drop small-shaped objects into a container.

therapist may need to help a nursing team identify appropriate opportunities during routine activities such as feeding and dressing to encourage the child's fine motor development. Once this groundwork has been established, families and nursing teams will be able to identify numerous strategies for encouraging such play. Table 13-5 includes activities for nursing teams to encourage a young child's fine motor development.

Incorporating Functional Movements Into Routine Caregiving

Functional movements such as coordinated sucking and swallowing, holding a bottle or spoon, and chewing are complex tasks that require the coordination of complex motor skills. A nursing team, in consultation with an occupational therapist, can incorporate into care plans appropriate feeding and dressing activities that further the motor goals of the individual child. Simple strategies such as using adaptive utensils and spending extra time incorporating self-feeding activities can promote the development

---

Motor Checklist

Positions the Child in the Most Normal and Stable Positions

☐ Supports the child's head if the child cannot yet maintain head control independently.
☐ Positions a child with reduced mobility in sidelying with supports along the back to enable the child to remain stable with arms forward to reach for toys.
☐ Places blanket rolls or other supports under the child's shoulders when placed in supine position to help the child reach for objects placed above.
☐ Uses own hands, body, or special equipment to help the child maintain trunk control needed for sitting.
☐ Uses blanket rolls to help align the child's body in sitting when necessary.
☐ Gradually reduces supports to encourage the use of head and trunk muscles to sit upright.
☐ Adjusts the amount of support needed to meet each child's individual needs.

Gives the Child Plenty of Time in a Variety of Positions

☐ Varies the child's positions throughout the day (in prone, sidelying, supported sitting, and supine position)
☐ Places child in supine position at various times throughout the day if medically appropriate.
☐ Assists the child in tolerating increased periods in supine position by using a toy or voice to distract the child.

Promotes the Child's Use of Hands and Fingers

☐ Assists the child in reaching and grasping by placing the child in a stable position with the arms forward in midline.
☐ Encourages the child to handle a variety of objects such as rattles, toys with moveable parts, spoons, cups, and equipment.
☐ Encourages the child to participate in feeding.
☐ Encourages the child to use hands to participate in dressing and other routines.

FIGURE 13-2. Motor checklist.

of important motor skills. For example, beginning dressing skills require the ability to push and pull with one's arms to put on a shirt, pants, or socks. These skills can be encouraged by promoting increased participation of a child in these activities and by incorporating appropriate positioning techniques discussed above. Physical and occupational therapists can guide home nurses to enable them to identify and incorporate effective strategies into the nursing care plan to promote many aspects of a child's motor development.

● CONCLUSION

The Motor Checklist shown in Figure 13-2 can be used by home care nurses and families working with therapists to promote the incorporation of basic motor development strategies into a child's nursing care plan. By reviewing the items in the checklist and by working with a therapist to identify a child's specific motor needs, the home nursing team will be better prepared to develop and implement interdisciplinary nursing care plans that provide for the optimal health and development of young children.

Ongoing staff development is needed for home health personnel to promote an understanding of and strategies for promoting the overall development of young children. Table 13-6 lists examples of video tapes that can be used by home health nurses. Home nursing teams who understand the importance of integrating a child's motor goals into everyday care plans can work with a child's therapist to identify specific goals and strategies for achieving those goals. The integration of developmentally appropriate strategies

TABLE 13-6 ● **Staff Development Videos**		
Title and Producer	**Description**	**Distributor**
Positioning for infants and young children with motor problems; University of Colorado Health Sciences Center School of Nursing	Demonstrates techniques for handling and positioning children with motor problems	Learner Managed Designs, Inc., (800) 467-1644
Encouraging motor development, Family-centered home health services for young children; Georgetown University Child Development Center	Video in a four-part series for home health nurses that demonstrates the principles of encouraging motor development described in this article.	Child Development Media, Inc., (800) 405-8942
Feeding and swallowing video series; Meyer Rehabilitation Center, University of Nebraska Medical Center	A series of seven videotapes for professionals and parents working with children with feeding difficulties	Child Development Media, Inc., (800) 405-8942
Infant motor development— A look at the phases; Goudy & Fetzer	Demonstrates normal motor development from birth through 12 months demonstrating the progression of skills.	Communication/Therapy Skill Builders, (800) 228-0752

into routine caregiving will provide a child with greater opportunities to achieve overall developmental gains.

● AUTHORS' NOTE

The authors have produced the video series, *Family-Centered Home Health Services for Young Children,* which is designed to be used with home health personnel. Individual video titles include: Responding to Families, Encouraging Communication and Play, Encouraging Motor Development, and Building Family-Centered Care Coordination. The video tapes are available through Child Development Media, Inc., (800) 405-8942.

● ACKNOWLEDGMENT

The authors thank Melmedica Children's Healthcare, Inc., Country Club Hills, Illinois, for the support and expertise they provided in the development of this article.

REFERENCES

Bailey, D. B. (1996). An overview of interdisciplinary training. In D. Bricker & A. Widerstrom (Eds.), *Preparing personnel to work with infants and young children and their families: A team approach* (pp. 3–21). Baltimore, MD: Paul H. Brookes.

Brown, D., Wyne, M. D., Blackburn, J. E., & Powell, W. C. (1979). *Consultation: Strategies for improving education.* Boston: Allyn and Bacon.

Dunn, W. (1996). Occupational therapy. In R. A. McWilliam (Ed.), *Rethinking pull-out services in early intervention* (pp. 243–265). Baltimore, MD: Paul H. Brookes.

Goldson, E. (1996). The micropremie: Infants with birth weight less than 800 grams. *Infants and Young Children, 8*(3), 1–10.

Hack, M., Friedman, H., & Fanaroff, A. A. (1996). Outcomes of extremely low birth weight infants. *Pediatrics, 98*(5), 931–937.

Hanft, B., & Place, P. (1996). *The consulting therapist: A guide for OTs and PTs in schools.* San Antonio: Therapy Skill Builders.

Hanft, B., Sippel, K, & Pokorni, J. (May, 1994). OTSG Case Management for Children with Disabilities Course. Atlanta, GA.

La Pine, T. R., Jackson, J. C., & Bennett, F. C. (1995). Outcome of infants weighing less than 800 grams at birth: 15 years' experience. *Pediatrics, 96,* 479–483.

Lippitt, G., & Lippitt, R. (1978). *The consulting process in action.* San Diego: University Associates.

Maternal and Child Health Bureau. (1994). *Standards of nursing practice for the care of children and adolescents with special health and developmental needs.* Washington, DC: U.S. Department of Health and Human Services.

McEwen, I. R., & Shelden, M. L. (1996). Preparing physical therapists. In D. Bricker & A. Widerstrom (Eds.), *Preparing personnel to work with infants and young children and their families: A team approach* (pp. 135–159). Baltimore: Paul H. Brookes.

Rainforth, B., & Roberts, P. (1996). Physical therapy. In R. A. McWilliam (Ed), *Rethinking pull-out services in early intervention* (pp. 243–265). Baltimore: Paul H. Brookes.

Singer, G. H. (1996). Introduction: Trends affecting home and community care for people with chronic conditions in the United States. In G. H. Singer, L. E. Powers, & A. L. Olson (Eds.), *Redefining Family Support* (pp. 3–38). Baltimore: Paul H. Brookes.

Ventura, S. J., Martin, J. A., Taffel, S. M., Mathews, T. J., & Clarke, S. C. (1994). Advance report of final natality statistics, 1992. *Monthly Vital Statistics Report. 43*(5) (suppl.).

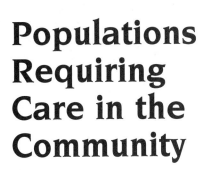

Roberta Hunt

Roberta Hunt

Roberta Hunt

Roberta Hunt

Populations Requiring Care in the Community

There is no "typical" client requiring community-based nursing care. For example, an elderly woman requiring follow-up care after hospitalization for a hip fracture, a premature infant requiring monitoring after months in the neonatal intensive care unit, an elderly man with diabetes and congestive heart failure, a young person with schizophrenia all require ongoing monitoring and assistance with medication adherence in community settings.

Chronic illness is a major health problem in the United States, affecting more than 31.5 million people. The management of chronic illness poses a major challenge for individuals and families as well as health care systems and society in general. Because most persons who suffer from chronic illness live with, rather than recover or die from that condition, typical therapeutic approaches are not often appropriate. Health care professionals are usually educated to cure rather than to only care for the ill. Consequently, they often find it frustrating to work with those who may never recover or experience a gradual or quick downhill trajectory.

If one member of a family has a chronic illness, the impact of the condition is experienced by all family members. Several years ago I was giving a lecture on the effect of chronicity on the individual, family, and community. One of my students raised his hand and shared the following: "My dad had a kidney condition that significantly affected his health all the years I was growing up. Our whole life revolved around my dad's illness. Over the years, people would ask my mother, 'How is your husband?' or ask me 'How is your dad feeling?' Just once I wish someone had asked me, 'How are you doing?' or ask my mom, 'How are you coping with your husband's illness?' "

When a family member has a chronic illness the entire family experiences the challenges of that illness. The key to successful nursing care is grounded in the nurse's ability to assess and work with the individual and family and promote their individual and collective coping styles.

Other populations requiring care in the community include those who are particularly vulnerable, whether because of age, health, socioeconomic factors, or life events. Examples include the elderly, children and infants, and those who are homeless.

This article discusses the work of Corbin and Strauss and provides a framework for assessing and developing interventions for chronic illness. Central to the Corbin and Strauss model is placing responsibility on the individual with chronic illness and their family members. The trajectory of the chronic condition is described in terms of past, present, and future perspectives, which all must be considered when planning care.

How are approaches for chronic conditions different from approaches for acute conditions? According to Corbin and Strauss, what are the factors that must be considered to manage chronic illness? What are some variables that influence the management of chronic illness? How can the nurse apply the trajectory framework to the nursing care provided for clients?

Nolan, M., & Nolan, J. (1995). Responding to the challenge of chronic illness. *British Journal of Nursing*, 4(3), 145–147.

Responding to the Challenge of Chronic Illness

MIKE NOLAN, JANET NOLAN

According to Funk et al (1993):

> Arthritis, cancer, diabetes, stroke, heart disease, respiratory illness, neuromuscular disorders, dementia and AIDS are but a few of the major chronic illnesses facing us today.

Chronic illnesses pose significant health problems and represent a major challenge for both health care systems and society in general (Asvoll, 1992). However, although such conditions lie outside the realms of traditional medical science (Funk et al, 1993), they still suffer from the inappropriate application of therapeutic approaches designed primarily for use in acute conditions (Pott, 1992). While the medical model is appropriate where cure is the aim, it can be counter productive in other circumstances (Reed and Watson, 1994). Moreover, interventions designed for palliative and terminal care are equally inappropriate because most people live with, rather than die from, chronic illness (Verbrugge and Jette, 1994).

An increasing number of nursing authors believe that the profession has a key role to play in meeting the health needs of people with chronic illness (Baines and Oglesby, 1991; McBride, 1992; Miller, 1992; Funk et al, 1993), with this challenge being variously described as lying "at the heart of nursing" (Funk et al, 1993) or as being "central to the mission of nursing" (McBride, 1992).

However, it has been known for some time that nurses do not appear to value working with patients whose conditions are not amenable to cure. For example, Kratz (1978), in describing the nursing care given to what she termed the "long-term sick in the com-

Mike Nolan, is Senior Lecturer in Nursing Research, Health Studies Research Division, and Janet Nolan is Lecturer in Nursing Studies, School of Nursing and Midwifery Studies, University of Wales (Bangor), Fron Heulog, Ffordd Friddoedd, Bangor, Gwynedd LL57 2EF.

munity," considered that nurses generally did not know about or value the care needed by patients who were not getting better. As a consequence, nursing interventions had little direction and became "aimless."

Similar conclusions have been reached by those studying the care of hospital patients, particularly elderly patients with chronic conditions (Evers, 1991; Reed and Bond, 1991; Reed and Watson, 1994). Working with patients with ongoing needs seems to offer nurses little job satisfaction, as they are generally unable to sustain a sense of therapeutic optimism (Reed and Watson, 1994). Yet McBride (1992) believes that managing chronicity should not be viewed passively as a failure of technology, but rather as an active process, representing the most exciting challenge currently facing nursing.

If the profession is to respond to this challenge, and truly assist people to live with chronic illness, then:

> A comprehensive, multidimensional model is urgently needed to serve as a guide for both research and service programs for persons with chronic conditions and those people who assist them (Baines and Oglesby, 1991).

Such a model must not merely focus on managing the acute exacerbations of chronic conditions; it must also provide a framework for promoting health (Kaplun, 1992) and empowering sufferers (Miller, 1992). This was explicitly recognised in a recent publication by the Royal College of Nursing (RCN, 1994) on the standards of care in rehabilitation nursing. It noted that, in the past, rehabilitation tended to focus on disability and illness at the expense of health and wellness, an approach that has limited the extent to which clients have been enabled to manage their own health and care.

● THE CORBIN AND STRAUSS NURSING MODEL

Woog (1992) contends that there is a need to:

> . . . engender a significant change in how we regard chronic disease and the betterment of health.

He advocates that nurses adopt the Corbin and Strauss (1992) model of nursing. This little known model appears to offer a valid approach, although in reality it was never intended as a nursing model per se but rather as a framework which could be used "by any discipline in whatever manner might correspond to its purposes and functions" (Corbin and Strauss, 1992).

Corbin and Strauss have developed what they term a "trajectory model" which they believe reflects the diversity, multiplicity and complexity of chronic illness.

They contend that most nursing interventions in chronic illness have been limited by the absence of an appropriate theoretical approach with which to underpin care. They argue that what is needed is a model that is based upon the experiences of individuals with chronic illness, and which can be used to provide the integration and cohesion that is needed to guide practice, teaching, research and policy. The framework they outline has evolved over 30 years, being based on both a series of research studies and the accounts and experiences of nurses working with chronic illness. The research they conducted includes the narratives and histories of patients with chronic illness cared for both in hospital and at home.

Trajectory Framework

The basic principle underpinning the Corbin and Strauss (1992) framework is the belief that chronic illness varies over time, i.e., it has a trajectory, and that its course, which can be divided into various sub-phases, is capable of being shaped and managed. However, in order to shape and manage any chronic illness successfully, a number of factors should be considered. Examples of these are highlighted in Figure 14-1. Corbin and Strauss believe that the most important variables are:

1. The stage or phase of the illness
2. Its biographical impact
3. Its impact on everyday life

They postulate that it is the careful analysis of the reciprocal interaction between the above three components that provides the key to success in the management of chronic illness. The central features of the model therefore concern the choices made about biographies (the impact of the illness on an individual's life course and self-image) and everyday activities. Within this context, the trajectory of the illness should be seen as having both a past and a future, which need to be taken into account when planning present care.

Nursing Intervention

A number of types of nursing intervention are advocated within the model, including direct care, teaching, counselling, referring, arranging and monitoring. However, central to the entire philosophy of the model is placing prime responsibility with the sufferer and his/her family, with nursing activities complementing and augmenting these efforts.

Conditions influencing the management of chronic illness

Type/amount/complexity/duration of technology and treatment

Resources available, both human and financial

Patient's experience of the illness

Motivation of patient and family

Setting of care

Lifestyle and beliefs

Interactions and relationships between participants in care

Type and stage of illness

Symptoms

Political and economic factors

Adapted from Corbin and Strauss (1992)

FIGURE 14-1.

In applying nursing interventions, Corbin and Strauss suggest an approach very similar to the nursing process (Figure 14-2). They also suggest that nurses should evaluate the practical value of their model, using four criteria based on those of Glaser and Strauss (1967):

1. Does the model "fit" with the area of interest?
2. Is it readily understandable?
3. Is it general enough to be applied to a variety of circumstances?
4. Does it allow the user to maintain some control as things develop and change over time?

In describing the application of this model, Woog (1992) has little doubt about its value, considering that:

> The model centers on the patient and affirms that his/her perceptions and beliefs about what is and may be happening to him/her are paramount to predicting the nature of the trajectory. This model is rich. It is client focused, conceptually sophisticated. It engenders research, care plans and policy changes which improve health (Woog, 1992).

These are bold claims indeed. On the other hand, Corbin and Strauss (1992) encourage nurses to use and adapt the model to their own purposes by adding and refining concepts as the model develops. A number of authors have considered the usefulness, or oth-

Applying the trajectory framework to nursing

Step 1	Determine the client's and family's response and their present management of the illness using • Illness • Biography • Everyday activities
	Establish goals of intervention
Step 2	Assess conditions influencing management (see *Table 1*)
Step 3	Define and refine the focus of the intervention using steps 1 and 2
Step 4	Provide interventions which may include: • Direct care • Teaching • Counselling • Referring • Arranging • Monitoring
Step 5	Evaluate effectiveness of the intervention — this may need a long-term perspective in taking into account factors identified in steps 1 and 2.

Adapted from Corbin and Strauss (1992)

FIGURE 14-2.

Key Points

● Chronic illnesses represent one of the major health challenges facing society.
● Interventions in chronic illness are still dominated by approaches more appropriate to acute conditions.
● Historically nurses give a low priority to patients with chronic illness.
● Models to help plan care in chronic illness do exist, e.g., Corbin and Strauss (1992).
● Nurses should apply and evaluate such models to determine which are the most useful.

erwise, of the model for the following: cancer recovery (Dorsett, 1992); cardiac illness (Hawthorne, 1992); human immunodeficiency virus/acquired immunodeficiency syndrome (HIV/AIDS; Nokes, 1992); chronic mental illness (Rawnsley, 1992); multiple sclerosis (Smeltzer, 1992); and diabetes mellitus (Walker, 1992).

However, little appears to have been written about the model in the UK. While it is by no means the only approach to meeting the needs of individuals with chronic illness (e.g., Miller, 1992; Rolland, 1988), it nevertheless merits closer attention. It is hoped that this brief article will prompt others to apply and critically appraise the value of the Corbin and Strauss (1992) model in planning their nursing interventions.

REFERENCES

Asvoll JE (1992) Foreword. In: Kaplun A, ed. *Health Promotion and Chronic Illness: Discovering a New Quality of Health.* World Health Organization (Europe), Copenhagen: IX–X

Baines EM, Oglesby FM (1991) Conceptualization of chronicity in aging. In: Baines EM, ed. *Perspectives on Gerontological Nursing.* Sage, Thousand Oaks: 251–74

Corbin JM, Strauss A (1992) A nursing model for chronic illness management based upon the Trajectory Framework. In: Woog P, ed. *The Chronic Illness Trajectory Framework.* Springer, New York: 9–28

Dorsett DS (1992) The trajectory of cancer recovery. In: Woog P, ed. *The Chronic Illness Trajectory Framework.* Springer, New York: 29–38

Evers HK (1991) Care of the elderly sick in the UK. In: Redfern SJ, ed. *Nursing Elderly People.* 2nd edn. Churchill Livingstone, Edinburgh: 417–36

Funk SG, Tornquist EM, Champagne MT, Wiese RA (1993) *Key Aspects of Caring for the Chronically Ill.* Springer Publishing Company, New York

Glaser B, Strauss A (1967) *The Discovery of Grounded Theory.* Aldine, Chicago

Hawthorne MH (1992) Using the Trajectory Framework: reconceptualizing cardiac illness. In: Woog P, ed. *The Chronic Illness Trajectory Framework.* Springer, New York: 39–50

Kaplun A (1992) *Health Promotion and Chronic Illness: Discovering a New Quality of Health.* World Health Organization (Europe), Copenhagen

Kratz CR (1978) *Care of the Long-Term Sick in the Community.* Churchill Livingstone, Edinburgh

McBride AB (1992) Managing chronicity: the heart of nursing care. In: Funk SG, Tornquist EM, Champagne MT, Wiese RA, eds. *Key Aspects of Caring for the Chronically Ill.* Springer, New York: 8–20

Miller JF (1992) *Coping with Chronic Illness: Overcoming Powerlessness.* 2nd edn. FA Davis, Philadelphia

Nokes KM (1992) Applying the chronic illness trajectory model to HIV/AIDS. In: Woog P, ed. *The Chronic Illness Trajectory Framework.* Springer, New York: 51–58

Pott E (1992) Preface. In: Kaplun A, ed. *Health Promotion and Chronic Illness: Discovering a New Quality of Health.* World Health Organization (Europe), Copenhagen: XI–XV

Rawnsley MM (1992) Chronic mental illness: the timeless trajectory. In: Woog P, ed. *The Chronic Illness Trajectory Framework*. Springer, New York: 59–72

RCN (1994) *Standards of Care: Rehabilitation Nursing*. RCN, London

Reed J, Bond S (1991) Nurses' assessment of elderly patients in hospital. *Intern J Nurs Studies* 28(1): 55–64

Reed J, Watson D (1994) The impact of the medical model on nursing practice and assessment. *Intern J Nurs Studies* 31(1): 57–66

Rolland JS (1988) A conceptual model of chronic and life threatening illness and its impact on families. In: Chilman CS, Nunnally EW, Cox FM, eds. *Chronic Illness and Disabilities. Families in Trouble Series 2*. Sage, Thousand Oaks: 5–68.

Smeltzer SC (1992) Use of the Trajectory Model of nursing in multiple sclerosis. In: Woog P, ed. *The Chronic Illness Trajectory Framework*. Springer, New York: 73–88

Verbrugge LM, Jette AM (1994) The disablement process. *Soc Sci Med* 38(1): 1–14

Walker EA (1992) Shaping the course of a marathon: using the Trajectory Framework for diabetes mellitus. In: Woog P, ed. *The Chronic Illness Trajectory Framework*. Springer, New York: 89–96

Woog P (1992) *The Chronic Illness Trajectory Framework: The Corbin and Strauss Nursing Model*. Springer, New York

Both the individual and the family experience challenges when a family member has a chronic illness. Identifying and facilitating the development of coping strategies with chronic illness must include the individual and family. The key to successful nursing care is grounded in the nurse's ability to assess and work with the family's coping style. This article discusses goals of care and coping tasks common to chronic illness.

What are some characteristics of chronic illness? What are some of the challenges that must be faced by the individuals and families experiencing a chronic condition? What are some of the goals of working with persons and families experiencing chronic conditions?

Martin, S. D. (1995). Coping with chronic illness. *Home Healthcare Nurse* 13(4), 50–54.

Coping With Chronic Illness

SHARON DEZZANI MARTIN

Families suffer in many ways when a member is stricken with chronic illness. Nurses frequently feel a sense of frustration when working with the chronically ill because cure is not possible. The author reviews the goals of care and coping tasks common to the chronically ill. Family coping styles are reviewed with suggestions for effective nurse behaviors with each style.

Working with a family who has a chronically ill member is one of the greatest challenges facing any home care nurse. Even when the nurse admits a patient in the hospital for an acute problem, it is imperative that other chronic problems are not ignored. It is also imperative for nurses to recognize that chronic illness in one family member affects the entire family unit. Thus the real client, when working with the chronically ill, is the entire family.

Home care nurses can work more effectively with families of the chronically ill by learning to assess and work accurately with the family's coping style. Once that style is determined, the nurse can tailor actions to ensure optimal effect. The following fictional Ross family illustrates important factors for working with the chronically ill.

● CHRONIC ILLNESS

More than 31.5 million people currently experience chronic illness (Table 15-1) in the United States, making it the number one health problem. As Americans age, the percentage of those with chronic illness increases from 6.9% for those younger than 45 years old to 24.1% for those 65 years or older.[1,2] In the future, it is expected that the average life expectancy will continue to increase, resulting in a greater number of elderly and chronically ill in the population.[3] But chronic illness is by no means a problem only for families with elders. Approximately 300,000 children and youth younger than 21 years

Sharon Dezzani Martin, RN, C, MSN, is an assistant professor of nursing, St Joseph's College, Windham, ME.

Case Study

The nurse arrived for her weekly visit to assess Mr Ross, a 66 year old who looked 80 years old. He had been seen on and off for the past 5 years for exacerbations of debilitating emphysema that had forced him to quit his work as a forester 6 years ago. The family, Mr Ross and his wife of 40 years, survived on disability payments, Medicare, and the meager amount his wife made as a part-time waitress.

As the nurse entered the rundown home, she sighed. Although they kept their appointments, the Ross' never seemed interested to learn about emphysema or its treatment. Compliance with the medication regime was questionable. Despite repeated warnings, they continued to heat their home with a smokey, coal-burning stove. Although they denied it, the nurse suspected Mr Ross or his spouse still smoked. The family had been discussed several times at professional advisory meetings, but the nurse continued to feel a deep sense of frustration and failure with the family.

Almost every nurse has endured the frustration of working with a family like the Ross', the family who seems uninterested, noncompliant, or perhaps even openly hostile when faced with a member who is chronically ill. These are the families who make us question our ability to teach or interact therapeutically. In addition, because chronic illness is involved, cure is not possible. The sense of accomplishment one feels when the patient recovers and leaves your care just never happens.

---

old are estimated to have limitations in physical functioning and require care.[4] The effect of a chronically ill member on the family can be devastating, no matter what the age.

● EFFECT OF CHRONIC ILLNESS ON THE FAMILY

A family member with a chronic illness affects the entire family unit. When working with a patient with chronic illness, the real client is the entire family.[5]

Although research can be inconclusive and even contradictory regarding the effect of chronic illness on the family, one fact seems clear, maintaining a chronically ill family member is hard work that may have negative physical, emotional, and financial effects, especially on the primary caregiver.[6-8] Family members endure many problems while caring for one who is chronically ill; they may not identify a specific problem but may simply

---

TABLE 15-1 ● Characteristics of Chronic Illness

According to the National Conference on Chronic Disease,[1] a chronic illness is defined as an impairment or deviation that has one or more of the following characteristics:

It is permanent
It leaves residual disability
It is caused by nonreversible pathologic alterations
It is requires special training of the ill individual or the family for rehabilitation
It may be expected to require an extended period of supervision, observation, or care

TABLE 15-2 ● **How Families Suffer**

According to Stuifbergen,[3] families suffer problems in the following categories when caring for a member with chronic illness:

Multiple social needs
    Lack of transportation, inadequate food, role changes, etc
    Social isolation (including loneliness and emotional strain)
    Few visitors, inability to leave home secondary to need for 7 day/week care needs, lack of phone, etc

Sexual activity changes (including illness-imposed changes or impotence)
    Impotence related to diabetes, feelings of undesirability related to altered body shape, etc

Financial insecurity
    Loss of income or health insurance, extraordinary medical bills, etc

identify total caregiving responsibilities as the stressor.[9] Other research identifies four general categories of difficulty as most common: unmet social needs, social isolation, sexual changes, and financial insecurity[3] (Table 15-2).

● THE GOAL OF CARE

In acute care settings, the nurse is more likely to see patients afflicted by acute illness, illnesses where the goal my be cure. This is the type of patient who provides a sense of reward to the caregiver. The patient improves, and transfers or leaves the facility. A goal has been reached, an accomplishment made. But what happens when we work with patients/families with chronic illness? The goal of cure is no longer appropriate. What, then, is the goal?

Care may be that goal for the chronically ill. It is a constellation of activities that not only helps the patient/family but also helps the nurse to identify required actions and, very importantly, to feel a sense of accomplishment[10] (Table 15-3).

TABLE 15-3 ● **Care Activities**

According to Thompson,[10] the goal of working with the chronically ill includes the following:

Prevention of other diseases
Early detection and treatment of exacerbations
Helping the patient/family determine and meet needs
Helping the patient/family make realistic goals and maintain hope
Boosting self-esteem by listening to and validating feelings
Pointing out positive gains and accomplishments
Showing genuine interest in the patient/family
Offering information and teaching as appropriate
Providing technical, hands-on care as needed
Helping the patient/family regain or maintain control over their lives

● COPING TASKS

Throughout life, we are faced with tasks to accomplish. The challenges and effects of chronic illness that must be faced by patients and families are called coping tasks (Table 15-4). Of the many coping tasks, maintaining a sense of being in control stands out as more critical.[11,12] Without a sense of self-control, it is difficult to complete many of the other coping tasks.

You might relate this to yourself for a moment. If you feel out of control, how well do you cope, interact, or adjust? We all hope that our actions help patients/families feel in control, but a reality check may alert us to behaviors or situations that have stripped patients of control.

Examine the caring behaviors in Table 15-3 and compare them with the coping tasks of Table 15-4. Many correlate highly, and one stands out distinctly. Helping the patient/family maintain a sense of control is critical to caring and coping. If this coping task is not met by appropriate caring behaviors of the nurse, the patient/family may have difficulty reaching any of the other coping tasks.

Recent research also is focusing on the critical task of maintaining hope. Factors that have been identified as supporting hope in chronic illness are family, religion, and friends.[13]

● HOW FAMILIES COPE

How do families manage and survive under the stress of a member who is chronically ill? The range of responses that you may have already seen in your practice includes families who manage stress well through those who descend into chaos. Some families are in chaos *before* anyone is ill thus making them even more vulnerable when a member becomes sick. What can you possibly do to help a family that is not coping well or to work most effectively with one that is coping well? What makes the difference between a family that can cope and one that cannot? We will look at some answers to these questions as we explore coping.

TABLE 15-4 ● Coping Tasks of Chronic Illness
Miller[16] identifies the following challenges that must be faced by the chronically ill:
Maintaining a sense of being in control
Maintaining hope despite an uncertain or downward course
Striving to feel normal (normalization)
Modifying lifestyle and daily routine
Obtaining information or skill to effect self-care
Maintaining positive self-concept
Adjusting to altered social relationships
Grieving over the losses of chronic illness
Dealing with role changes
Dealing with pain/discomfort
Adjusting to prescribed regimen
Confronting the inevitability of death
Dealing with the social stigma of illness or disability

Coping is defined as a dynamic process that is used to manage external or internal demands perceived to be exceeding the individual's resources.[14,15] Coping strategies are the "specific techniques a sick person selects to deal with the illness and its consequences," "The aim of coping is mastery, control, or resolution" (16, p 16). Note the concept of *control* arising again. In other words, families use a variety of techniques to deal with (cope with) stress in the hope of either resolving the stress or at least feeling in control of themselves in the stressful situation.

Another critical coping strategy emerging in research is the concept of normalization, that is "the process by which family members come to define their ill member and their family life 'as normal'. . . . (13, p. 6) Families moving toward normalization acknowledge the chronic illness but minimize its social and personal significance.[14] Normalization allows the family to emphasize abilities rather than focus on deficits and problems.[17,18]

Families experiencing life stress use a variety of other coping strategies as well, some are effective, some not. How might you determine if a family's coping is effective? Simply stated, coping is effective when *the family* feels that

(1) distress is within manageable limits;
(2) some hope has been preserved; and
(3) a sense of personal worth has been maintained.[16]

A fourth criterion might be that coping is effective when the family notes that *they feel in control* of the situation.

Remember that some families do not meet these four criteria even before anyone is sick or things go wrong. It may appear to the nurse that the family has an apparent inability to cope with chronic illness, in fact they may have had an inability to cope with life in general prior to the illness. Families with chaotic coping prior to illness may need special referrals and an interdisciplinary approach for effective care.

● COPING STYLES

A step that is important for the nurse working in the homecare setting is to identify the *general coping style* of the family and design nursing interventions that work effectively with that style. A simple Continuum of Coping Styles has been suggested as follows:[16]

Approach—Nonspecific Defenders—Avoidance

The family's coping style is determined by observing how the person/family *repeatedly responds to threats* of any kind.

Behaviors exhibited by patients/family using the *Approach style* of coping would include:

Tackling—energetic fighting of illness and compliance with therapy.
Vigilant focusing—great alertness to information and interest in details of illness and therapy.
Sensitizing—ready acknowledgment of negative and positive feelings.

The style is called *Approach* because the family will seek (approach) the knowledge necessary to control the disease. Some authors call this information-seeking strategies, that is behaviors designed to actively find solutions to problems.[19] Working with families using this coping style can be an enjoyable, productive experience for the nurse. The family is interested and actively participates in care.

Behaviors associated with the *Avoidance* coping style include:

Repression—excluding bad thoughts and feelings from consciousness.
Denial—denying the presence of a thought or feeling.
Projection—assigning one's own undesirable characteristics to others.
Selective inattention—hearing what one wants to hear.
Rationalization–unconsciously distorting reality by assigning some plausible explanation in order to mask unrecognized motives.
Minimizing—down-playing importance of a sign or symptom.

(Definitions of the above coping styles are from Garland and Bush.[20])

This style is called *Avoidance* because the family will seem to avoid information, deny the illness, or reject efforts to deal directly with the illness. Working with families who use the *Avoidance* style can be a frustrating experience unless you recognize that this is their coping style and decide to alter your own behavior to work with them effectively. If this has been the family's coping style throughout life the chances that you will be able to change that style during the crisis of chronic illness is minimal. Accepting them "as is" goes a long way toward successfully helping these families.

Nonspecific Defenders are those who may use either *Approach* or *Avoidance* coping styles depending upon the situation. Working with these families can be a real challenge as it necessitates that the nurse alter her approach to match the situation and clues offered by the family.

● WORKING WITH THE FAMILY'S COPING STYLE

You may not be able to change the family's coping style but you can identify and work with that style effectively. The following are behaviors that the home care nurse might use to effectively work with both the *Approach* and the *Avoidance* styles. The nurse can alter her behavior on a situational basis to match the style of the *Nonspecific Defender*.

Family Exhibits Approach Style of Coping

The nurse can:

Keep them informed
Allot plenty of time for talking, questions and answers
Use consistent technical approach to procedures
Encourage full participation in care
Engage in mutual goal setting
Let the family know that they are in control by word and action
Teach, teach, teach

Family Exhibits Avoidance Coping Style

The nurse can:

Teach and inform in a general, nondetailed way watching for signs of interest and exploiting all teachable moments
Be prepared to take as much more time for information sharing as teaching will be in much smaller doses

Listen, listen, listen

Be prepared to do more of the hands on care for a longer period of time

Listen carefully for the family goals

Never press the family to learn or do or to share feelings as it may result in resistance

Be patient. Don't allow your own feelings to interfere with your technique of working with these families. Don't succumb to self-pity or feelings of failure because they don't respond "like they should"

● THE ROSS FAMILY

Look again at the frustrating Ross family. What were some of the effects this family has suffered because of Mr. Ross' chronic illness? What coping tasks were they trying to meet? How could the homecare nurse effectively "care" for this family?

Based upon the information provided we might conclude that the Ross' cope using the Avoidance style. Accepting them "as is" would go a long way toward decreasing the nurses' frustrations as well as improving the ability to care for the family effectively.

Teaching should be general, non-detailed and applied in small doses. The nurse should listen more than talk and never press the family to share or do what they do not wish to do. Extra patience is required. Families progress at their own speed which may be different than our own speed. Finally, let the family stay in control, accept their decisions and statements even when we may not agree with those decisions.

Working with a family like the Ross' may not be textbook, feel-good nursing but nursing isn't meant to help the nurse, it is meant to help the patient/family. When working with the chronically ill the best care may require that we change our behavior rather than that the patient/family change theirs.

REFERENCES

1. Conference on Chronic Disease. *Preventive Aspects, Chicago, 1951: Conference Proceedings, Preventive Aspects of Chronic Disease.* Baltimore: Commission on Chronic Illness, 1952.
2. US Bureau of Census. *Statistical Abstract of the United States: 1981,* Ed 102. Washington, DC: Government Printing Office, 1982.
3. Stuifbergen AK. The impact of chronic illness on families. *Fam Community Health* 1987; 4:43–51.
4. Newacheck P, Fox H, McManus M. Home care needs of chronically ill children. *Caring* 1988; 7:4–10.
5. Bullough V, Bullough B. *Nursing in the Community.* St Louis: Mosby, 1990, pp 494–496.
6. Lubkin I. *Chronic Illness Impact & Interventions.* Monterey: Jones & Bartlett, 1986, pp 150–164.
7. Schulz R, Visintainer P, Williamson GM. Psychiatric and physical morbidity effects of caregiving. *J Gerontol Psychol Studies* 1990; 45:181–191.
8. Neundorfer MM. Family caregivers of the frail elderly: Impact of caregiving on their health and implications for interventions. *Fam Community Health* 1991; 14:48–58.
9. Hull M. Coping strategies of family caregivers in hospice homecare. *Oncol Nurs Forum* 1992; 19:1179–1187.
10. Thompson L. When caring is the only cure. Managing the chronically ill patient. *Nursing* 1987; 17:58–59.
11. Cohen C. Patient autonomy in chronic illness. *Fam Community Health* 1987; 1:24–34.
12. James M. Starting from scratch; Living with chronic illness. *Caring* 1989; 8:26–29.
13. Raleigh EDH. Sources of hope in chronic illness. *Oncol Nurse Forum* 1992; 19:443–448.
14. Lazarus RS. Stress, coping and illness. In Friedman H (ed). *Personality and Disease.* New York, NY: John Wiley, 1990, pp 97–120.

15. Lazarus RS, Folkman S. *Stress, Appraisal and Coping.* New York, NY: Springer, 1984, p 141.
16. Miller J. *Coping With Chronic Illness: Overcoming Powerlessness,* Ed 2. Philadelphia: FA Davis, 1992, pp 19–47.
17. Robinson C. Managing life with a chronic condition: The story of normalization. *Qualitat Health Res* 1993; 3:6–28.
18. Knafl KA, Deatrick JA. How families manage chronic conditions: An analysis of the concept of normalization. *Res Nurs Health* 1986; 9:215–222.
19. Call JG, Davis LL. The effect of hardiness on coping strategies and adjustment to illness in chronically ill individuals. *Appl Nurs Res* 1989; 2:187–188.
20. Garland L, Bush C. *Coping Behaviors & Nursing.* Clearwater: Reston Publishing, 1982, pp 13–23.

This article traces the movement of the care of the mentally ill from community to institution and back to community. The role of the psychiatric nurse as a case manager is discussed. Case studies are used to highlight issues typical to home care for clients with mental illness.

What are advantages to psychiatric home care? What are the typical intervention strategies used by the nurse? Describe the case manager role of the psychiatric nurse.

Quinlan, J., & Ohlund, G. (1995). Psychiatric home care: An introduction. *Home Health-care Nurse*, 13(4), 20–24.

Psychiatric Home Care: An Introduction

JUDITH QUINLAN, GAIL OHLUND

Healthcare has undergone many changes in the past 5 years. Hospitalization has become extremely expensive to the consumer and the payor. Alternative healthcare services are being considered and used, with the emphasis on cost containment and cost and clinical effectiveness. Psychiatric home care is clinically effective and less costly.

Care of the person who is mentally ill has come full circle in the United States. In Colonial times, the mentally ill were kept at home by parents or reluctant family until they became so violent or socially unacceptable that they were placed in institutions. These institutions, horrendous in nature, continued to increase in number in the 18th and 19th centuries. By the late 20th century, they had evolved into "humane warehouses." Treatment was minimal, and the setting was extremely restrictive.

During the 1970s, patient rights legislation came into effect. Most county and state institutions were required to release their patients into ill-prepared communities that had limited mental health services. Consequently, county health systems expanded services by increasing hospital beds and community clinics, but were never able to fully "gear up" for the overwhelming number of clients.

Out-of-control healthcare costs are forcing states and counties to decrease mental health services to patients who were never served adequately. In an effort to control costs, Medicare, health maintenance organizations, and private insurers also are decreasing mental health services and hospital length of stays for patients. As a result, acute psychiatric hospitals and units now are being used primarily for crisis-patient episodes, requiring discharge for patients before they are completely stabilized, thus increasing the chances for destabilization and a quick return to the hospital. Rather than minimizing costs, this cycle of episode, hospitalization, discharge/episode, hospitalization, discharge has perpetuated the escalation of costs of healthcare providers.

Judith Quinlan, RNC, is the interim director, St. Mary Medical Center Home Health Agency, Long Beach, CA. Gail Ohlund, RN, is the director of Ohlund & Associates, a psychiatric home care consulting firm, San Clemente, CA.

117

These hospital stays not only are costly in dollar amounts, but also have a negative impact on the patient who is mentally ill. General well-being, self-esteem, and opportunity for recovery tend to decrease during stays in hospitals, thus reducing the patient's overall functioning baseline.[1] Psychiatric hospital units should not be eliminated, however, because they provide a safe haven for those patients whose illnesses exacerbate to such an extent that they are no longer safe at home. It is not possible to avoid readmissions to hospitals entirely.[5] The nature of mental illness, with its remissions and exacerbations, precludes this. Therefore, treating the patient at home is again proving to be the least restrictive and most cost-effective holistic model of care.[3,4]

Psychiatric home care services are relatively new to Medicare-certified home care agencies. Although some agencies have had psychiatric patients on their services, they have treated them within the medical-surgical program. Today, agency personnel who are interested in providing care for the psychiatric patient see the need and efficacy for developing specialized programs similar to home infusion and hospice programs. Because psychiatric patients can be difficult and exhausting to treat, some agencies elect to refer their patients only to those agencies that provide specialty psychiatric services.

● LITERATURE SEARCH

Very little literature is available on psychiatric home care in the United States. British Commonwealth countries have reported research confirming the supposition that psychiatric home care not only is cost effective by decreasing hospital admissions and length of stays when patients are readmitted to the hospital, but also improves patients' quality of life by maintaining and/or increasing the baseline of functioning.[2,3,5,6]

The literature substantiates the positive outcomes of psychiatric home care. The psychiatric home care nurse is in a unique position to operationalize the processes that ensure committed, quality patient care and assist in these positive outcomes. In addition to help from psychiatric home care services and the patient's physician, the caregiver and/or family must receive education and available community resources and understand the patient's illness to ensure successful outcomes.[1,6]

● PSYCHIATRIC REGISTERED NURSES AS CASE MANAGERS

Medicare-reimbursed psychiatric home care, and private-pay and managed-care companies, use a managed-care model modified so that the psychiatric registered nurse case manager is the primary "hands-on" nurse. The psychiatric nurse plays a vital role in the patient's transition from the hospital to the community. Her or his role is to collaborate professionally with the psychiatrist to stabilize the patient and decrease frequent hospitalizations, thereby enhancing the patient's quality of life.

Because psychiatric patients are not stabilized completely when discharged from the hospital, they have a tendency to decompensate mentally and physically on arrival home. Frequently, the hospital discharge planner has not had sufficient time to implement all the discharge plans. The patient may need equipment for safety or treatment. They may be unable to obtain the ordered medications. They are often anxious and confused. These high-risk patients are frequently the ones without social supports, or they may lack the energy or sophistication to link into support systems. This is where the psychiatric home care nurse can make a real difference.

The nursing process lends itself to home care nursing. The psychiatric nurse case manager visits the patient within 72 hours (but usually the day after the referral) to assess the patient's mental status and make a head-to-toe physical assessment. The nurse then evaluates the data, and in professional collaboration with the psychiatrist and the patient's other physicians develops a medical care plan. The nurse's ability and skills to describe to the physician the patient's psychiatric, medical, and psychosocial status at home allows the psychiatrist a glimpse of the "whole" patient within his or her own environmental setting, and, therefore, improves physician-patient understanding and patient outcomes.[6]

The medical care plan that was initiated on the inpatient unit can be modified and completed during home care services. The psychiatric nurse makes referrals to appropriate members of the interdisciplinary psychiatric home care team. This team consists of a social worker, home health aide, physical therapist, dietitian, occupational therapist, and speech therapist. It is valuable to the team and patient if members of these disciplines have had experience with psychiatric patients.

The nurse ensures and monitors patient compliance with physician visits and medications. Patient status and medical care plans are evaluated during the bimonthly interdisciplinary treatment team conference, but the psychiatric nurse initiates and encourages communication between team members at any time.

The psychiatric registered nurse is the only home care nurse who must have credentials approved by Medicare before practicing in the setting.[8] The approval is needed primarily because the psychiatric nurse engages the patient in a therapeutic alliance, and is considered a therapist.[9] The nurse is caring, supportive, knowledgeable, and accessible. She or he listens, counsels, and teaches. The nurse works on practical solutions to immediate problems, and unites the treatment team in managing the patient's economic, housing, health, and justice system deficits.[7,10] The nurse is the key link in the connection between community and home.

Social interventions and education of the caregiver/family results in a significant increase in positive patient outcomes.[11] Recognizing that the patient's home is the patient's power base and that the home care nurse is a visitor, the psychiatric nurse skillfully works within those parameters. The psychiatric nurse has the skills necessary to assess and understand the burden of mental illness on the caregiver/family and to educate and assist the patient and caregiver/family to cope more effectively with mental illness.[12] Establishing a therapeutic relationship with the patient and caregiver can promote earlier disclosure of recurring symptoms by the patient and facilitate interventions and education. Patient and caregiver satisfaction with home care services is related directly to their perception of the skilled nurse's care.[4]

● CONCLUSION

The American Nurses Association states that case management optimizes a client's self-care capability and promotes efficient use of resources.[13] The psychiatric home care nurse uses the nursing process within the case management model to optimize cost-effective, quality patient care. This holistic approach not only includes collaboration with the professional disciplines, but also reaches out to the caregiver, family, neighbors, and community. The approach also empowers the patient and caregiver to become more independent, resolve problems more assertively, and return to the community with greater strength.

The physician, nurse, social worker, home health aide, dietitian, occupational and physical therapist, and caregiver play important roles in reconstituting the patient. Including the decreased hospitalizations and length of stays and the increase in medication and physician visit compliance, quality psychiatric home care services are not only cost-effective but also the least costly service to date.[5,6]

Case Study

The following case studies describe patient demographics, psychiatric and medical history, psychiatric home care assessment, special issues, and case management.

Mrs A is a 70-year-old patient with a diagnosis of paranoid schizophrenia, anorexia with associated weight loss, a history of congestive heart failure, and insomnia. During the past 20 years, she had multiple admissions to acute psychiatric facilities. On her last admission, conservatorship was considered, but she stabilized on haldol decanoate medication. Her hospitalization lasted for 1 month. On discharge, she was referred for follow-up psychiatric home care.

The results of the initial mini-mental status examination stated that the patient was alert and oriented, looked younger than her age, and had paranoia, auditory hallucinations, depression, and isolative behavior, but with no evidence of suicidal ideation.

The physical assessment showed a weight loss of 20 pounds with accompanying anorexia, and insomnia with interrupted sleep patterns. Mrs A also had a history of congestive heart failure, but was not in acute distress at the time.

Case management goals were to decrease paranoia and hallucinations, restabilize medications, increase body weight, increase socialization skills, stabilize sleep patterns, decrease readmissions to hospital, and organize the household, which was in disarray.

The patient's support network consisted of a neighbor and the psychiatrist. A referral was made to the social worker, who found a part-time homemaker to assist with household chores and organization and meals, and provide some companionship.

The psychiatric nurse managed medications; gave haldol decanoate injections; provided supportive therapy; instructed the patient in reality-based thinking, medication usage, and side effects; and ensured doctor-visit compliance. The nurse collaborated with the psychiatrist in restabilizing medications, and monitoring efficacy of sleeping medications, and signs and symptoms of the psychiatric disease process. The nurse administered 25 mg of haldol decanoate intramuscularly every 2 weeks, and managed extrapyramidal symptoms.

The patient was taught signs and symptoms of congestive heart failure, and to notify her doctor if her feet and/or hands swelled with edema, breathing became difficult, or a sudden weight gain occurred, or she became fatigued easily.

The patient was weighed each visit and was taught to use journal entry to track food intake and ensure appropriate nutrition. The neighbor was supported in increasing socialization time and decreasing helpful time, which increased the patient's independence and socialization.

The patient has not been readmitted to the hospital in the past 2 years.

Muijen et al[6] states that once psychiatric home care is discontinued, the patient eventually returns to the costly care of hospitals and communities. This is a quality and cost-effective concern that needs more exploration, research, and resolution. Other areas needing more study include psychiatric nurse visits to the elderly who are not homebound; identification of high-risk patients appropriate for long-term care; and employment of appropriate, unique psychiatric home care nurses.

Psychiatric home care nursing is an exciting practice, and is especially suited to the knowledgeable psychiatric nurse who desires collegial, professional relationships with physicians and can manage cases autonomously.

Case Study

Mr B is a 74-year-old patient with a diagnosis of major depression with anxiety and acute congestive heart failure. During the past year, the patient had one psychiatric hospital admission, and numerous medical and emergency room admissions for anxiety with panic attacks associated with acute congestive heart failure.

The patient was referred to psychiatric home health by the psychiatrist to reduce the emergency and hospital readmissions.

The results of the initial mini-mental status examination showed that the patient was alert and oriented; looked his age; had moderate to severe anxiety and depressed mood; and was hopeless and despondent about decreased health issues, poor coping skills, and impaired insight. The patient had no evidence of suicidal ideation.

The physical examination showed a thin, anxious man who weighed 140 pounds, was 5 feet 10 inches, and had congestive heart failure symptoms of shortness-of-breath, right and left pedal edema +1, crackles in right lobes, and poor appetite. The patient was on multiple heart medications, and anti-depressant, antianxiety, and sleep medications.

Case management goals were to stabilize anxiety attacks; elevate mood; stabilize the patient and instruct him in disease processes of depression, anxiety, congestive heart failure, and the relationship between these illnesses (eg, increased anxiety equals difficulty breathing equals increased anxiety); teach coping/relaxation skills; decrease readmissions to emergency room and hospital; secure a more structured, independent living arrangement; increase independent activities of daily living management, safety, and energy conservation; and refer the patient to a partial in-hospitalization program when his condition was stabilized.

The patient lived alone in an apartment. His only support system was a relative living close by. The house was cluttered, and living alone increased his level of anxiety. Safety during activities of daily living was impaired because of his anxiety and congestive heart failure. A referral was made to a social worker, who relocated the patient to a high-functioning retirement/assisted living arrangement.

The patient refused a home health aide, but was willing to have occupational therapist visits for instruction in safety management when performing activities of daily living, and energy conservation. The psychiatric nurse managed psychiatric and medical medications, and instructed the patient in medication usage for anxiety attacks, depression, and edema associated with congestive heart failure. The patient was taught about disease processes, to recognize signs and symptoms of exacerbation of depression and anxiety; and about congestive heart failure, to notify his doctor if swelling of the feet or hands increased, breathing became more difficult, or a sudden weight gain occurred. Verbalization of feelings was encouraged; supportive therapy was provided; and desensitization techniques, deep breathing, diversional activities, relaxation, and imagery were taught to decrease anxiety. The patient was instructed to keep a log to identify periods of anxiety so that he would recognize precipitating events.

The patient was weighed each visit. Through support and nutritional screening and education, no additional weight loss or episodes of anorexia occurred.

The patient received psychiatric home care services for 4 months and then was referred to a partial in-hospital program, which he attended for 1 year. The patient had one hospital admission for acute congestive heart failure during the 16 months he was monitored by home health services and the partial program.

Case Study

Mrs C is a 70-year-old patient with a diagnosis of bipolar disorder, depressed phase, dependent personality, congestive heart failure, osteoarthritis, and a neurogenic bladder. During the past 5 years, she has had multiple admissions to psychiatric hospitals when she was in the depressed phase of her bipolar's mood disorder. The hospitalizations usually lasted 1 month or longer. The patient's mood cycled, or changed, every 3 to 4 months, but during the depressed phase she became extremely dependent, anxious, agoraphobic, and fearful of being alone, and had self-care deficits.

The results of the initial mini-mental status examination showed an alert, oriented, agoraphobic patient with a depressed, despondent, and anxious mood. There was no evidence of suicidal ideation, although the patient was extremely hopeless.

Through physical examination, pain, an unsteady gait secondary to osteoarthritis, continuous stress incontinence from the neurogenic bladder, and a sleep pattern disturbance were seen. The patient had a history of congenital heart disease, but was in no acute distress at this time.

Case management goals were to stabilize/instruct on new antidepressant medication, teach assertion techniques, increase independence, desensitize her agoraphobia, stabilize sleep patterns, decrease pain, increase safe ambulation, decrease readmissions to hospital, and instruct patient/caregiver in disease management.

The patient's support network was a homemaker/assistant who had been with the patient for years. A referral was made to a social worker to evaluate the home environment for safety, to instruct and support the patient/caregiver in exercising housing options, and to assist them with community resources.

The psychiatric nurse managed medications, provided supportive therapy, taught assertion techniques to decrease dependency, and instructed patient/caregiver on disease processes (management of the depressed and manic phases of patient's illness, congenital heart disease, arthritis, stress incontinence) and importance of medication compliance. The psychiatric registered nurse instructed the patient in relationships between manic phases of the illness and exacerbation of congenital heart disease such as increased exhaustion, edema, and shortness of breath. She instructed the patient on pain management with medications, deep-breathing and relaxation skills (imagery, relaxation tapes and videos), and importance of verbalizing feelings and thoughts. The patient also was instructed in desensitization techniques to decrease isolative and agoraphobic behavior. She refused occupational and physical therapy, so the nurse instructed her on activities of daily living; safety, management, and energy conservation; safe ambulation; and use of cane for assistance when walking.

The patient received psychiatric nursing services for 4 months, refused a partial in-hospital program, and was referred to an adult day center at the Senior Center on discharge. She has not been readmitted to any psychiatric hospitals for the past 2 years.

REFERENCES

1. Kane C: The outpatient comes home. *J Psychosoc Nurs* 1984;22:19–25.
2. Gillis LS, Koch A, Jarji M: The value and cost-effectiveness of a home-visiting programme for psychiatric patients. *S Afr Med J* 1990;77:309–310.
3. Lear G: Managing care at home. *Nurs Times* 1993;85:26–27.
4. Van Dongen CJ, Jambunathan J: Pilot study results: The psychiatric RN case manager. *J Psychosoc Nurs* 1992;30:11–14.

5. Dean C, Gadd EM: Home treatment for acute psychiatric illness. *Br Med J* 1990;301:1021–1023.
6. Muijen M, Marks I, Connolly J, et al: Home based care and standard hospital care for patients with severe mental illness: A randomized controlled trial. *Br J Med* 1992;304:749–753.
7. McDaniel C: Reorganization of community psychiatric services by professional nurses. *Issues Ment Health Nurs* 1990;11:397–405.
8. Health Care Financing Administration: *Medicare Home Health Intermediary Manual* Pub 13. Baltimore, MD: Health Care Financing Administration. 1979.
9. Kozlak J, Thobaben M: Treating the elderly mentally ill at home. *Perspect Psychiatr Care* 1992; 28:31–35.
10. Aponte HF, Zarski JJ, Bixentine C, et al: Home/community-based services: A two tiered approach. *Am J Orthopsychiatry* 1991;61:403–408.
11. Leff J, Kuipers L, Berkowitz R, et al: A controlled trial of social intervention in the families of schizophrenic patients: Two year follow-up. *Br J Psychiatry* 1985;146:594–600.
12. Gerace L, Tiller J, Anderson J, et al: Development of a psychiatric home visit module for student training. *Hosp Community Psychiatry* 1990;41:1015–1017.
13. American Nurses Association. *Nursing Case Management*. Kansas City, MO: American Nurses Association, 1988.

Congestive heart failure is a common chronic condition affecting a large percentage of the elderly population. For these individuals, rigorous attention to self-care is necessary to maximize their ability to maintain and perform activities of daily living. Thorough assessment provides the key to effective intervention.

How is chronic congestive heart failure assessed and managed in community-based settings? What is the nurse's role in the management of medications for persons with congestive heart failure? What are the three essential elements of the typical nursing care plan for individuals with congestive heart failure?

Singh, P. (1995). Managing chronic congestive heart failure in the home. *Home Healthcare Nurse*, 13(2), 11–15.

Managing Chronic Congestive Heart Failure in the Home

PAMELA SINGH

Appropriate management of the patient with chronic congestive heart failure by the home health nurse is critical. Thorough assessment of the patient during the nursing visit can detect subtle changes in the patient's condition. Knowing what to look for and how to respond can improve the patient's quality of life significantly.

Your patient, Mr Stone, has just been discharged from the hospital with a diagnosis of congestive heart failure. You arrive at his home to begin the case. He appears to be comfortable, but tells you that just a few days ago he was so sick that he thought he was going to die. As you prepare to assess Mr Stone, you need to understand the complexity of his illness to mobilize his ability to manage his congestive heart failure at home.

Despite medical advances for the treatment of patients with chronic congestive heart failure, their prognosis is not good. In stable patients with mild symptoms, the annual mortality rates are approximately 10%, whereas in patients with advanced, progressive symptoms, mortality rates are 50%.[1] Furthermore, 40 to 50% of patients with heart failure endure sudden cardiac death related to ventricular dysrhythmias.[1] Knowing these statistics, and understanding that many patients will live with congestive heart failure for years will help you plan your management strategy with Mr Stone.

Pamela Singh, RN, MS, is the director of quality improvement, The Visiting Nurse Association of San Diego, Carlsbad, CA.

● ASSESSMENT

To begin your assessment of the patient, you need to determine the type and severity of the underlying disease that has caused the heart to fail.

Many different conditions, including hypertension, valvular heart disease, myocardial ischemia, and myocardial infarction, can impair the heart's ability to pump efficiently.[2] Mr Stone tells you that he is 70 years old, and had a heart attack 5 years ago. His physician told him that it affected the left side of his heart. You know that left ventricular failure increases the workload on the right side of the heart, because the right ventricle must contract more to overcome increased pressure in the pulmonary vessels.

Therefore, during his initial stages of heart failure, his heart tried to compensate for its decreasing efficiency via tachycardia, ventricular dilatation, and myocardial hypertrophy to increase cardiac output.[3] However, because chronic congestive heart failure develops gradually, these initial compensatory mechanisms become inadequate and other organ systems become involved as well.

Initial signs and symptoms of chronic congestive heart failure affecting multiple organ systems include pitting, dependent, or peripheral edema and fatigue.[3]

With disease progression, liver enlargement and tenderness may occur, as well as ascites, neck vein distention, pulmonary edema, pleural effusion, exertional dyspnea, persistent hacking cough with or without frothy sputum, crackles, angina pain in patients with coronary artery disease, and anxiety.[3]

Because Mr Stone has congestive heart failure, you must focus on the cardiovascular and pulmonary systems, and relevant aspects of gastrointestinal and skin assessment.[4] Observe his level of consciousness. Reduced cardiac output can diminish cerebral blood flow and oxygenation.[5] Make a visual inspection of the chest, observing for movements, pulsations, and exaggerated lifts or heaves. Determine the rate, rhythm, and character of his pulse. The pulse rate is usually elevated, compensating for a low cardiac output. Alternating pulse (pulsus alternans), characterized by an alternating strong and weak pulse with a normal heart rate and interval, may be present.[4] It is associated with left ventricular malfunction, causing a variance in left ventricular preload.

Increased heart size is common in congestive heart failure. This enlargement can be detected by precordial palpation, with the apical impulse displaced laterally to the left and downward.[4] Heart failure patients will have a third heart sound (S3), which indicates a pathologic condition. A fourth heart sound (S4) can occur as well, and is a reflection of decreased ventricular compliance associated with ischemic heart disease, hypertension, or hypertrophy.[4] If Mr Stone's heart rate is rapid, more than 100 beats per minute, S3 and S4 may merge into a single gallop. The neck should be assessed for jugular vein distension, carotid pulse, and bruits.[5]

Pulmonary artery pressures that are continuously elevated cause fluid to move into alveolar spaces.[4] The fluid that builds up results in crackles. In the initial stages of congestive heart failure, crackles are detected usually at the bases of the lungs, but as pulmonary congestion increases, crackles may be heard throughout the entire chest.

Next, assess Mr Stone's feet, ankles, and sacral area for dependent edema. Color and temperature of the skin should be assessed for findings of pallor, decreased temperature, cyanosis, and diaphoresis.[4]

Heart failure may result in hepatomegaly.[4] The liver span may be increased, and palpated well below the right costal margin. Spleen enlargement also may be present in advanced stages of the disease.

Your findings at this time indicate that Mr Stone is stable. His blood pressure is 140/80; heart rate, 82; respiratory rate, 22; and temperature, 98.2. His heart sounds are regular, but he does have an S3. He has no edema, and reports fatigue only with exertion. There are no exaggerated lifts or heaves on inspection of his chest wall. He is alert and oriented with no other signs of disease progression. His lungs are clear to auscultation bilaterally, and his weight is 170 lb.

● MEDICATIONS

Your next area of concern is medications. Mrs Stone is the primary support system for Mr Stone. They have no children, and have adequate insurance and income to pay for his medications, which play a major role in management of heart failure. Digitalis glycosides and other positive inotropic agents, diuretics, vasodilators, and angiotensin-converting enzyme inhibitors are some of the drugs used to improve cardiac functioning.[2]

Mr Stone currently is taking the following medications: digoxin, 0.125 mg by mouth once daily; Lasix (Hoechst-Roussel, Somerville, NJ), 20 mg by mouth once daily; and Capoten (Squibb, Princeton, NJ), 12.5 mg by mouth three times a day. You explain to Mr. Stone that it is necessary for him to take his medications as prescribed by his physician. You also tell him that the digoxin can slow his heart rate, and that he must take his pulse before taking this medication each day, and to hold the dose and call his physician if his heart rate is less than 60 beats per minute.

Digoxin strengthens and prolongs the myocardial contraction, allowing the ventricles to empty more completely.[2] Digoxin toxicity is a potential problem. Monitoring for nausea and vomiting, cardiac arrhythmias, and vision changes will be part of the patient's ongoing assessment. The physician may order periodic blood testing to assess the patient's digoxin level.

Loop diuretics such as Lasix are used to treat the edema associated with congestive heart failure.[2] This drug will block chloride reabsorption in the loop of Henle, and will interfere with the reabsorption of sodium and water.[2] The effect will decrease the amount of blood returning to the heart.

Capoten is an angiotensin-converting enzyme inhibitor that interferes with the renin-angiotensin-aldosterone system. By blocking the conversion of angiotensin I to angiotensin II, this drug will prevent vasoconstriction, sodium, and water retention to reduce stress on the heart further.[2]

● DIET

Mr Stone had been placed on a special diet. He was told in the hospital to eat a low sodium, fat, and cholesterol diet. This diet should be expanded to include foods high in potassium and fiber to prevent hypokalemia and constipation. Developing constipation can decrease the patients heart rate by stimulating the vagus nerve (Table 17–1).

● DEVELOPING A PLAN

Your plan to assist the patient to manage his heart failure at home now can be developed. You must assess the patient's knowledge level before any teaching plan can be developed. However, there are some essential elements that must be included in the plan.

First, all medications must be taken as the physician ordered.

TABLE 17-1 ● Assessment and Intervention Checklist

Assessment

Cardiac history
Level of conciousness
Blood pressure, pulse characteristics
Neck vein distension, bruits
Chest auscultation for adventitious sounds
Cough, shortness of breath on exertion
Orthopnea
Edema
Skin characteristic
Cyanosis, pale
Weak, dizzy, tired
Low urine output
Liver enlargement, ascites

Interventions

Make breathing easier
Promote rest
Elevate feet
Rising from lying to standing position
Provide emotional support
Monitor weight
Instruct on skin care
Provide nutritional education
Monitor elimination
Instruct on and monitor medications

Second, the amount of sodium consumed must be limited to prescribed amount, and fluid intake should not exceed that which was ordered.

Activity level must be controlled. Mr Stone must get enough rest during the day, and should only do the specific amount of activity ordered by the doctor. Daily weight should be recorded with the patient weighing himself at the same time each morning using the same scale. He should be instructed to call his physician if he gains 2 lb or more overnight.[6] If oxygen was prescribed, then instruction regarding this therapy would be necessary. Mr Stone does not need supplemental oxygen at this time.

Most importantly, the patient needs to know what can cause his disease to exacerbate. This includes not taking medications as ordered, consuming too much sodium, drinking too much fluid, having fever or infection, engaging in too much activity, and having rapid or irregular heartbeat or strong emotional reactions.[6] Warning signs will develop if Mr Stone's heart failure is worsening. These include increased dyspnea during activity or rest, unusual fatigue, tight shoes or swollen ankles, cough without other symptoms, swollen hands or tight rings, swelling in back or hip area, 2-lb weight gain overnight, feelings of overwhelming anxiety, and cold skin or a cold sweat.[6]

Your visit with Mr. Stone has ended. Before leaving, make sure that he knows who to call in case of an emergency and has his physician's phone number close at hand. Assessing, planning, implementing, and evaluating the nursing care plan for the patient with chronic congestive heart failure can be challenging for the patient, nurse, and patient's family. By using a strong nursing knowledge base and good communication skills, the patient can live his or her life to the fullest.

REFERENCES

1. Massie BM, Sokolow M. Cardiovascular Disease. In Tierney L, McPhee S, Papadakis M, Schroeder A (eds). *Current Medical Diagnosis and Treatment.* East Norwalk, CT: Appleton & Lange, 1993, pp 263–351.
2. Solomon J. Managing a failing heart. RN 1991; 8:46–51.
3. Fukuda N. Outcome standards for the client with chronic congestive heart failure. *J Cardiovasc Nurs* 1990;4(3):59–70.
4. Laurent-Bopp D. Pathophysiology of heart failure. In Underhill S, Woods S, Silvarajan Froelicher E, Halpenny J (eds). *Cardiac Nursing,* ed 2. Philadelphia: JB Lippincott, 1989, pp 220–227.
5. Jackson B. Performing a rapid assessment of the heart. Nursing 1992; 2:32C–32D.
6. Majorowicz K, Hayes-Christiansen CV. Congestive heart failure: Disease process & home care. *Cardiovascular Nursing.* Springhouse, PA: Springhouse, 1989, pp 291–296.

With the advent of health care reform, earlier discharges from acute care facilities have become standard among the elderly. Consequently, greater numbers of older adults are cared for in their own homes by nurses or by members of their family. Regardless of the age of the person, these factors create a tremendous demand on caregivers and family members. These demands may create stress and strain on the family and caregiver. The potential for elder abuse must be assessed and strategies implemented to minimize the likelihood of abuse.

What are characteristics of the elderly who are abused? What are characteristics of the abuser? Identify strategies to detect elder abuse. How can the nurse intervene to prevent elder abuse? What are the goals of intervention? What professional and legal responsibility does the nurse have to report elder abuse?

Allan, M. A. (1998). Elder abuse: A challenge for home care nurses. *Home Healthcare Nurse*, 16 (2), 103–110.

Elder Abuse: A Challenge for Home Care Nurses

MARY ANN ALLAN

Healthcare practitioners are aware that elder abuse exists in our society, and in light of present economic conditions, its prevalence may be increasing. This problem often goes undetected because abuse frequently is not acknowledged by the abused or the abuser. Home care nurses are in a prime position to recognize elder abuse and to intervene accordingly. This article addresses the characteristics of abused older adults, their abusers, strategies to detect elder abuse, and interventions that home care nurses can use to manage or to prevent the problem.

The influence of healthcare on our society has created a new awareness of problems related to the older adult. With advances in medical technology, people are living longer. Therefore, the number of dependent elderly with a high rate of chronic illness is increasing. The elderly are likely to be dependent on others due to physical or cognitive impairment. Healthcare reform is encouraging more community-based care for older adults and earlier discharges from acute care facilities. This often places an increased burden on the caregiver. Increasingly, home care nurses will care for greater numbers of older adults in their own homes or in the homes of their families. Consequently, nurses need to be aware of the impact that these changes may have when delivering care to the elderly population.

Mary Ann Allan, MSN, RN, CS, GNP, MAED, is a recent graduate of the University of Mary, Bismarck, ND.

The purpose of this article is to facilitate detection of the abused elderly client by assimilating knowledge about the characteristics of abused older adults and their abusers, strategies to detect elder abuse, and management and prevention of elder abuse. By applying knowledge of elder abuse when working with the older adult, the home care nurse can recognize potential problems and intervene accordingly. Although emphasis is placed on abuse of the elderly in the community, it should be recognized that elder abuse may exist in other settings such as acute and long-term care facilities.

● DEFINITION OF ABUSE

All discussions of elder abuse include physical violence: acts carried out that cause physical pain or injury. The most common acts are slapping, hitting, and striking with objects. Psychological abuse is defined as an act carried out against the elder adult with the intention of causing emotional pain or injury; it often accompanies physical abuse. Examples include threats, insults, and statements that humiliate or infantilize the elder.

Neglect of the elderly is often referred to as the failure of a caregiver to meet the needs of the dependent elderly person. It may be intentional (e.g., willfully withholding food or medications or refusing to take the elder to seek medical advice). Neglect may also be unintentional and could result from ignorance or from genuine inability to provide care (Lachs & Pillemer, 1995). For example, the caregiver may be unable to perform caregiving duties such as bathing or changing an incontinent elderly person. Therefore, an elderly person with poor hygiene, skin breakdown, and urine burns may be neglected either intentionally or unintentionally (Lachs & Fulmer, 1993).

Many definitions of abuse include acts of material or financial exploitation. Some of these include theft of pension checks, threats to enforce the signing or changing of wills or other legal documents, and coercion involving any financial matters (Lachs & Pillemer, 1995). In some situations, the money may be used for the family, thus resulting in neglect of the elder's basic needs. Exploitation may also occur in the form of fraud schemes: someone may persuade the elderly person to withdraw their life savings in a "get rich quick" scheme which, ultimately, may leave the elderly person penniless. In other cases, the elderly person is a target for less than reputable contractors who insist that house repairs are essential–at great cost to the elder.

● CHARACTERISTICS OF THE ABUSED ELDER

Several theories of causation have been used to identify and test risk factors for elder abuse, but a consistent profile of the elderly person at risk has not emerged (Lachs & Fulmer, 1993). Some studies suggest that those at risk are most likely to be female, widowed, frail, cognitively impaired, and chronically ill (Jones, Dougherty, Schelble, & Cunningham, 1988; Rounds, 1992; Shiferaw et al., 1994). The Pillemer and Finkelhor (1988) study revealed similar findings. However, the one exception was that elderly men were most often the recipients of abuse.

Although it has been suggested that the frail elderly are the most likely to be abused, some studies have not found a direct relationship between abuse and poor health, functional impairment, or excessive dependence on the abuser (Homer & Gilleard, 1990; Pillemer & Finkelhor, 1988). However, Lachs and Pillemer (1995) reported the great likelihood that increased frailty does play some part in mistreatment. Problems of physical health may increase vulnerability of the elderly in the presence of other risk factors. Some of these include cognitive impairment and a living arrangement shared with the abuser (Homer & Gilleard, 1990; Jones et al., 1988; Pillemer & Finkelhor, 1988). Home care nurses providing for the elderly client with dementia, incontinence, or impairments in performing activities of daily living (ADL) should be alert to assessing risk factors for elder abuse.

● CHARACTERISTICS OF THE ABUSER

Who abuses the elderly? It is most likely to be the person with whom he or she resides. Often an adult child is the abuser (Owen & Owen, 1995). Middle-aged or elderly relatives with mental illness or substance abuse problems are likely to be abusive (Lachs & Pillemer, 1995). In one study, the abuser was a spouse in 58% of the cases (Pillemer & Finkelhor, 1988). Family members who depend on the elder for financial assistance, housing, or other necessities have a higher risk of becoming abusive (Jones et al., 1988).

Kosberg (1988) identified several factors that increase the risk of the caregiver becoming an abuser. These include alcohol and drug abuse, cognitive impairment, economic stress, caregiver inexperience, a history of family violence, a blaming personality, unrealistic expectations, and economic dependence on the elder. O'Malley, Everitt, O'Malley and Campion (1983) pointed out that family characteristics related to abuse include lack of family support, overcrowding, isolation, marital conflict, and the increased burden placed on the caregiver.

● DETECTION OF ABUSE

Home care nurses must be aware that elder abuse exists and that in the face of the present economic conditions, its prevalence may be increasing. Because abuse is frequently not acknowledged by the abused or the abuser, it is important that home care nurses remain alert to its presentation (Jones et al., 1988; Lachs & Fulmer, 1993). Reasons for the reluctance of victims to report abuse include denial, shame, and fear of retaliation (Fulmer, McMahon, Baer-Hines, & Forget, 1992). For some of the elderly, reporting an abusive situation may lead to placement in a nursing home or other institution. Older adults with a family history of domestic violence may feel that they are receiving treatment similar to what they once displayed toward their children.

Concerns surrounding detection of elder abuse have been well documented in the literature. Lack of knowledge regarding detection on the part of healthcare practitioners has been reported. Fulmer et al. (1992) reported that abuse often is confused with normal age-related changes or signs and symptoms of disease. Similarly, clinical criteria for abuse and neglect may be interpreted differently among health practitioners (Clark-Daniels, Daniels, & Baumhover, 1990). Cultural values and beliefs may play a role in defining abuse or neglect, adding to the complexity of the issue (Hanson Frost & Willette, 1994). In addition, many older adults have subtle signs of abuse and neglect (dehydration or poor hygiene) that can go undetected (Jones et al., 1988).

The epidemiology of injuries is not understood, including the situations that surround false-positive and false-negative diagnoses. Presently, there are major gaps in knowledge about the many clinical presentations of elder abuse (Lachs & Fulmer. 1993). Many professionals refer to the lack of standard protocols for determining abuse (Clark-Daniels et al., 1990; Fulmer et al., 1992; Sanders, 1992). Notwithstanding the lack of available data, there are guidelines that the home care nurse can use to recognize elder abuse (Lachs & Fulmer, 1993).

● STRATEGIES TO DETECT ELDER ABUSE

Home care nurses are in a critical position to detect and intervene in suspected cases of elder abuse. Although elder abuse occurs in institutions as well as in community nursing stations, it may be less obvious in private dwellings in the community unless home care nurses recognize it. Hence the only opportunity for assessing elder abuse arises when the home care nurse visits a patient at home for an acute or chronic problem (Rounds, 1992). Another opportunity for detection presents itself when the older adult visits a primary care setting or an emergency department.

In order to intervene, the nurse needs to be aware of normal age-related changes as well as the demographic and social backgrounds of the abused and the abuser (Criner, 1994). Assessment data should be obtained from the elderly patient, caregiver, family members, neighbors, and community agencies if necessary (All, 1994). A multidisciplinary approach is of utmost importance. Lachs and Pillemer (1995) emphasized the importance of careful documentation (description of events and drawing of injuries) because the medical record may be used in the event of legal action later. If possible, consent should be obtained to investigate elder abuse. In addition, Lachs and Fulmer (1993) suggested that the use of a standardized assessment protocol is an excellent policy for ensuring that a thorough assessment is performed.

History Taking

Routine questions surrounding elder abuse and neglect should be incorporated into the home care nurse's daily practice (Bruce, 1994). The potential victim of elder abuse should be interviewed alone to avoid intimidation by the presence of the alleged abuser. Elderly persons may be hesitant to report in front of others that they are victims of abuse. Exploring medical complaints can be a method of screening for domestic violence (Jones et al., 1988). In addition to eliciting information about the present illness and past medical history, the home care nurse should assess functional status. Is the patient able to perform activities of daily living? Who performs instrumental activities of daily living? Who prepares the meals? Who handles the finances? If abuse is suspected, the home care nurse may ask the elder, "Does anyone ever hit you?" "Do you spend a great deal of time alone?"

It is equally important to determine the patient's social and financial resources. Are friends or other family members involved in the caregiving process? Does the elder have access to community and religious activities? Are the financial resources meeting the patient's needs, or is financial exploitation a concern? The home care nurse may ask the elderly patient, "Do you know how much money you have?" If interventions are necessary, it is crucial that the financial status be known so appropriate resources for the patient can be accessed (Lachs & Pillemer, 1995).

The suspected abuser should be interviewed alone as well. A nonjudgmental approach is best because confrontation yields less information. Empathy and understanding are essential in obtaining an accurate history. The home care nurse may say, "Caring for your father with his dementia must be difficult. Do you ever lose control?" The identification of specific stressors is important. For example, any history of recent stressful events in the family such as bereavement, job loss, or family problems should be discussed (Lachs & Fulmer, 1993). The history should include lifestyle, family structure, caregiving skills, and personality. Is the caregiver financially dependent on the elder? What is typically involved in providing care? Does the caregiver have support systems to assist? What community resources, if any, are being utilized to assist with providing care for the elder?

Other clues of elder abuse may include a pattern of "physician hopping," unexplained delay in seeking treatment, explanation of past injuries inconsistent with present findings, previous unexplained injuries, and previous complaints of similar injuries. The interaction between the patient and the caregiver is an important observation as well. A caregiver who insists on providing the medical history may be a clue. Does the caregiver appear to be overly concerned with the patient's care? Does the patient appear to be fearful of the caregiver? The behavior of both parties must be noted (Bloom, Ansell, & Bloom, 1989).

Objective Data Collection

Abuse should be suspected when the older adult is seen with multiple injuries in various stages, when injuries are not explained, or when the explanations are not possible given the type of injury. The most common physical injuries include unexplained bruises, lacerations, abrasions, head injury, and unexplained fractures. Dehydration and malnutrition are the most common manifestations of neglect (Jones et al., 1988).

A thorough physical examination is crucial in detecting elder mistreatment. One may begin the assessment with an observation of behavior and appearance. Is the patient appropriately attired and neatly groomed? Is there evidence of anxiety, withdrawal, or depression? Anetzberger et al. (1993) emphasized that the skin is the most valuable and exposed organ in detection. It is essential that the examination include assessment for signs of dehydration, unusual distribution of bruises, ecchymoses in various stages, bruises or burns that suggest improper use of an object or signs that the hands and/or feet may have been improperly immersed in hot or boiling water by the abuser. The clinician should examine for skin breakdown and burns from urine, which may be signs of neglect. Table 18-1 shows physical findings in the detection of elder abuse.

Appropriate imaging and laboratory tests follow the physical examination as indicated by the assessment. Are laboratory values consistent with the history? For example, low-serum albumin results may reflect underlying medical problems or malnutrition from withholding of sustenance. Radiograph studies such as x-rays may be indicated when the examination is suggestive of fractures (Lachs & Fulmer, 1993).

In addition to the thorough physical examination, a formal mental-status test should be performed. Cognitive impairment may indicate possible delirium or suggest underlying dementia, which may be a risk factor for abuse. The patient may not be able to give an accurate history. Also, if the cognitive impairment is severe, the patient will not be able to make decisions regarding interventions that require informed consent (Lachs & Pillemer, 1995).

Costa (1993) emphasized that an awareness of the problem of elder mistreatment and a high index of suspicion are the most important elements in diagnosing elder abuse. The differential diagnoses of many common geriatric presentations may be a result of elder abuse and neglect (Lachs & Fulmer, 1993). For example, a fracture may indicate either osteoporosis or physical force. Although depression is not uncommon among the elderly, it may be a response to an abusive environment. Other subtle signs such as malnutrition, failure to thrive, dehydration, and oversedation may be indications of abuse (Criner, 1994). Similarly, inappropriate high- or low-serum drug levels may mean either noncompliance of the patient or withholding of medications or overmedication by the caregiver (Lachs & Fulmer, 1993).

TABLE 18-1 ● Physical Findings in Detecting Elder Abuse	
Focus Area	Items to be Noted
General appearance and vital signs	Hygiene; cleanliness; appropriateness of dress; posture affect; mental status; withdrawal; signs of malnourishment
Integument	Bruises; scars; abrasions; decubitus ulcers; multiple skin lesions in various stages; skin color, turgor and other signs of dehydration; discolored skin (healed burns); whiplash burns (use of rope or cord)
Head and neck	Trauma (hematomas, lacerations); traumatic alopecia; facial; bruises, scars, whiplash injuries (from shaking)
Eyes and ears	Hyphema; subconjunctival hemorrhage; detached retina; black eyes; ruptured tympanic membrane with blood or fluid trapped behind
Nose and mouth	Epistaxis; bruises and lacerations of lips (forced feeding or gagging to silence)
Thorax and lungs	Rib fractures; bruises to breasts
Abdomen	Bruised or punctured viscera; extreme tenderness (palpate organs carefully)
Genitalia/rectal	Rectal and vaginal bleeding; poor sphincter tone; infestations; vaginal infection; excoriated perineum
Extremities	Limited ROM (note crepitations which may indicate fracture); wrist or ankle lesions (restraints) immersion burn (stocking—glove distribution); cigarette burns on hands
Neurologic—Psychiatric	Anxiety; depression; cognitive impairment; delirium (may be sign of neglected UTI, malnutrition)

● INTERVENTION

Prevention of elder mistreatment is a challenge for the home care nurse. A proactive response to the problem is essential, and nurses should be contributing to the formulation of plans to safeguard older people (Owen & Owen, 1995). Diagnosis, management, and prevention of elder abuse should involve the interdisciplinary team consisting of nurses, physicians, social workers, and others. The focus of treatment should be disease prevention, education, and health promotion. All aspects of elder care should be evaluated before the elderly person leaves the acute care setting, then regularly during home visits. It is crucial that caregiver stress be addressed before it leads to mistreatment (Criner, 1994). Therefore, the importance of family involvement cannot be overemphasized.

Two goals of intervention are safety of the elder and breaking the cycle of mistreatment. If mistreatment is suspected, the home care nurse must consider an important question related to safety. Is there an immediate threat of danger to the elderly person or to anyone else in the environment? If there is, interventions must center around immediate medical needs and/or removal of the victim to the hospital, if appropriate. Hospitalization provides the opportunity to address the needs of the elder and to arrange for necessary services (Jones et al., 1988).

Williams-Burgess and Kimball (1992) warned healthcare practitioners that denial of the problem by family members is likely to occur. The family must recognize that a problem exists before any changes can be implemented. Anxiety, shame, and guilt can have a paralyzing effect on the family. The home care nurse who supplies support and validation can assist the members to a stage of recognition and action. This may be a slow process. The goal of the nurse is to offer alternatives appropriate for the situation.

Fulmer (1989) pointed out that "family as client" is an important construct in elder abuse. The situation is seldom unidimensional and, therefore, requires resources to assist all of the individuals in the situation. Costa (1993) stressed that an important goal is to make the elder as functional as possible, thereby decreasing dependency on the caregivers. This author supports the use of aids to assist with ADL as well as community resources such as both physical and occupational therapy.

In the event that the abused elder decides to remain in the situation, the home care nurse may involve support services such as homemaker services, religious organizations, counseling, and respite care. Resources such as social assistance may be necessary to facilitate these services. If the family does not qualify for home care services, the home care nurse should attempt to improve the situation by involving other family members in caregiving to decrease the burden on the caregiver and refer to community resources. In some circumstances, interventions aimed at the psychopathology of the abuser may be warranted. Counseling or job training may be appropriate strategies for improving the situation (Lachs & Fulmer, 1993). However, alternative living arrangements such as foster care or nursing home care should be explored with the patient and family, especially if the abuser's behavior cannot be modified. The importance of monthly contact between the elder and the home care nurse is emphasized to decrease isolation and to increase the awareness that concerned healthcare providers are interested in and are monitoring progress in the situation (Hyde-Robertson, Pirnie, & Freeze, 1994). The emphasis is on accessing help to stop the abuse rather than punishing the family and the elderly patient.

Castillo (1994) emphasized that elderly persons should be treated as adults. Their independence and right to make decisions must be considered in the formulation of a management plan. The elderly person must be given an opportunity to choose an acceptable approach to improve the caregiving situation and to meet the needs for self-determination (Hyde-Robertson et al., 1994). Therefore, the importance of assessing cognitive status and decision-making abilities by home care nurses cannot be overemphasized.

Competent older adults have the right to make decisions regarding their personal care. Therefore, if they choose to remain in the abusive situation, their wishes must be respected (All, 1994). The role of the home care nurse is to emphasize that there is no need to remain in the present situation, to offer interventions, and to institute a follow-up plan (Lachs & Pillemer, 1995). Names and telephone numbers of community services should be given to the elder in the event that an emergency arises. Unless a court determines that there is incompetence and appoints a guardian, the elder is assumed to be capable of judging his or her own needs (Jones et al., 1988).

If the elder in a situation is deemed to be incompetent, intervention may include petitioning the court for a conservator. In this circumstance, the home care nurse can provide an opinion with regard to competency, along with documentation of elder abuse, ensuring that the abuser does not become the conservator. Similarly, if the abused elder wishes to be removed from the abusive environment, the home care nurse may be instrumental in obtaining a court order to facilitate this proceeding (Lachs & Fulmer, 1993).

Several states have mandatory reporting laws that require practitioners to report suspected elder abuse to an agency such as Adult Protective Services. In many states, the suspicion of abuse is grounds for reporting; the practitioner does not have to prove it. In most situations, the reporter remains anonymous. Rather than being perceived as an investigation, the home visit from Adult Protective Services may be viewed as an opportunity to gather information about the patient in his or her own environment and to identify services that may be of benefit to the elder (Lachs & Pillemer, 1995).

Clark-Daniels et al. (1990) expressed concern about the "informational gap" that exists regarding the resources available to intervene in situations of elder abuse. All practitioners must be aware of existing state laws and the importance of establishing protocols for detecting and reporting abuse. If agencies such as Adult Protective Services are not available, the home care nurse should contact the local law enforcement agency to determine the proper procedure. Practitioners need to know if their state law protects them from liability when they report suspected abuse, and they should check if this is so. Healthcare providers need to be educated in the recognition and treatment of elder abuse and must be knowledgeable about what strategies work well in each situation (Bruce, 1994; Hyde-Robertson et al., 1994; Penhale & Kingston, 1995).

As leaders in healthcare, home care nurses are in a position to educate the public through community meetings and the media. Community collaboration is essential to protect the elderly population. Home care nurses can assist by gaining access to the political arenas and working with others to formulate policies against elder mistreatment. They can accomplish this by lobbying Congress and presenting their concerns related to elder abuse. Furthermore, practitioners must mobilize other legislators and colleagues to increase the awareness of this problem (Hyde-Robertson et al., 1994).

● IMPLICATIONS FOR HOME CARE NURSES

Home care nurses are in a unique position to evaluate potentially abusive situations. With the shift in healthcare from institutionalization to community-based care, many elderly people with chronic health problems and increased dependency on others will be cared for in the home. Caregivers are thus likely to face greater burdens.

Home care nurses may intervene in several ways. It is imperative that home care nurses recognize signs of elder abuse such as mental confusion, incontinence, dehydration, and unexplained injuries. Because more than one type of abuse may exist, the nurse must be attentive to both verbal and nonverbal communication of the elder as well as to the interaction between the elder and the caregiver. It is important to consider both the elder's and the caregiver's perceptions of caregiving. Although the history and physical findings are a major focus of the assessment, the home care nurse also should assess the level of illness and level of care that is required. It is equally important to assess the caregiver's ability to perform care. In some situations, it may be necessary to ask both the caregiver and the elder direct questions about the existence of abuse. This may be viewed as an opportunity to seek help (Rounds, 1992).

In addition to assessing the physical, cognitive, psychosocial, and economic status, the home care nurse should address environmental factors that may create safety concerns. Does the elder live in an environment free from hazards such as clutter, poor lighting, and unsafe stairways? Home visits provide the nurse with the opportunity to assess the entire situation surrounding the elder and the caregiver. In this way, the home care nurse can intervene early by identifying stressors in the home situation and by providing community resources and support systems to assist with caregiving.

Education is a key to prevention of elder abuse. Home care nurses are in a position to empower elderly patients by discussing ways to promote healthful behavior and thereby decrease dependency on others. Suggestions include maintaining a strong family, social, and community network. The importance of maintaining contact with friends and neighbors when moving in with a family member should be emphasized. It could be suggested that personal matters such as finances and legal affairs be managed by professionals, thus avoiding conflict with caregivers.

In addition to educating the public and other healthcare professionals, the home care nurse can educate caregivers about the uniqueness and the many needs of the elder. Understanding the declining health and resultant increased needs of the elderly population are potential keys to preventing elder abuse (Rounds, 1992).

Home care nurses need to be aware of laws related to reporting elder abuse in their states. They must also be aware of the community resources and support groups available to assist the elder and the caregiver. Home care nurses are in a strong position to prevent, detect, and intervene in abusive situations. Insightful and objective home care nursing practices can provide a valuable front-line defense against the continuation of any abuse to which an elderly patient may have been subjected.

● ACKNOWLEDGMENT

The author acknowledges Professors Mary Leetun and Joanne Gladden, Nursing Division, University of Mary, Bismarck, North Dakota, for their guidance in the preparation of this article. The author also acknowledges Dr. Betty Ann Rambur, Chairperson, Nursing Division, for her encouragement to publish.

REFERENCES

All, A.C. (1994). A literature review: Assessment and intervention in elder abuse. *Journal of Gerontological Nursing, 20*(7), 25–32.

Anetzberger, G.J., Lachs, M.S., O'Brien, J.G., O'Brien, S., Pillemer, K.A., & Tomita, S.K. (1993). Elder mistreatment: A call for help. *Patient Care, 27*(11), 93–130.

Bloom, J.S., Ansell, P., Bloom, M.N. (1989). Detecting elder abuse: A guide for physicians. *Geriatrics. 44*(6), 40–56.

Bruce, C.H. (1994). Elder abuse. *Journal of the American Academy of Physician Assistants, 7*(3), 170–174.

Castillo, P.A. (1994). Elder mistreatment: A common yet elusive problem. *Physician Assistant, 3,* 34–40.

Clark-Daniels, C.L., Daniels, R.S., & Baumhover, L.A. (1990). Abuse and neglect of the elderly: Are emergency department personnel aware of mandatory reporting laws? *Annals of Emergency Medicine, 19*(9), 970–977.

Costa, A.J. (1993). Elder abuse. *Primary Care, 20*(2), 375–389.

Criner, J.A. (1994). The nurse's role in preventing abuse of elderly patients. *Rehabilitation Nursing, 19*(5), 277–297.

Fulmer, T.T. (1989). Mistreatment of elders: Assessment, diagnosis, and intervention. *Nursing Clinics of North America, 24*(3), 707–716.

Fulmer T., McMahon, D.J., Baer-Hines, M., & Forget, B. (1992). Abuse, neglect, abandonment, violence, and exploitation: An analysis of all elderly patients seen in one emergency department during a six-month period. *Journal of Emergency Nursing, 18*(6), 505–510.

Hanson Frost, M., & Willette, K. (1994). Risk for abuse/neglect: Documentation of assessment data and diagnoses. *Journal of Gerontological Nursing, 20*(8), 37–45.

Homer, A.C., & Gilleard, C. (1990). Abuse of elderly people by their carers. *British Medical Journal, 301,* 1359–1362.

Hyde-Robertson, B., Pirnie, S. M., & Freeze, C. (1994). A strategy against elderly mistreatment. *Caring Magazine, 13*(11), 40–44.

Jones, J., Dougherty, J., Schelble, D., & Cunningham, W. (1988). Emergency department protocol for the diagnosis and evaluation of geriatric abuse. *Annals of Emergency Medicine, 17*(10), 1006–1015.

Kosberg, J.I. (1988). Preventing elder abuse: Identification of high risk factors prior to placement decisions. *Gerontologist, 28*(1), 43–50.

Lachs, M.S., & Fulmer, T. (1993). Recognizing elder abuse and neglect. *Clinics in Geriatric Medicine, 9*(3), 665–675.

Lachs, M.S., & Pillemer, K. (1995). Abuse and neglect of elderly persons. *The New England Journal of Medicine, 332*(7), 437–443.

O'Malley, T.A., Everitt, D.E., O'Malley, H.C., & Campion, E.W. (1983). Identifying and preventing family-mediated abuse and neglect of elderly persons. *Annals of Internal Medicine, 98:* 998–1005.

Owen, A., & Owen, S. (1995). Tackling abuse of older people. *Health Visitor, 68*(12), 493–495.

Penhale, B., & Kingston, P. (1995). Recognising and dealing with the abuse of older people. *Nursing Times, 91*(42), 27–28.

Pillemer, K., & Finkelhor, D. (1988). The prevalence of elder abuse: A random sample survey. *The Gerontologist, 28*(1), 51–57.

Rounds, L. (1992). Elder abuse and neglect: A relationship to health characteristics. *Journal of the American Academy of Nurse Practitioners, 4*(2), 47–52.

Sanders, A.B. (1992). Care of the elderly in emergency departments: Conclusions and recommendations. *Annals of Emergency Medicine, 21*(7), 830–834.

Shiferaw, B., Mittelmark, M.B., Wofford, J.L., Anderson, R.T., Walls, P., & Rohrer, B. (1994). The investigation and outcome of reported cases of elder abuse: The Forsyth County aging study. *The Gerontologist, 34*(1), 123–125.

Williams-Burgess, C., & Kimball, M. J. (1992). The neglected elder: A family systems approach. *Journal of Psychosocial Nursing, 30*(10), 21–25.

In some communities, 85% of persons living on the streets are addicted to alcohol or other drugs, or they have some form of mental illness. Nationally, the fastest growing segment of the homeless population is women with children. This article discusses homelessness and its relationship to mental illness.

What factors commonly precede homelessness? Identify interventions and treatments related to homelessness. How can nurses assume a role of advocacy on behalf of persons who are homeless and mentally ill or disabled?

Walker, C. (1998). Homeless people and mental health: A nursing concern. *American Journal of Nursing*, 98(11), 26–32.

Homeless People & Mental Health: A Nursing Concern

CHARLES WALKER

Whether homelessness precipitates mental illness or vice versa, it's clear that life on the streets exacerbates the condition. Here's how you can help.

*I*t's a cold winter morning: A chilling wind nudges your patient, a 46-year-old war veteran, from sleep. Crouching over the sidewalk grate where he has spent the night, he cradles the faded army-green duffel bag that doubles as his pillow. If there were a thermostat in his open-air "home," it would read 35° F.

As a steady, biting snow assaults what's left of his dreams, he stands up, swaying slightly in the rush-hour din of downtown. His layered sweatshirts and socks are soiled and torn. The shadow of his tall, thin figure is reflected on the icy ground as he brushes soot and snow from his beard and jacket. He tugs at his wool ski cap so that it covers his ears, then he fingers the buttons of his jacket and pulls up his collar. That ritual completed, he slings the duffel bag over his shoulder and proceeds with a deliberate gait down the street and away from you.

He's a war veteran, a high school graduate, a panhandler. He may be mildly developmentally disabled, schizophrenic, or functionally illiterate. Perhaps he's a father of four, unskilled and jobless. The woman waking on the next grate? Maybe she's a teenage single parent, a high school dropout. She might even be a former corporate manager, laid off, her success turned sour.

● A STARTLING STATISTIC

Homeless people are not simply victims of unemployment, recession, racism, or governmental indifference; about 85% are on the streets because they are addicted to alcohol or

Charles Walker is an assistant professor in the Nursing Department at Tarleton State University, Stephenville, TX, and a doctoral candidate in nursing at Texas Woman's University, Denton, TX. He is also a volunteer with Habitat for Humanity.

other drugs or have some form of mental illness. So say policy analysts Alice S. Baum and Donald W. Burnes, authors of *A Nation in Denial: The Truth About Homelessness*. Baum and Burnes began studying the problem of homelessness from the inside in 1986, when they worked at a community organization for the poor and homeless. They saw people frustrated and angered by personal lives out of control—lives addled by alcoholism and drug addiction, mental illness, lack of education and skills, or self-esteem so low that it often seemed more like self-hatred. The authors' firsthand observations contradicted many economic and social theories held by advocates for this population.

Long-term solutions to homelessness in America, then, must begin with redefining the problem (see *The Homelessness Epidemic*). Homeless people are not a monolithic and homogeneous group. Calling them simply "the homeless" is misleading; the term implies sameness and doesn't broaden our understanding of the complexities of contemporary homelessness. Rather, when people are on the streets because of problems that can be addressed by current social and health care services—addiction, mental illness, AIDS, postwar trauma, sexual abuse, physical disability, to name a few—they are in effect our patients and clients. We need to stop stigmatizing life's difficulties and diseases. Continuing to do so prevents the people who most need treatment from asking for and getting it.

We must confront the mistaken notion that homelessness is a choice. Who would willingly choose to become disengaged from every available source of social support? Who would choose to live a life estranged from family, friends, and society? It's important to understand the connection between homelessness and chronic mental illness, for with understanding can come the sensitivity and compassion necessary to serve this population.

One of the strengths of nursing is its enormous diversity of skills, perspectives, and approaches to human matters. Nurses, by virtue of our broad education and dedication to promoting health and relieving suffering, have a significant role in addressing the homelessness epidemic. This article will explore the phenomenon of homelessness among those with disabling mental illness, discuss its antecedents, and specify possible interventions. I'll also consider legal and ethical concerns, and make recommendations for nursing practice.

● A COMPLEX PHENOMENON

To understand these patients, it helps to become familiar with the demographic descriptors and psychiatric symptomatology that characterize them. The phenomenon of homelessness among people with mental illness can be confusing because of its complexity.

Demographic portrait. When the number of people living on the street first swelled in the early 1980s, little reliable information existed on the size of the homeless population nationwide. This remains difficult to gauge; estimates now range from 350,000 to six million people. This population's growth has resulted, in part, from demographic shifts. As the number of young to middle-aged adults at risk for chronic mental illness has risen, for instance, there has been an appreciable increase in the absolute number of homeless people living with mental illness.

Apart from homelessness and psychopathology, no single characteristic applies uniformly to members of this group. Although both men and women are homeless, men appear to be disproportionately represented in most places. Research by Neal L. Cohen and colleagues reports that 60% of homeless people with mental illness are Caucasian, 29% are African American, and 7% are Hispanic.

The Homelessness Epidemic

"What we have found in this country . . . is one problem that we've had, even in the best of times, and that is the people who are sleeping on the grates [who are] homeless, you might say, by choice."—President Ronald Reagan, January 31, 1984

Although there has long been homelessness in the United States, the problem has increased in magnitude during the past three decades. Homeless people have become more visible, eliciting greater public awarenes and concern.

The precise extent of this major national problem is difficult to determine. Minority women with young children are the fastest growing segment of the homeless population. The physical and mental suffering of these single-parent families is great: more than three-fourths of families seeking shelter either have no kindred network or have exthausted all potential sources of social support before turning to public shelters. Homeless children are particularly vulnerable. The loss of cherished possessions and the inherent instability and uncertainty in their lives lead these children to seek a sense of self through friendships and fantasies. And homeless children also share many of the same risks (such as poor nutrition) as other American children reared in poverty.

Homelessness is not just an urban phenomenon. Although the population is more concentrated and thus more visible in large cities, rural communities are now reporting growing numbers of—and more diversity among—homeless people. In past eras, the town's alcoholic or "hobo" might have been the only visibly homeless person; today, the rural homeless are often families with children, with both parents looking for permanent or temporary employment and shelter. The needs of these families are complex and more difficult to satisfy because of limited social welfare and health care services.

People with low incomes are targeted as a high-risk population for many of the health problems identified in Healthy People 2000, a national agenda for health promotion and disease prevention. Poverty is among the chief contributors to homelessness. Homelessness, however, is not regarded as a "health" problem worthy of consideration in this agenda. Despite this omission, several objectives relate—directly or indirectly—to the phenomenon of homelessness among people disabled by physical or mental illness. These include:

Health status objective. Reduce the prevalence of mental disorders (excluding substance abuse) among adults living in the community to less than 10.7%. (Baseline: one-month point prevalence of 12.6% in 1984).

Risk reduction objective. Increase to at least 30% the proportion of people aged 18 and older with severe, persistent mental disorders who use community support programs. (Baseline: 15% in 1986).

Services and protection objective. Increase to at least 50% the proportion of primary care providers who routinely review with patients their cognitive, emotional, and behavioral functioning and the resources available to handle any problems that are identified.

Though the commonly cited causes of homelessness include scarce low-income housing and inadequate income supplements for the nation's poor, policy analysts agree that homelessness is closely linked to such social and health concerns as mental illness, alcoholism, and drug abuse.

Source: U.S. Department of Health and Human Services, *Healthy People 2000: National Health Promotion and Disease Prevention Objectives* (DHHS Pub. No PHS 92-50212). Washington, DC, The Department, 1991.

The High Cost of Homelessness

Most health care professionals can attest to the burden placed on hospitals by the lack of resources for homeless patients, many of whom would not be admitted for their condition if they had a place to live or receive care. But just how expensive is this stand-in for appropriate social services?

New York City investigators compared the diagnoses and lengths of stay of 18,864 homeless individuals to those of 383,986 low-income patients. Length-of-stay data were compared after adjusting for diagnosis. Among admissions for homeless patients, 51% were treated for psychiatric illness or substance abuse, compared to 22.8% of the low-income group. Another 19.7% of admissions were for trauma, respiratory disorders, skin disorders, and infectious diseases excluding AIDS, many of which investigators say could have been treated on an outpatient basis. There were significantly higher rates of coexisting substance abuse, mental illness, and AIDS among the homeless patients; a full 80.6% had a pimary or coexisting diagnosis of mental illness or substance abuse.

Lengths of stay for homeless patients averaged 4.1 days longer than those of the other patients, even after adjusting for severity of illness, coexisting illnesses, infection with HIV, and demographic characteristics. In 1997 dollars, the cost of the additional days per discharge averaged $4,094 for psychiatric patients, $3,370 for patients with AIDS, and $2,414 for all other patients.

Why do these admissions—many of which could have been prevented—accrue such high costs? The leading reason hospital staff cited was placement problems. Hospitals are under court order to place homeless patients in housing upon discharge. If shelters are full, discharge is held up. Medically speaking, there is often a reluctance to discharge patients who require follow-up care because of concern that they won't be able to obtain it or won't adhere to treatment. Admissions for many conditions that would otherwise be treated on an outpatient basis are permitted because clinicians believe the patient's condition will worsen on the streets.

The authors call for an increase in supportive housing, which is in extremely short supply, for the mentally ill.

Source: Salit, S. A. et al., *N Engl. J. Med.* 338;1734–1740. June 11, 1998.

These patients comprise a variety of diagnostic groupings, including schizophrenia, bipolar-affective disorder, and personality disorders. Some have histories of psychiatric treatment involving stays in state mental health hospitals. In many communities, though, increasing numbers have never been in state institutions. Homeless mentally ill patients show higher levels of positive symptoms, such as vivid hallucinations, delusional thinking, and odd behavior, than the general population; from birth through age 18, they experience greater family discord, and they are less likely than their never-homeless counterparts to have sustained long-term commitment to any sort of therapy.

While some spend their entire lives in one neighborhood or region, substantial numbers exhibit varying degrees of mobility. Those who travel do so by established routes and are often attracted to medium-sized cities in warm climates. Certain circumstances occur frequently enough to warrant special mention: for example, the existence of impoverished and highly stressed social networks, revolving-door use of mental health services, a high prevalence of physical illness, and a strong resistance to traditional treatment interventions.

Psychiatric manifestations. The mentally disabled homeless are commonly characterized by the media and our collective imagination as disheveled and dirty; wearing clothes inappropriate to the season; pushing their possessions in a shopping cart; urinating or defecating in public; shouting and gesturing animatedly to trees, store windows, or passersby; or remaining mute and withdrawn when approached. All, some, or none of these behavioral indicators may actually apply. Attempts to preserve one's identity under the strain of homelessness can produce bizarre behavior. Peculiar and highly idiosyncratic behaviors inevitably contribute to a progressive disaffiliation with the larger society. And although personal behavior has significance, its meaning must be understood within a larger social context.

So which comes first: homelessness or mental disturbance? Some investigators have studied how psychiatric disorders can lead to homelessness. For example, chronic mental illnesses such as schizophrenia tend to interfere with a person's efforts toward economic security. These patients often lack a regular income—because of unemployment or an inability to apply for assistance—and a lack of other material resources. Such deficiencies can eventually cause homelessness. As nurse authors Candy Dato and Margaret Rafferty note, "homelessness has become a dimension of mental illness." Other researchers have concentrated on how life on the streets exacerbates or precipitates mental illness. Ellen Baxter and Kim Hopper, in their classic 1981 anthropological study of homelessness among severely mentally ill men and women in New York City, state plainly that "were the same individuals to receive several nights of sleep, an adequate diet, and warm social contact, some of their symptoms might subside."

Conceptual confusion. Words with imprecise definitions and uncertain referents abound in the mental health field. The concept of "the homeless mentally ill" is no exception; it's generally used to describe those who are at once chronically mentally ill and without a permanent residence.

The "chronically mentally ill" are widely defined today as people with major mental disorders whose illnesses are severe, persistent, and cause social and vocational dysfunction. In the face of transience and deinstitutionalization, chronicity of illness must be established using a combination of diagnostic and functional indicators, rather than institutional tenure. Moreover, there are inherent difficulties in confirming chronic mental illness in this population. Homeless people tend to be shy and frightened or wary, are frequently alcohol and drug abusers, and may possess different values from those of nurses and other mental health professionals. In short, the problem of defining mental illness, particularly for a homeless population, is considerable.

By comparison, defining homelessness would seem simple. While it is widely agreed that homelessness implies both a lack of fixed abode as well as a dimension of disaffiliation or social isolation, the absence of permanent shelter cannot stand as the sole criterion. For instance, it would be hard to assert that members of the Kickapoo Indian tribe, who live in reed huts under a bridge across the Rio Grande at Eagle Pass, Texas, are homeless. Although the Kickapoo have been portrayed on national television as having no permanent shelter, they do share a rich tribal affiliation. And whether a reed hut constitutes adequate shelter in the climate of the Rio Grande Valley is open to question.

Further, home is a concept with deep existential implications. The word *home* evokes a complex set of meanings for each individual. Homelessness, therefore, is more than having no address or phone number; it's a disengagement from mainstream society—from friends, family, neighborhood, community. Homelessness means being disconnected from the social support systems that usually provide help in time of crisis; it means being without structure, being utterly alone. The boundaries of the concept of homelessness are not fixed, and definitions are tentative. Strategic planning and intervention should therefore be approached judiciously and evaluated as they proceed.

● ANTECEDENT FACTORS

Several factors precede or cause homelessness among people living with mental illness. Let's consider the most publicized of these—deinstitutionalization—as well as the reformist ideals that produced it and explanations for its failure.

Deinstitutionalization. Perhaps the greatest irony in the present plight facing people with chronic mental disability is that it's the direct result of our society's 35-year flirtation with the seductive optimism of reform—a reform broadly known as deinstitutionalization. Behind the legislation that drove this reform was a concern for the civil rights of psychiatric patients.

The 1950s heard frequent professional critiques and public outcries over the deplorable warehousing and abuse of psychiatric patients in state hospitals. Major breakthroughs in treatment, such as the advent of psychoactive drugs and group therapy, promised a cure for mental illness. These, along with a growing philosophy that patients would improve and receive more humane care within the community, led to the opening of institution doors. Most chronic psychiatric patients were released.

This was not the solution some had hoped for. To understand how such a laudable concept could go wrong, it's necessary to examine two factors: individual characteristics, and the inadequacy of community resources.

Individual characteristics. Profound lack of trust, fear of closeness, and the desire for autonomy cause some people to avoid giving their real names and to refuse social services. The dehumanizing effects of institutional living may cause others to display submissiveness and excessive dependence. In part, though, such characteristics are probably due to the psychotic process itself. Many patients express their psychiatric vulnerability by becoming attached to homelessness as a way of life, one that demands minimal social expectations and few interpersonal contacts. They may share the same sidewalk; their cardboard boxes may abut; yet they tend not to interact. They remain isolated from each other and from society at large. A survey by Charles Grigsby of 166 homeless people in Austin, Texas, revealed progressive disaffiliation among those with moderate to severe mental dysfunction, which led to their entrenchment in homelessness.

In addition, homeless people with mental illness suffer from a high incidence of depressive symptoms such as apathy, reduced activity, and indecisiveness. Whether the depression is a chronic condition or an acute reaction to extreme life stressors is unclear. A small but notable minority suffer from unresolved grief about the scarcity of primary relationships in their former and present lives. And because they dwell in public places, exhibit detachment, and may have the slowed reactions secondary to depression, they are frequent victims of theft, mugging, sexual assault, and homicide.

Inadequate resources. Deinstitutionalization was accelerated in 1963 by two significant federal developments. First, Aid to the Disabled (now known as SSI) became available to the mentally ill. Second, the Community Mental Health Centers Construction Act was passed. As it turned out, in the community care network to be underwritten by the federal government, only 700 of a planned 2,000 centers were built. Nevertheless, since

1955, state mental hospitals have discharged significantly more inpatients than in previous decades, while the number of people with mental illness has doubled.

It's important to note that although after-care stabilization and rehabilitation were among the services eligible for funding, an agency didn't have to offer such services in order to qualify as a fundable comprehensive community mental health center. Further, most mental health professionals prefer to treat people who are more like themselves— the "worried well"–rather than "street people" or "transients." People with serious chronic mental illness constitute less than one-fourth of all admissions to community mental health centers today.

● STRATEGIC INTERVENTIONS

Intervention and treatment require a thorough analysis of the alternatives. Case management addresses holistic human needs within the context of managed-care outcomes measurement and dwindling resources, while temporary shelter and reinstitutionalization are only short-term solutions. (See *Ethics of Serving the Homeless*, for definitions of some of the terms discussed below.) Several interventions follow.

Stop-gap measures. Loosely following the ethical principle of *distributive justice*, some cities have provided mentally ill homeless people with one-way bus tickets to their states of origin in an effort to distribute the financial burden they create more equitably throughout the nation. Other cities have instituted stiffer vagrancy laws, making rummaging through garbage or sleeping on the sidewalk criminal offenses. Police roundups, after which homeless people are dumped in jail or psychiatric detention wards, are political maneuvers that tend to occur in cities with too few publicly operated shelters. These actions support the ethical principle of *fidelity*, wherein elected officials fulfill campaign promises by maintaining climates that suit the sensibilities of their middle- and upperclass constituencies.

Ethics of Serving the Homeless

Homelessness among the mentally ill presents profound ethical considerations for nurses and nursing. Following are some principles you might use to determine an ethical course of action in treating homeless patients and families.

Principle of autonomy—the right of the individual to self-governance or self-determination. Includes freedom from confinement and the right to refuse treatment.

Principle of beneficence—the moral imperative to perform acts of kindness or charity. Often associated with another ethical principle, nonmaleficence, which is the refusal to do harm.

Principle of distributive justice—the effort to be morally just by sharing benefits or burdens equally. Encourages fair treatment and equity for all responsible parties.

Principle of fidelity—the fulfillment of one's duties or obligations. Implies a strict adherence to oaths, vows or promises made. Related to the ethical principle of veracity, or truthfulness.

Principle of utility—the conviction that the moral rightness or wrongness of an action is determined by its outcome. Most often identified by the maxim "The greatest happiness for the greatest number." In conventional usage, utilitarian means doing that which is most expedient or which will yield the maximum reward.

Considering the prevalence of such strategies as "Greyhound therapy" and "mercy arrests," it's hard to criticize the well intentioned who advocate for, if nothing more, "three hots and a cot" (three hot meals and a place to sleep). In fact, so many people with mental illness frequent city shelters that in some cases the shelters have become the alternative to state mental hospitals. Oddly enough, more austere accommodations tend to lengthen shelter stays. Since spartan shelters are also service-poor, they foster greater hopelessness and dependence among homeless people.

Board-and-care homes and single-room occupancy hotels, even when conditions are adequate, don't attract and keep homeless clients. Low-cost housing is often unavailable for those who are ready to leave the streets, because of arson, condominium conversion, or urban gentrification.

Reinstitutionalization. The mental health community expressed valid concerns about the therapeutic shortcomings of state hospitals during the 1950s. However, state hospitals were performing some crucial functions. The term *asylum* was sometimes appropriate; these institutions did offer sanctuary from a world that most of their patients were unable to cope with. They also provided health care, patient monitoring, respite for the patient's family, and a social network, as well as food, shelter, and much-needed daily support and structure.

Some professionals have responded to the growing disillusionment with deinstitutionalization by suggesting that everyone with chronic and severe mental illness be sent back to the state hospitals. Some, perhaps, romanticize the degree and quality of care that patients had received there. To many, reinstitutionalization seemed to be the simplest solution.

In the fall of 1987, Mayor Edward Koch of New York City undertook to place the city's most mentally disabled homeless people in a specially designated 28-bed psychiatric unit at Bellevue Hospital. Koch's maneuver, an act of *beneficence* intended to protect the most vulnerable people from the perils of winter street life, brought instant charges of demagoguery. Dismayed civil libertarians appealed on behalf of the patients, citing autonomy and the fundamental right to choose. But Koch's boldness also won praise from the American Psychiatric Association, which argued that maintaining a patient's constitutional rights to liberty sometimes took everything into account except illness. In effect, those who were left on the streets were being allowed to die with their rights on.

Reinstitutionalization is a costly choice. In some areas, community leaders have urged that state-funded regional hospitals be built close enough to cities so that patients could receive needed services and still see their families. But funding is scarce. In both the private and public sectors, promoters of managed care typically seek treatments for homeless patients, based upon the ethical principle of *utility*, that are consistent with the bottom line: profit.

Service coordination. Many professionals, such as the case managers who help their mentally ill clients cope with daily activities and who supervise their medical treatment, advocate coordination of services rather than reinstitutionalization. Their programs aim to serve as links to reality for those who have been repeatedly hospitalized and continue to resist standard treatment. Studies have shown that when they are placed in more permanent housing and are given assistance from a cadre of caseworkers, they can learn to manage their money, buy clothes and food, untangle red tape for their share of social security benefits, and reconnect with social goals and functions. This approach is not only more humane but more cost effective. On average, according to a report by Carl O. Helvie and Betty B. Alexy, hospitalization costs for each program participant drop by over $5,900 per year. Although not all clients respond to such thorough intervention, the value of the lives redeemed by such projects can't be measured in dollars.

Believing that shelters are only a temporary solution to homelessness, Department of Housing and Urban Development Assistant Secretary Andrew Cuomo suggests more controversial solutions such as funding job training programs, providing health care services, and making affordable housing available. Such services will probably best be dispensed by private nonprofit agencies specializing in after-shelter case management. Cutting-edge approaches such as these, which integrate administrative, financial, and clinical resources, need your expertise and leadership.

● ASSUME A LEADING ROLE

Nurses have long served the needs of psychiatric patients who are released into the community. By designing and staffing programs patterned after National Institute of Mental Health demonstration projects, nurses can emphasize several aspects of service for these men and women, such as providing supportive care for those who once loaded the case registers of public agencies, arranging short-term shelter or more permanent housing, and directing outreach toward clients living on the streets.

The needs of homeless people go beyond mental health treatment. Clinicians have argued persuasively that mental health needs are best met within a context of meeting basic survival needs—food, clothing, shelter, housing, employment, and entitlements. Many have found that creating a climate of credibility and trust may mean departing from clinical norms. Outreach workers often begin by "hanging out" with homeless people in a series of unscheduled and unstructured visits, offering a cup of coffee or a sandwich, listening to concerns, and attending to urgent physical problems such as open sores. This nonthreatening approach helps develop trusting relationships that are critical to long-term gains.

Mental health assessment presents a challenge for clinicians as well as for program managers. Because it's important to develop familiarity and build trust, assessing a homeless person's mental health status is often gradual. Information may have to be gathered piecemeal during many short conversations in soup kitchens, back alleys, and shelters. And because outreach is broad in scope, relationships may develop with people who can't ultimately be served: for example, a client who isn't willing to enter a program, or one who is found not to be significantly mentally ill. When possible, assessment of mental health should be conducted in conjunction with assessment of physical health.

Outreach providers emphasize that most homeless people with mental illness will accept mental health and other services as long as they are presented as nonthreatening and supportive. When people are too ill to care for themselves, or are dangerous to others, involuntary hospitalization may be necessary. In those cases, the hospitalization period may be an opportunity to establish a supportive relationship. A clinician who accompanies a patient during an involuntary admission or visits him while he is hospitalized sometimes finds the patient willing and able to accept help after he's discharged.

Nurse managers can assist in planning and implementing programs for this population. Outreach and case management programs that attempt to contact and link large numbers of individuals to existing services, with relatively brief after-care, however, can probably expect limited long-term success. Many communities don't have sufficient resources, and their existing programs may have to develop new services. It helps to be realistic about human nature, too. Referring someone for services doesn't necessarily mean that he'll follow through. And linking patients to treatment and housing doesn't guarantee that they'll stay connected. There are no quick fixes.

It's also relevant to look at the extent to which chronically ill psychiatric patients are dependent on others. Some patients may need more than what their nurses and other caregivers can provide. For instance, a homeless patient who requires psychoactive medication may be unable to follow detailed instructions. Some patients can benefit from depot doses of long-acting medications given at monthly intervals (see *Depot Dose Pharmacotherapy*), but others don't respond well to large doses of neuroleptic medications administered all at once. You would arrange with shelter personnel to ensure that such patients receive daily medication with their guidance, accurately and on time.

Successful intervention is possible. Sometimes success lies in helping someone return to society's mainstream; at other times, in raising his level of functioning just a little, allowing him to work in a sheltered workshop. Often, success may mean simply engaging with people, stabilizing their living situations, and helping them to lead more satisfying, dignified, and less oppressed lives.

You can assume a leading role on behalf of homeless patients who are mentally ill or disabled in the following ways.

- Offer direct care, including comprehensive health assessment, medication monitoring, and first aid treatment or referral for identified illnesses and injuries.
- Meet emergency needs for food, shelter, and minor medical care through voluntary efforts and political intervention.
- Coordinate community resources, ensure resource availability, and eliminate duplication through case management.
- Develop and support comprehensive social policies affecting the homeless.
- Plan and implement housing rehabilitation programs.
- Recommend significant improvements in the current state hospital system for those needing temporary "asylum."
- Encourage legislation to support involuntary commitment to outpatient treatment facilities.
- Conduct research to illuminate more comprehensively the nation's mentally disabled homeless population.

Depot Dose Pharmacotherapy

Depot dosing of neuroleptic medications permits clients to visit the clinic as infrequently as every four to six weeks. At the clinic, a single injection of the prescribed medication is administered, which effectively alleviates psychotic symptoms for up to a month or more.

Haloperidol decanoate is given in doses 10 to 15 times the previous daily dose, but not to exceed 100 mg initially. Over several months, the dose may be increased incrementally to as much as 300 mg/month.

Fluphenazine decanoate (or fluphenazine enanthate) is administered in doses ranging from 12.5 to 25 mg every two weeks. The dose may be slowly increased until a maximum dose of 100 mg every three to six weeks is achieved.

Periodically throughout pharmacotherapy, judge the efficacy of prescribed medications by assessing the patient's mental status. And in order to be alerted to possible side effects or adverse reactions, monitor blood pressure, CBC, and liver functions; evaluate bowel and bladder elimination; and observe for extrapyramidal symptoms, tardive dyskinesia, and neuroleptic malignant syndrome.

Caring for Women in Temporary Housing

What are the health care needs of homeless women and children who reside in transitional shelters? Research data concludes that homeless women have numerous physical and psychological concerns, and they underuse the health care services available to them. Thirty homeless women residing in a transitional shelter were interviewed regarding their health and how they decided to seek treatment. The women ranged in age from 20 to 30 years old, and were African American, Caucasian, or Hispanic; all but two had children in the shelter as well. The health concerns these women most often mentioned were: mental health, sexually transmitted diseases, and substance use.

When asked to describe their health, the women usually specified mental health concerns such as drug use, bipolar disorders, depression, suicidal behaviors, self-mutilation, and anxiety related to abuse from their partners. Themes that emerged from the narrative data included shame, fear, need for information, eligibility for services, managing health concerns, and surmounting their troubles on their own. Shame was associated with drug and alcohol abuse, STDs, and psychiatric disorders. The women feared either being "locked up" in a psychiatric facility or being unable to retain custody of their children.

The respondents had limited information about their own and their children's health, preventative health practices, and community-based services. Because of ineligibility for services such as Medicaid, many of the women said that they couldn't afford treatment—even medications. The fragmented health care system also complicated their ability to manage their health. For example, many women recounted having to wait for long periods in emergency rooms or clinics because so many private physicians don't accept Medicaid. Finally, their worries about "overcoming it alone" existed before the women reached the shelter. They often ignored signs and symptoms of illness in themselves and their children, hoping the problems would subside without treatment. Several of the women had stopped trying to obtain health care because of their past experience or their shame, fear, and lack of information.

This study sheds light on how women in shelters perceive their health, and what inhibits them from managing it more effectively. Women with children may stay in shelters for long periods, providing nurses an opportunity to intervene by promoting health management. Future research may expose how nurses can assist such women more practically, both in the shelter and once they leave.—*Abstracted by Judith A. DePalma, MSN, RN, director, Nursing Research, AUH-Allegheny General, Pittsburgh, PA*

Source: Hatton, D.C. Managing health problems among homeless women with children in a transitional shelter. *Image: J. Nurs. Schol.*, 29(1), pp. 33–37. 1997.

● HELP IS ON THE WAY

Homeless people, particularly those with disabling mental illnesses, live under precarious circumstances in an environment characterized by resource scarcity. By understanding the causes and treatments of severe mental illness, you can assist in the creation of social policies that will enhance residential stability and promote access to care in the least restrictive settings possible. To achieve these goals, you'll also need to work with housing advocates who can offer direction for increasing the availability of decent, affordable housing. This task demands personal and professional commitments from all of us within the nursing community.

SELECTED REFERENCES

Arce, A.A., and Vergare, M.J. Homelessness, the chronic mentally ill and community mental health centers. *Community Ment. Health J.* 23:242–249, 1987.

Baum, A.S., and Burnes, D.W. *A Nation in Denial: The Truth about Homelessness.* Boulder, Westview Press, 1993.

Baxter, E., and Hopper, K. *Private Lives/Public Spaces: Homeless Adults on the Streets of New York City.* New York, Community Service Society of New York, 1981.

Dato, C., and Rafferty, M. The homeless mentally ill. *Int. Nurs. Rev.* 32:170–173, Nov. 1985.

Hopper, K., et al. *The 1986–1987 NIMH-funded CSP Demonstration Projects to Serve Homeless Mentally Ill Persons: A Preliminary Assessment.* Rockville, MD, National Institute of Mental Health, 1989.

Hunter, J.K., ed. *Nursing and Health Care for the Homeless.* Albany, State University of New York Press, 1993.

Jezewski, M.A. Staying connected: The core of facilitating health care for homeless persons. *Public Health Nurs.* 12:203–210, June 1995.

Jones, A., and Scannell, T. Outreach interventions for the homeless mentally ill. *Br. J. Nurs.* 10:1236–1238, Nov. 1997.

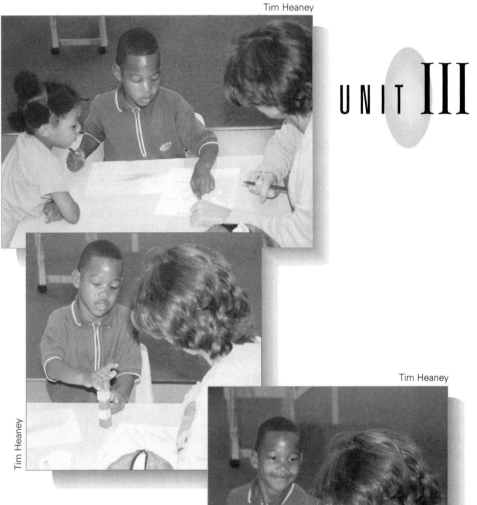

U N I T III

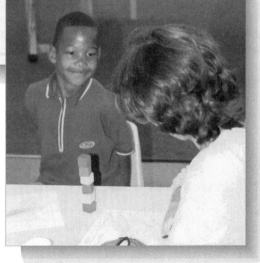

Skills for Community-Based Nursing Practice

A s the role of the nurse has evolved so have the clinical skills necessary for successful nursing practice. Professional nursing in community-based settings requires skills and knowledge in communication, assessment, psychosocial care, teaching, case management, and ethical decision-making.

COMMUNICATION SKILLS

Skills and knowledge in the area of communication require building trust and strengthening therapeutic communication, comprehensive documentation, and discharge planning. Building trust between the nurse and the client is essential because nurses are increasingly required to accomplish more in less time. It has become imperative that a productive working relationship be established with the client beginning with the first visit to facilitate mutual goal setting between the client and nurse. Strengthened communication skills may result in improved client satisfaction, greater success resolving potential problems, and improved satisfaction for both nurse and client.

ASSESSMENT SKILLS

Comprehensive assessment is the cornerstone of effective community-based care. Following the practice of holistic care, the psychosocial, physiologic, and spiritual dimensions of the client and family are assessed. Further, community-based care embodies self-care, family, community, and culture within this process. Assessment of capacity for self-care begins with a functional assessment. Basic assessment of physiologic functioning includes screening of nutritional intake, condition of the skin, and knowledge of prescribed medications. Community-based nurses are also responsible for assessment of the client's home environment to assist the nurse and client to consider aspects of the home environment in planning. Community assessment, which is used to determine the health status and needs of a group of individuals, is another technique used by nurses in community care.

SKILLS IN PSYCHOSOCIAL CARE

Psychosocial care requires the nurse to function as a client advocate and to demonstrate caring. Nurses working in community-based nursing are in a unique position to facilitate incorporation of the client's psychosocial needs in the plan of care. This may be accomplished by blending activities the client enjoys with activities of daily living or by listening to the client's concerns about soul and spirit. Numerous studies show that religious practices are correlated with greater health and longevity.

TEACHING SKILLS

As health care enters the 21st century, more care will be provided outside the acute care setting. Clients are discharged from the hospital "quicker and sicker" or they are not being admitted at all to an acute care facility. Consequently, teaching has assumed increasing importance as a cost-saving intervention. Sometimes a creative but simple teaching strategy will lead to successful learning. Often, it is important to assess a client's learning style as the first step to effective teaching. Other times, more complex assessment and instructional design are necessary to enhance learning.

CASE MANAGEMENT SKILLS

Although a frequently used term, case management is not easily defined. Typically, the elements of case management are assessment, coordination, integration, and evaluation of appropriate health and supportive care services over a length of time. Translated to community-based care, case management includes assessing client needs, planning and coordinating services, referring to other appropriate providers, and monitoring and evaluating progress. To understand case management, it is helpful to be familiar with different types of case management models and the diverse roles of the case manager.

ETHICAL DECISION-MAKING SKILLS

Ethical decision-making in community-based settings is influenced by different factors and logistical considerations from those in the acute care setting. Influencing factors include lack of time for decision-making, the setting itself, the client's support system, the need for interdisciplinary communication, and the frequent lack of an institutional ethics committee. These factors create different challenges that require creative problem-solving by nurses working with clients in community-based settings.

An essential component of community-based care is building trust between the client and the nurse. Trust-building techniques allow the nurse to both establish trust at the first meeting and build trust in subsequent visits. Trust enhances mutual goal-setting.

How is trust defined? What can we learn from research on trust? What are some trust-building strategies?

Wendt, D. (1996). Building trust during the initial home visit. *Home Healthcare Nurse*, 14 (2), 92–98.

Building Trust During the Initial Home Visit

DEBORAH WENDT

Building trust between the client and nurse is an essential component of home healthcare nursing practice. As home healthcare nurses struggle to accomplish more in less time, they need to rapidly gain the confidence of new clients and their caregivers. This article describes trust-building strategies that home healthcare nurses can use to establish productive working relationships with clients beginning with the first visit.

● CLINICAL PROBLEM

Jean Smith, RN, made the first home visit to the Jenkins family. Mary Jenkins, 74 years old, was just discharged from the local hospital after treatment for a stroke. The hospital referral stated that Mary was to be staying at her daughter Carolyn's home until she was able to be independent. Jean arrived at the home while Carolyn was at work. She introduced herself to Mary, collected the baseline assessment data, explained the agency's services and had Mary sign all the admission forms. Early the next day, Carolyn Jenkins called the agency office and said that the family decided they do not need nursing services.

What went wrong? Possibly, Jean neglected the most important part of the first visit—establishing a trusting nurse–client relationship.

An effective nurse–client relationship based on trust is essential to the practice of nursing. Without such an alliance, nursing care cannot be delivered successfully. In home healthcare, unless rapport between client and nurse develops rapidly, the nurse may not even be allowed into the clinical setting (Stulginsky, 1993a).

Because clients in the home setting control the clinical environment, the early cultivation of a helping relationship is urgent. Of all the tasks that a nurse must accomplish

Deborah Wendt, RN, MS, CS, is an Assistant Professor of Nursing, College of Mount St. Joseph, Cincinnati, OH.

during the first home visit—gathering baseline assessment data, starting therapeutic interventions, informing the client about agency routines and procedures, reporting to the physician or referring agency—the establishment of the nurse–client relationship is the most important. Keating and Kelman (1988) compared this budding relationship to the bonding process that occurs between mother and child. How this relationship starts and how it develops determines the effectiveness of future nursing interventions and, ultimately, the health of the client. In many instances, nurses not only help to create a healing environment, but their relationship with the client also becomes the healing environment itself (Quinn, 1992).

Critical to the formation of a healthy nurse–client relationship is mutual trust. Trust between nurse and client does not develop automatically or by chance. Experienced community health nurses consciously and deliberately use trust-building techniques to ensure that trust between client and nurse begins with the first contact.

As home healthcare practice moves toward a prospective payment system, nurses will need to accomplish more with fewer visits. Emphasizing the establishment of a nurse–client relationship during the first visit will make subsequent visits more productive. Effective nurse–client relationships also result in increased client satisfaction—an important indicator of quality care. Home care clients rarely write comments on evaluation surveys about how skillfully a nurse inserted a catheter or redressed a wound. Instead, clients comment about the interpersonal skills of the nurse (Harris, 1994). Today's healthcare consumer demands a nurse who is not only competent but who is also caring (Ludwig-Beymer et al., 1993).

● THE CONCEPT OF TRUST

To use trust-building techniques, nurses need to understand the concept of trust. Most resources define trust as "having confidence in someone or something." Within the nursing literature, trust is defined by Meize-Grochowski as "An attitude bound to time and space in which one relies with confidence on someone or something. Trust is further characterized by its fragility" (Meize-Grochowski, 1984).

Consistency, empathy, and confidentiality are frequently cited as elements of a trusting relationship (Meize-Grochowski, 1984).

An interpersonal helping relationship contains four phases: orientation, transition, working, and termination (Leddy, 1993; Pender, 1987). Trust between client and nurse develops in the orientation phase and then is tested during the transition phase. This may be illustrated by the newly admitted client who makes frequent calls to the office to ask questions, checking to see if the nurse is really available for consultation. If the relationship survives transition, the nurse and client move to the productive working phase (Pender, 1987).

Because trust is an attitude, it is difficult to observe or measure. But the presence of trust becomes apparent by its consequences (Meize-Grochowski, 1984). After a trusting relationship is established, clients communicate openly and honestly with the nurse. They share feelings and are not afraid to display anger and frustration. Families tend to be available for home visits and usually keep the nurse informed about changes in their schedule or residence. Although gaining a client's trust does not ensure absolute compliance with the plan of care, clients openly discuss deviations from prescribed treatment. When nurse and client mutually trust one another, the client becomes a partner in care. The nurse relies on the family for accurate data and collaborates with the family on healthcare decisions (Morse, 1991).

● RESEARCH ON TRUST BUILDING

In one research study (Morse, 1991), data from 86 interviews with hospital-based nurses were analyzed using grounded theory to describe the evolution of nurse–client relationships. Grounded theory is a qualitative research technique in which data collection, data analysis, and theory development occur simultaneously. The researcher interacts with the research subjects in a social setting until a testable theory emerges (Roberts & Burke, 1989). In this study, trust emerged as a significant characteristic of nurse–client alliances. Clients developed two types of trust in the nurse: trust in the nurse's technical competence and trust in the nurse as a person. Sometimes, clients tested the trustworthiness of a nurse by sharing a small confidence. The nurse who handled this secret appropriately gained the client's trust.

A second study (Thorne & Robinson, 1988) used interview data from 77 chronically ill clients to examine the client's perception of trust in healthcare relationships. Using grounded theory, a three-stage process of trust development emerged. Clients initially placed a naive, almost absolute trust in the healthcare provider. This level of trust quickly dissolved, and the client entered an angry distrustful stage. Resolution soon followed as the clients reconstructed a "guarded alliance" with health professionals in one of four ways. Some clients trusted certain health professionals almost absolutely while distrusting all others. Some clients trusted most health professionals because of certain identified norms or behavioral patterns. A third group of clients distrusted all health professionals, whereas the final group carefully negotiated intimate relationships with selected professionals.

Data from both of these studies indicate that trust is reciprocal. In other words, as nurses work to gain the client's trust, nurses also are learning to trust or distrust the client. Some clients reported that they used specific strategies to gain a nurse's trust. These strategies included being knowledgeable about their illness and care, expressing concern and interest in the nurse as a person, and giving gifts to the nurse (Morse, 1991; Thorne & Robinson, 1988).

The final study (Zerwekh, 1991) which provides insight into building trust with clients examined anecdotal data from interviews with 30 public health nurses. These nurses executed maternal/child home visits. The comparative analysis and interpretation of these interviews revealed 16 family care-giving competencies. One of the competencies was building trust. These nurses described six strategies used to build trust with clients: getting through the door, backing off, listening, discovering and affirming strengths, not judging, and persisting.

The results of these studies lead to several conclusions. First, trust and trust building are significant components of the nurse–client relationship. Secondly, trust building is not a simple process but one that occurs in stages, fluctuates over time, and involves reciprocity. Lastly, nurses working in the community already use a variety of trust-building strategies.

● IMPLICATIONS FOR PRACTICE

The following trust-building strategies are based on the cited resources and clinical experience. These strategies are intended to be used by the home healthcare nurse who works with acute or chronically ill clients. These strategies are summarized in Table 20-1.

Begin Cultivating the Client's Trust with the First Contact

Most nurses contact clients for the first time by phone. Because consistency is one of the elements of trust, the nurse who will see the client most often should be the one to make

TABLE 20-1 ● **Trust-Building Strategies**
1. Begin cultivating the client's trust with the first contact.
2. Establish credibility with the client.
3. Use an empathetic, nonjudgmental approach.
4. Guard the client's privacy.
5. Expect testing behavior from clients.
6. Learn to trust the client.
7. Persevere with the nurse–client relationship.

this call to negotiate the home visit. The family, especially the main caregiver, should be included in this orientation visit (Keating & Gelman, 1988). This ensures that all concerned family members receive the same information at the same time.

If more than one nurse will be caring for the client, this should be explained to the family. The number of nurses that visit a particular client should be limited so that the client and nurse are not constantly negotiating new relationships (Morse, 1991). One or two nurses or, if necessary, a team of nurses should work with a consistent caseload of clients. These strategies are summarized in Table 22-1.

Consistency also requires that a nurse's words and actions match. Appointments must be kept and the client must be informed about the results of any consultations or referrals. Observation of the nurse's style and behavior over time induces the client to trust the nurse (Wilson & Kneisl. 1992).

Establish Credibility with the Client

Though research indicates that some clients immediately trust health professionals, this type of trust is fragile and temporary (Morse, 1991; Thorne & Robinson, 1988). Some clients and families also may initially distrust a nurse based on negative experiences, whereas others may not even understand what nurses actually do (Stulginsky, 1993b). In any of these scenarios, nurses need to prove their competence quickly. The nurse can accomplish this by performing some concrete activity that the client is not able to do but that is perceived as beneficial. This is sometimes called "hooking" the client (Zerwekh, 1991).

Venipuncture, catheterization, or the performance of any technical skill may be the "hook." Calling the physician to adjust medications or quickly obtaining home care equipment also may effectively validate the nurse's credibility and usefulness.

Use an Empathetic, Nonjudgmental Approach

Home health nurses are invited into homes as guests (Stulginsky, 1993a). This suggests that the nurse provides identification, asks permission before washing hands or using the phone, and addresses the client formally as "Mrs. Smith" or "Mr. Jones." If the family is uncomfortable with this level of formality, they will usually say so. It is safer to move from formality to informality than to assume familiarity and possibly offend the client. Entering as a guest also means acknowledging that the client controls the clinical setting. The nurse may try to persuade or negotiate with the family for change, but the client ultimately has the right to accept or reject the nurse's advice (Stulginsky, 1993a).

Using effective communication skills such as appropriate eye contact, attentive listening, and paraphrasing lets the family know that they have been heard and understood. The amount of time for an initial visit must be individualized, but the client and family should not feel rushed. Most clients want to talk about their recent illness and healthcare experience. Allowing the client and family time to tell their story about the health problem and its impact on their lives provides useful assessment information and serves as the foundation for the nurse–client relationship (Stulginsky, 1993b).

Home health visits expose nurses to a variety of cultures and lifestyles. Nurses demonstrate acceptance of this diversity through verbal and nonverbal communication (Keating & Kelman, 1988). An attitude of respectful curiosity is usually most successful when discussing distinctive family routines and customs.

Guard the Client's Privacy

To receive good nursing care, clients must share intimate details about their lives and lifestyles. Nurses show respect for the client's privacy by discussing such information only with those involved with the client's care. The issue of confidentiality should be discussed thoroughly with the client during the initial home visit (Morse, 1991).

However, in some cases such as child or elder abuse, the nurse must report information about the client or family with or without their consent. This may destroy a trusting relationship. To try to mitigate this destruction, home healthcare nurses may inform the family about their legal obligation to report abuse explaining that the purpose of the report is to ensure that the family obtains needed help (Stanhope, 1992).

Expect Testing Behavior from Clients

Research suggests that clients will develop different types of trust at different stages in the relationship (Morse, 1991; Thorne & Robinson, 1988). This means that the nurse can expect some fluctuations in client behavior as the relationship progresses. To gain trust in the nurse, clients need to ask questions. First, these questions may focus on the nurse's technical competence: Where did you go to school? Have you performed this procedure before? Why do you do it that way? Later in the relationship, the questions grow more personal: Are you from around here? Do you have children? Do you like your job? Brief but honest responses to these inquiries facilitate the development of trust (Morse, 1991).

Clients or families may test the relationship by trying to bribe or provoke the nurse. They may be confrontational, try to give the nurse money or gifts, or call the nurse repeatedly. Effective nurses confront each of these behaviors using a calm, problem-solving approach. By establishing ground rules while not rejecting the client, the nurse remains compassionate and consistent. If this testing period is negotiated successfully, trust develops, and the family becomes open to change and intervention.

Learn to Trust Clients

Trust in nurse–client relationships is reciprocal. Because home health nurses visit intermittently, they must rely on the client or the client's caregiver for full implementation of the care plan. Although clients and families may not always follow the medical treatment plan precisely or report health observations in clinical terminology, they are the authority on their perception of the situation. When nurses treat clients as competent collaborators, clients gain confidence and develop more trust in the nurse (Morse, 1991).

Just as some clients have had negative experiences with the healthcare system, some nurses have learned through experience not to trust clients (Morse, 1991). Nurses need to be aware of their own biases and the effect they have on the development of trust (Wilson & Kneisl, 1992). Constantly searching for the client's ulterior motives may greatly hinder the development of reciprocal trust (Morse, 1991).

Persevere with the Nurse–Client Relationship

Trust building is a complex process that varies to some extent with each client. If a client is slow to develop trust, the nurse must persist in contacting and supporting the family even in the presence of confrontation and resistance (Morse, 1991). This demonstration of commitment and acceptance may in itself produce a trusting relationship. If a client refuses nursing visits, efforts should be made to discuss and evaluate the reasons for visit termination.

When visiting a home places a nurse at risk of injury or if a client is so noncompliant that the nurse and agency might be held legally liable for participating in an unsafe care situation, the nurse may have to end the relationship. However, personality conflict and inconvenience usually are not acceptable reasons for the nurse to abort a nurse–client relationship. If one nurse is experiencing difficulty in establishing trust with a family, a second nurse can be assigned to the case. Sometimes a change in personal style is all that is needed. For example, a new graduate visited an elderly woman twice and found the woman to be extremely cold and distant. When a different nurse made the third visit, she reported that the client was friendly and warm. After comparing notes, the new graduate realized that she had been all business during her visits, whereas the second nurse had "warmed up" the client by listening and engaging in small talk.

Sometimes a family does not refuse visits but is consistently busy, absent, or noncompliant. This behavior should be confronted gently. The nurse should explain the effects of the client's behavior nonjudgmentally. For example, a nurse might confront a client who was not at home by stating, "Mrs. Jones, this is the third day that I have gone to your house and there was no answer. This means that I have had less time to care for my other clients because I spent an hour each day driving back and forth to your home. I want to continue to see you, but we will have to work out a way to be sure that our appointments are kept."

All community nurses have occasionally had the unsettling experience of knocking at a client's door, hearing people inside, but not being admitted. Some clients never develop trust in the nurse, and stop nursing visits. However, if this happens repeatedly to the same nurse, that nurse may need to review her interpersonal skills and trust-building techniques. Some sources suggest that bonding with 90% of clients is an acceptable average for a home care nurse (Stulginsky, 1993b).

● SUMMARY

The practice of nursing requires a healthy nurse–client relationship. In home healthcare, this relationship begins with the first client contact and must be secure enough after the initial home visit for clients to want nursing care to continue. Trust, as one of the central components of the nurse–client relationship, needs to be cultivated actively with each newly admitted client. Nurses can use practical strategies to build trust in relationships. The outcome of constructive use of these strategies will be increased client well-being and satisfaction with care.

● CLINICAL PROBLEM RESOLUTION

Jean Smith, RN, called Carolyn Jenkins and politely asked why she canceled further visits. Carolyn explained that her mother said the nursing visits would cost $88 each and that she had signed a number of forms that she did not understand. Jean arranged a meeting with Mary and Carolyn to review the forms and the method of payment. During this visit, she listened carefully as Mary and her daughter shared their frustrations and their perception of Mary's illness. They both wanted Mary to regain her independence, so Jean designed a plan of care that would achieve this. Jean called the physician from the home for consultation and to obtain an order for physical therapy. At the end of this visit, Mary and Carolyn were eager for nursing visits to continue.

Although Jean originally made some mistakes (she did not meet with the main caregiver nor did she establish credibility), she persisted in the relationship and effectively established trust with the Jenkins family.

REFERENCES

Harris, M.D. (1994). Home healthcare nursing is alive, well, and thriving. *Home Healthcare Nurse, 12,* 17–20.

Keating, S.B., & Kelman, G.B. (1988). *Home health care nursing: Concepts and practice.* Philadelphia: JB Lippincott Co.

Leddy, S., & Pepper, J.M. (1993). *Conceptual bases of professional nursing* (3rd ed.). Philadelphia: JB Lippincott Co.

Ludwig-Beymer, P., Ryan, C.J., Johnson, N.J., Hennessy, K.A., Gattuso, M.C., Epsom, R., & Czurylo, K.T. (1993). Using patient perceptions to improve quality care. *J Nurs Care Qual, 7,* 42–51.

Meize-Grochowski, R. (1984). An analysis of the concept of trust. *J Advanced Nurs, 9,* 563–572.

Morse, J.M. (1991). Negotiating commitment and involvement in the nurse–patient relationship. *J Advanced Nurs, 16,* 455–468.

Pender, N. (1987). Health promotion in nursing practice (2nd ed.). Norwalk, Connecticut: Appleton & Lange.

Quinn, J. (1992). Holding sacred space: The nurse as healing environment. *Holistic Nurs Pract, 4,* 26–36.

Roberts, C.A., & Burke, S.O. (1989). *Nursing research: A quantitative and qualitative approach.* Boston: Jones and Bartlett Publishers.

Stanhope, S.B., & Lancaster, J. (1992). *Community health nursing: Process and practice for promoting health.* St. Louis: Mosby Year Book.

Stulginsky, M.M. (1993a). Nurses' home health experience part I: The practice setting. *Nurs Health Care, 14,* 402–407.

Stulginsky, M.M. (1993b). Nurses' home health experience part II: The unique demands of home visits. *Nurs Health Care, 14,* 476–485.

Thorne, S.E., & Robinson, C.A. (1988) Reciprocal trust in health care relationships. *J Advanced Nurs, 13,* 782–789.

Wilson, H.S., & Kneisl, C.R. (1992) *Psychiatric nursing* (4th ed.). Menlo Park, CA: Addison-Wesley Publishing Co.

Zerwekh, J. (1991) A family caregiving model for public health nursing. *Nurs Outlook, 5,* 213–217.

Inadequate communication can lead to misunderstandings, client and provider dissatisfaction, and inappropriate interventions. Effective therapeutic interactions recognize and interpret verbal and nonverbal techniques accurately. Proficient communication paves the way for building trust through open and honest exchange between the nurse and client. Comprehensive assessment allows mutual decision-making and planning among the nurse, client, and family members.

What are some guidelines for better communication? How can the nurse assess how the client and family are involved in care? What behaviors reaffirm trust? What questions promote empathy and understanding?

Heineken, J. (1998). Patient silence is not necessarily client satisfaction: Communication problems in home care nursing. Home Healthcare Nurse, 16(2), 115–121.

21

Patient Silence Is Not Necessarily Client Satisfaction: Communication Problems in Home Care Nursing

JAN HEINEKEN

Although we may believe we are inviting client feedback about care, it is clear from a recent study surveying home care providers and older adult care recipients that failures in communication continue to plague us. Inadequate communication can lead to misunderstandings, client and provider dissatisfaction, and even termination of the home care provider–client relationship. By strengthening communication skills, staff can see changes in client satisfaction, have greater success in resolving potential problems, and may ultimately experience more job performance satisfaction.

Silence on the part of a client cannot necessarily be interpreted as satisfaction with the care received. Home care supervisors, nurses, and patients indicate that failures in communication continue to exist. In a recently completed 3-year study funded by the National Institutes of Health and the National Center for Nursing Research (No. 1 R15-NRO3190-01) that examined successful and failed caregiving relationships, the theme of flawed communication emerged as an important area to examine and attempt to improve.

Jan Heineken, PhD, RN, is Professor, School of Nursing, San Diego State University, San Diego, CA.

This article elaborates on only one issue identified in the study: the reasons why staff may need to improve communication techniques and the strategies for accomplishing this. A more complete report of factors underlying successful and failed caregiving relationships is available by contacting the author. Findings do indicate that there is a need to guide, encourage, and teach clients to speak up and speak out more clearly and directly. In so doing, they will become empowered and nursing staff will have more information on which to address problems in staff–client relationships. In these times of working harder and faster to meet the demands and constraints of changing healthcare delivery systems and resources, a focus on improving communication can increase nurse efficiency, improve client satisfaction outcomes, and improve nurse satisfaction in the workplace.

● CLIENT SCENARIO

As part of the study, an interview was scheduled with Dr. T, an articulate 66-year-old PhD school psychologist receiving home care. Although partially paralyzed in one leg since birth, she had always lived independently. After an on-the-job injury, at which time she sustained a compound fracture of the tibia and fibula, she was hospitalized for surgical pinning. Recovery and rehabilitation were slow. In the process, she was transferred from the acute hospital to a skilled nursing facility.

After 2 months, Dr. T was ready to be discharged to her two-story townhouse where she lived alone. The discharge planner arranged for Dr. T to have a rented hospital bed, installation of safety aids, and home visits by registered nurses (RNs) to draw blood, monitor correct placement of her support TED hose, and change dressings. Routine personal care was provided by a certified nurse's aide visiting 4 hours a day, 3 days a week. These services and equipment were funded through Workman's Compensation funds. After funding ended, the client arranged for more aide visits by paying out of her own pocket for these expenses.

In the interview, Dr. T said she was "generally pleased" with the home care, but this statement was made with little enthusiasm in her voice. When encouraged to explain "if or how things could have been improved," she became animated. The more she disclosed, the more emotional she became:

- She disliked the lack of care provider consistency. In one particularly disruptive week, she was cared for by three different home care aides.
- Care providers had different approaches, causing her to feel anxious and uncertain if staff communicated with each other about the specifics of her care. She felt obliged to direct the staff in the "proper way to do the procedures because they didn't seem to know exactly the right way."
- One aide was constantly rough and hurried with her. According to Dr. T, "She showed no verbal or nonverbal signs of caring" and "ignored my requests." Dr. T thought the aide's approach and behaviors were inexcusable.

Upset as she was, Dr. T admitted that she chose to remain silent about most of her complaints until long after the fact. At no time did she discuss these issues with her care providers. She did call the nursing supervisor to request that the uncaring aide be replaced. The request was honored immediately. The client acknowledged that stifling her complaints caused her to feel frustrated, anxious, and resentful. When asked why she did not call about *all* her concerns, she answered:

No! I've learned not to do that. In most situations I'm assertive, even aggressive sometimes. But, not in this situation. No. Confrontation between patients and paid caregivers is not easy.

Apparently, this otherwise articulate, assertive, well-educated psychologist could not bring herself to give direct feedback to the people who most needed to hear it. When asked a second time why she did not report these concerns, she could not give a clear answer.

Possible explanations for her inability to discuss these issues with her home care providers include the following:

- Although never stated, and perhaps never even silently acknowledged within herself, it is likely Dr. T found herself confused and at a loss to know how to respond. Needing home care was a unique situation for her, one in which she had lost personal control and endured a shift of power—away from herself to a state of dependence on others. In this state of dependence, she was forced to rely on the kindness of others. As Wendy Lustbader (1991) affirmed, the "one who gives help is more powerful than the one who receives it" (p. 34). Perhaps, such a shift of power and control was so stressful that Dr. T's usual methods of coping and relating to the world were at risk. This shift may have caused her to remain uncharacteristically silent and immobilized.
- By all appearances, Dr. T seemed to be a very considerate, kindly individual, dedicating her life to helping others. Perhaps she did not want to cause "trouble" for the home care personnel.
- Dr. T may have also had concerns about possible repercussions from the care providers if she complained. Perhaps she feared her care would be compromised.

Had Dr. T presented herself as a "submissive, compliant older client" not wanting to be a "bother" and feeling overwhelmed or intimidated with complicated care delivery services, her reluctance to act would have been more predictable and understandable. However, her silence raises an important question. If a client with her skills and professional background hesitates because "speaking up" is too difficult, then how many other less independent and/or less articulate home care clients remain silent and dissatisfied?

● GUIDELINES FOR BETTER COMMUNICATION

One goal of the self-care/self-responsibility movement is "to empower the public for increased control over their own health" (Bohny, 1997, p. 283). Johnson (1989) in restating Dorothea Orem's self-care model believes that every adult has both the "right and responsibility to care for self" (p. 175). Enabling or empowering the client to speak up for what he or she needs is an important aspect of self-responsibility. In so doing, the client will help the staff identify better and perhaps more efficient ways of delivering care viewed as satisfying to the patient. However, clients have different abilities, potentials, and motivations when it comes to being able to speak out in this manner.

To avoid silence, achieve open two-way communication, and empower clients, home care providers may wish to adopt the following guidelines for better communication:

1. Establish and reaffirm trust and empathy.
2. Examine client and family sick role beliefs.
3. Directly ask for client feedback.

● UNDERSTAND HOW THE CLIENT AND FAMILY ARE INVOLVED IN THE SICK ROLE

Coming to know the client includes appreciating how strongly he or she embraces or minimizes the dependent sick role. Meleis (1988) explained that the sick role evolves from the interactions between the patient, significant others, and the social system. These interactions shape and modify client behaviors occurring with illness or injury. A person's perspective about the sick role may differ for short-term illness compared with chronic long-term conditions. The extent to which a person relinquishes or is able to modify sick role behavior depends in part on her or his own expectations and perceptions, and may also be influenced by the expectations and perceptions of significant others.

An example taken from the study involves an independently employed nurse's aide employed by a privately paying patient. Within a 3-week period, the aide terminated employment with her client. The client was Mrs. J, a 70-year-old woman diagnosed with partial paralysis after a cerebral vascular accident. In coming to know and understand the client, the aide became increasingly frustrated because even though Mrs. J was physically capable of performing some aspects of her physical care, she wanted the nurse's aide to do it all. This attitude was supported by a protective, hovering husband who explained to the aide that "his little princess deserved all the best care and shouldn't have to lift a finger." Even after the importance of rehabilitation was stressed, the aide believed her goals for patient improvements differed from those held by the couple. As a result, she terminated employment because other private paying clients wanted to work toward increased independence and improvement, and the aide believed she would find more job satisfaction working with such clients. Although it is clear that not all staff have choices about retaining or terminating home care patients, exploring client and family beliefs about illness and recovery will likely lead to better success at setting mutually realistic treatment goals and approaches.

● REAFFIRM TRUST AND EMPATHY

Achieving open, honest communication begins with building trust. Experienced home care providers are able to establish trust, recognizing that trust is the basis for successful nurse–client relationships. Northouse and Northouse (1992) spoke of trust as "an individual's expectation that he or she can rely on the communication behaviors of others" (p. 37).

Trust creates the belief that events are predictable and that people are sincere, competent, and accepting. At key times within the relationship, it may be prudent to reaffirm the presence of trust, particularly if the relationship has not gone as smoothly as hoped. This reaffirmation can be accomplished by demonstrating the following behaviors:

- Following through on things you have promised
- Keeping appointments or calling to explain what has happened to make you late
- Showing warmth and caring, including use of appropriate eye contact and smiling
- Being an active listener, showing interest and confirmation
- Conveying a sense of calm, even if feeling hurried
- Talking about procedures before doing them
- Being honest and giving the patient complete information

The primary way of helping the patient to feel understood and affirmed is by communicating *empathy* (Brammer, 1979). This is done by thinking with the patient, rather than for or about the patient. When sports spectators find themselves leaning forward to watch racers cross a finish line, they are experiencing empathy because it is a "feeling into" or "feeling along with" the individual. With patients, empathy can be achieved by asking a series of questions, and with each patient response, trying to simulate what and how the patient is feeling by listening closely, then repeating or paraphrasing what the patient has just said. When this is done correctly, the patient knows the care provider has listened and understood. Questions that promote this kind of empathy and understanding include these:

- Describe your health and abilities before you became ill. Now?
- How were you involved with family and friends before? Now?
- How has this condition changed your life?
- How long do you think you will need home care?
- As you think ahead to your future, what kind of picture do you see?
- What concerns do you have?

Periodically throughout the relationship, the home care provider would be wise to reaffirm this bond of empathic understanding with the patient, particularly as physical and emotional changes occur. This reaffirmation is accomplished by asking some of these same questions about the patient's changes. This effort is usually rewarded by the client expressing appreciation at feeling the staff member is really listening and understanding (Arnold & Boggs, 1995).

● ASKING THE CLIENT OUTRIGHT AND GIVING POSITIVE REINFORCEMENT

When a therapeutic relationship has been reaffirmed using the described steps, the client may feel inclined to be more candid about evaluating his or her home care. However, this can be achieved only if the home care provider is sincere and ready to accept feedback. The client may have been asked to provide feedback to previous care providers, but in so doing was met by defensiveness or other perceived repercussions.

Patients in the study gave a number of accounts showing why they remained silent with caregivers. One 65-year-old woman had this to say about her care provider:

She can't understand me, she doesn't try. I get mad at her inside, but don't say things. This is hard on me, of course. I feel that she's temperamental and might walk out. Then where would I be?

Another patient said:

I really need somebody here, but I'm not pleased with her care. But it took me a long time to find anyone as nice as she is. I just can't come out and tell her what I want her to change because I'm afraid I'll hurt her feelings and she'll quit.

On the subject of asking for feedback, one nursing staff member said:

I prefer someone talk to me directly and say, "We'd rather have you do this way or that way." Then I can discuss it with them. Communication. That's what I want. So if they don't do that, and instead just say something to the agency, it doesn't accomplish much.

Another aide said:

> Those [patients] that are too timid to approach an individual are going to lose caregivers that are basically doing a good job for them. The patient loses out because they can't talk directly. Then they complain, the caregiver is replaced, and the whole process could start again.

Patients will need continuous reinforcement and encouragement, particularly when discussing feedback perceived as sensitive. One strategy described as "successful" in the study suggests that the care provider should mention early in the relationship that all feedback is important—both positive and negative. The staff member should explain that all such feedback is helpful in improving the care provider's ability to give better care, not only for this particular patient, but for future patients the care provider will come to know. Setting and maintaining the tone for successful open communication will be facilitated by saying things such as these:

- I very much want to be able to help you the best way I can. What do you want me to know about your care?
- Are there things you would like me to do differently?
- Are there things other nurses have done for you that you particularly liked?
- Not every patient feels comfortable giving care providers direct feedback about how care could be improved. I find I really need to hear this from my patients so I can do the best possible job. You would really be helping me by being honest.
- I plan to ask you to tell me at the end of visit how you would rate the care today on a scale of 1 to 10. Can I count on you to help me with this? (This question should be asked only if the patient is willing and able to answer it.)
- I appreciate and need you to be direct and open with me. Your suggestions and comments will help me better care for you and for other patients who may have similar needs.

Some of these same questions can be asked of the family members who specifically play a pivotal role in the patient's care. This effort at including the family in such client-centered communication will likely yield more direct feedback from them as well.

As one home care provider in the study said:

> I always try to create an environment with the patients where if they don't like something, they speak up. I need them to tell me.

The home care provider went on to say:

> If you don't tell me, then I'm not going to know what I'm doing isn't comfortable for you, or it's not the way you prefer it to be done. I can't read your mind and if you don't speak up and tell me, I'm just going to continue doing it the way you don't like. So you have to tell me. Then we can work it out.

● SUMMARY

Helping to guide and empower home care clients in speaking up clearly and directly continues to be a challenging task. The strategies mentioned are useful in caring for younger, chronically disabled clients as well as for older home care clients. A home care study by

Eustis and Fischer (1992) reaffirmed this common fact with the finding that "clients of all ages need help in negotiating relationships" with their care providers (p. 21). Encouraging open, truthful communication between home care providers and clients can be accomplished and may save nursing time in the end.

Success in achieving client feedback requires determination, trust building, empathy, patience, genuine acceptance, and continuous reinforcement on the part of home care staff. Achieving success also means taking a closer look at the nurse–client relationship to examine how the client and family view the sick role. If these healthcare provider–client communication guidelines are followed, the healthcare provider can be better assured that client silence is client satisfaction and not suppressed dissatisfaction that could be expressed at a later time.

REFERENCES

Arnold, E., & Boggs, K. (1995). *Interpersonal relationships: Professional communication skills for nurses.* Philadelphia: Saunders.

Bohny, B. (1997). A time for self-care: Role of the home healthcare nurse. *Home Healthcare Nurse, 15*(4), 281–286.

Brammer, L. (1979). *The helping relationship: Process and skills.* Englewood Cliffs, NJ: Prentice-Hall.

DeGraff, A. (1988). *Home health aides: How to manage the people who help you.* Cliffton Park, NY: Saratoga Access Publications.

Eustis, N., & Fischer. L, (1992). Common needs, different solutions? Younger and older homecare clients. *Generations, 16*(1), 17–22.

Johnson, R. (1989). Orem's self-care model for nursing. In J. Fitzpatrick and A. Whall (Eds.), *Conceptual models for nursing: Analysis and application* (pp. 165–184). Norwalk, CT: Appleton & Lange.

Melies, A.I. (1988). The sick role. In M. Hardy & M. Conway (Eds.), *Role theory: Perspectives for health professionals* (pp. 365–375). Norwalk, CT: Appleton & Lange.

Northouse, P., & Northouse, L. (1992). *Health communication: Strategies for health professionals.* Norwalk, CT: Appleton & Lange.

Many community-based services require specific assessments and documentation to receive reimbursement for services rendered. This article outlines the elements of a functional assessment, which meets the basic requirements of Medicare.

What are the two basic rules to consider when assessing function? What is included in the environmental assessment? What is assessed regarding neurologic and emotional status? What is assessed regarding cognitive and emotional status, integumentary status, and respiratory status? What is included in determining the client's ability to perform the activities of daily living?

Neal, J. (1998). Functional assessment of the home health client. *Home Healthcare Nurse*, 16(10), 670–677.

Functional Assessment of the Home Health Client

LESLIE JEAN NEAL

Since the collection of Medicare patient information through the use of the Outcomes and Assessment Information Set (OASIS) has become mandatory, it is increasingly important that home care nurses understand how to conduct a functional assessment. This article presents each element of function that should be assessed, explains how to assess each element, and describes some of the most common instruments used in performing a functional assessment. Additionally, tips are included for assessing the home environment and the client's safety.

The assessment of a client's ability to function is crucial to the delivery of high-quality appropriate home healthcare. Although many people regard function as related mostly to activities of daily living (ADL) and mobility, it actually encompasses much more. No haphazard determination must be made of the client's ability to function, which includes how the client functions, whether adaptive or assistive devices are necessary for independent functioning, and whether supervision, assistance, or complete care are needed for the client to remain at home. This determination or assessment is pivotal to the plan of treatment, the referrals made to other healthcare disciplines and community resources, the client's length of stay in home care, and the ultimate outcome of care.

Too frequently, it seems, the functional assessment is taken for granted or is conducted without guidelines or consistency among providers and between clients. This article describes each element of function that should be assessed, explains how to assess each element, and describes some of the most common instruments used in performing a func-

Leslie Jean Neal, PhD, RN, C, CRRN, is a rehabilitation clinical nurse specialist at Inova VNA Home Health, Springfield, VA.

tional assessment. In addition, tips are included for assessing the home environment and the client's safety in the home, because it is important that home care professionals be able to determine whether clients have the functional ability to navigate their environment safely.

The reader may note that the elements of functional assessment reviewed in this article correspond to questions asked by the Outcome Assessment Information Set (OASIS), although the MOO numbers (identifying numbers in the OASIS data set) are not listed. It should be noted that the answer to each corresponding OASIS question is not addressed here. Therefore, the reader should not use this article as a guideline for answering OASIS questions, but as a means of better understanding the intent of the OASIS questions and learning how to make clinical decisions in rating patients on the data set.

● STANDARD ELEMENTS OF FUNCTIONAL ASSESSMENT

It is important that the home care professional understand how to measure function and do it consistently over the course of the client's stay on service. This information will be instrumental in determining whether the client should be discharged or recertified. Before assessing the typical elements of functional status such as the ability to perform ADL and the instrumental activities of daily living (IADL), the professional must determine whether there are environmental, cognitive, or neurologic/behavioral barriers to independent function. It is important to acknowledge that societal and cultural barriers also can enforce limitations on function, but these barriers are not addressed here. In reading this article, two basic rules should be kept in mind:

1. Whether the patient needs the assistance of another person is key to assessing independent functional ability accurately.
2. In measuring function, the patient's ability to conceptualize an activity is just as important as the patient's physical ability to perform the activity.

● THE ENVIRONMENTAL ASSESSMENT

The home care patient may not be physically, cognitively, or emotionally disabled, yet may have functional limitations related to barriers in the home environment. Structural barriers and safety hazards must be pinpointed and removed if the patient is to function safely and as independently as possible within the home.

To determine whether structural barriers exist that limit the patient's independent mobility, the professional must first make a thorough assessment of the home. Absence of structural barriers means the client can navigate hallways, ambulate unassisted or with an assistive device or wheelchair, and get to all areas in the home that need to be accessed (e.g., bathroom, kitchen, bedroom) for full self-care, which involves getting help and being able to obtain such necessities as the toilet, the phone, or the fire extinguisher while in those areas.

The patient may need to use stairs to reach the toilet, bedroom, or kitchen. These are areas to which access is vital for clients who must take care of themselves during all or part of the day or night. If the patient can manage the required stairs unassisted or with an assistive device, but without the help of another person, then the patient can be regarded as independent within his or her environment.

It is important to determine the existence of stairs the patient does not need to use in getting to the kitchen, toilet, or bedroom, but may use for another purpose. This includes stairs that go from the inside of the house to the outside, whether the patient currently uses them or not. The patient may eventually use any of these stairways or need them in an emergency, and others in the home as well as visitors may use them. Consequently, these unused stairs too must be included in an evaluation of stairway safety during the first home visit. The stairway assessment includes lighting, the presence and stability of banisters, the stability and surfaces of the steps, and the slope or steepness.

Inadequate stair railings are those banisters that are not very stable and cannot support the patient's weight if the patient must lean on them while using the stairs. Any wobbling of the railings means they are unsafe. The railings should be safe for everyone who uses them.

It is also important to look for narrow doorways that do not permit a wheelchair, walker, or obese person (if applicable) to pass through or doorways that are blocked. All of these structural barriers must be eliminated or bypassed so the client has the potential to function independently within the home.

A floor is unsafe if no one, especially the patient, can walk on it without falling, slipping, or sliding. It is unwise to assume that the patient will always wear skidproof shoes. An inadequate roof is one that leaks or does not give protection from the weather. The same can be said of windows.

The home care professional should assess the lighting to determine whether it is adequate for the patient's safe movement within the home. The assessment should determine whether the patient has the lighting needed or wanted, not whether there is enough light for the professional to work.

Gas and electrical appliances may be safe for others in the home who use them correctly, but if the patient cannot demonstrate proper use of these appliances, then they must be considered unsafe. Inadequate heating or cooling is determined by the capability of the home to provide heat or cool air, and also by the patient's ability to turn the heat or cool air on and off. Fire safety devices include a working smoke detector (batteries must be checked) and a fire extinguisher that the patient can access, knows how to use properly and quickly, and physically is able to use.

Unsafe floor coverings can severely limit the patient's ability to function independently. If they prevent safe ambulation, then the patient cannot reach necessary areas to toilet, eat, and sleep. Floor coverings are unsafe if they slide or have borders (fringe or rubber) that can catch someone's foot or the tip of a walker or cane.

The home must be assessed for improperly stored hazardous materials including paint and other chemicals that emit toxic fumes, may ignite, or have not been tightly sealed and placed beyond the reach of children or cognitively impaired adults. These items are best stored in the garage or a shed. (For a more detailed description of environmental assessment, see Narayan, 1997.)

● NEUROLOGIC AND EMOTIONAL STATUS

Neurologic status includes perceptual, sensory, and cognitive function as well as emotional status. All are important factors in the assessment of functional ability.

Perceptual Function

The inability to perceive sensations of hot or cold and sharp or dull is likely to limit functional ability. Impairment of perceptual function can affect many ADL aspects as well as present significant safety concerns.

Sensory Function

If the patient has visual, hearing, understanding, or speech impairments, these must be considered in the assessment of overall functional ability. In addition, the presence of pain can significantly alter ability to function.

VISION

If the patient has impaired vision, then it is likely that function and mobility will be limited. To determine whether sensory deficits impair function, the patient's vision should be tested while he or she is wearing contact lenses or eyeglasses if these are customarily worn. The patient can be directed to read aloud from a section of newspaper, a paragraph from a book with regular type, or the bottles of medicine in use, then asked to explain the meaning. The patient's ability to understand what has been read can assist the professional in getting a sense of how significant cognitive deficits are to a particular client's impaired function.

If the patient cannot read the medication label or newspaper but can count fingers held at arm's length and point out objects on the floor, in far corners of the room, and above the head, then the client is probably safe within the environment with regard to structural barriers. If the client does not appear to understand directions, then the assessor should move about the room and watch to note whether the client's eyes follow the movement.

Inability to read instructions or medication labels is a significant impairment in function and must be addressed by ensuring that instructions and labels are written in large bold type. If the patient is legally blind, then the pharmacy should be asked to provide directions and labels in Braille type, or the Association for the Blind should be contacted for suggestions. Some medication cassettes can be obtained with raised Braille, but the caregiver may need to fill the cassettes with the prescribed dosages for the patient. Talking books should be suggested to the visually impaired patient who enjoys reading.

HEARING AND THE ABILITY TO UNDERSTAND SPOKEN LANGUAGE

How well a person hears and understands can significantly affect that person's ability to function within the environment. If the patient regularly wears a hearing aid, then the hearing should be tested with the hearing aid in the ear. The patient's understanding in his or her own language should be tested.

First, the patient's ability to hear and understand complex conversation can be tested by giving some teaching and then, after 10 to 15 minutes, asking the patient to explain what was taught. The teaching should include several steps to a procedure or a number of items to remember. It is important to perform the teaching for only about 10 minutes before moving on to another activity. The patient should then be asked 10 to 15 minutes later what was learned during the teaching. Within 24 hours, the patient should be asked in person or over the phone if he or she remembers the teaching session. In this way, it is possible to test several things that are important in assessing function:

- The patient understands complex instructions.
- The patient has immediate recall (remembering something after 15 minutes have elapsed).
- The patient has the ability to remember something that occurred in the last 24 hours.

Patients might hear and understand complex instructions, but may have a need for some prompting, for the assessor to speak louder, or for repetition. They might hear and understand only simple instructions such as "open your mouth" or "stand up," and may need to be prompted frequently when trying to explain what they understand. However, patients might not hear and understand even these simple commands, and may need continual repetition or demonstrations in order to understand.

Finally, patients might not respond at all or may lack ability to hear and understand familiar words or expressions such as their names, the song Happy Birthday (if the patient is an English-speaking American), or familiar expressions in their own language. If the patient has any difficulty hearing or understanding spoken language, referral should be made to an audiologist or speech–language pathologist.

SPEECH AND ORAL EXPRESSION OF LANGUAGE

If the patient is able to hold an appropriate conversation 10 to 15 minutes long, using clear pronunciation and appropriate pauses between words, then he or she is considered to be independent in oral communication. Professionals should judge a patient's verbal communication by comparing it with their own. The patient may speak very quickly, use words that do not make sense, speak very slowly, or use a tone of voice that is not appropriate to the topic of conversation.

It is helpful to ask patients why they think the nurse is visiting them, what they think their health needs are, and how they feel about the visit. These questions require clients to speak and express their feelings. If the patient cannot engage in complex conversation or uses only simple words or phrases to communicate, a referral to a speech–language pathologist should be considered.

The client incapable of communicating verbally may communicate without words. It is important to assess whether the patient can communicate in some fashion that would enable him or her to obtain help if necessary. If the inability to communicate verbally is a recent development, then the patient should be referred to a speech–language pathologist.

PRESENCE OF PAIN

Pain is a common culprit of impaired function. A client in pain is less likely to participate in ADL and IADL. Most homebound elderly patients have some form of chronic pain, typically arthritis. Although they may carry on with their activities or movements despite the pain, it is important to ask whether the pain exists. If the patient has pain, determine its frequency, intensity, and what methods provide relief. Evaluate whether pain prevents smooth and fluid movements and thus limits the patient's function. Consider placing the patient on a pain schedule so that functions important to the patient can be performed 30 minutes after the use of an analgesic.

● COGNITIVE AND EMOTIONAL STATUS

Cognitive ability is an important component of function. If the patient is unable to focus on the task, cannot remember the steps involved in the task, requires prompting, or is delirious or comatose, then independent function is unlikely. Also, feelings of depression can impair function because even though the impairment is psychological, the patient is unable to perform functional activities. Beginning with the greeting at the start of the first visit, the patient should be observed carefully for the following:

- The patient makes eye contact with the visitor (although in some cultures to do so is considered rude).
- The patient greets the visitor.

• The patient appears to be well groomed or has made an attempt or expressed the need to groom him- or herself.

The patient should be asked the following questions during the visit. An attempt should be made not to ask them all at once. It is helpful to work them into the conversation.

• Where are you now? OR, What is your address?
• What is the date (particularly the month and year)?
• What is my [nurse's] name?
• Do you know why I am here? OR, How do you feel about my being here?
• How many hours of sleep (average) do you get each night? (This should be asked of all patients because it will elicit clues about the patient's emotional status and the presence of pain.)

Finally, the patient should be asked to perform a simple task such as getting the visitor a drink of water or showing the nurse where the bathroom is. Again, this should be incorporated into the visit. It should not be obvious that the patient is being tested. (For a more detailed neurologic assessment see Neal, 1997.)

Any of the following observations are indicative of neurologic, emotional, behavioral, or cognitive impairment that may disrupt function:

• The patient is not alert and/or is unaware of his or her surroundings.
• The patient does not know who he or she is or who the visitor is (assuming the visitor has been identified as the nurse).
• The patient does not know what his or her situation is.
• The patient does not know the date, at least the month and year.
• The patient cannot shift attention from one person or thing to another appropriately.
• The patient cannot recall directions given 10 to 15 minutes ago or displays other signs of short-term memory loss.
• The patient expresses feelings of extreme sadness or thoughts of suicide.
• The patient is unable to stop his or her activities when they should be stopped (e.g., continual brushing of the hair or washing of the hands).
• The patient is incapable of self-protection because he or she commits unsafe acts. For example, the patient lights matches for no reason.
• The patient constantly interrupts with sexual comments, threats, childlike or paranoid behavior, or profanity.

● INTEGUMENTARY STATUS

This article does not discuss the assessment of skin integrity. However, it is important for the professional to know that wounds can be disabling and therefore affect functional ability (Neal, 1995). If the patient cannot perform ADL or IADL because of the wound itself, the dressings, or the accompanying pain, then the wound impairs the patient's functional ability, and appropriate steps should be taken to decrease the disabling effects of the wound.

● RESPIRATORY STATUS

The ability to breathe without effort determines whether the patient can perform ADL or IADL. Additionally, the need to perform nebulizer treatments periodically and to drag oxygen tubing, not to mention the safety hazard the oxygen and the tubing present, may severely limit where the patient can go and what the patient can do.

The patient should be assessed for shortness of breath or dyspnea while resting (sitting or standing), talking, eating, or engaging in mild activity such as toileting, or demonstrating a procedure. It should be determined whether the patient becomes short of breath (SOB) while walking, after climbing stairs, or after walking more than 20 feet (this must be measured by using the assessor's own foot to simulate 1 foot of distance). To assess for dyspnea or SOB, the patient should be observed for the following:

- slowing down or stopping the activity before it is completed
- sitting down midway through or immediately after finishing the activity
- breathing deeply or in quick shallow breaths
- complaining of chest tightness or pain.

● ADL AND IADLS

After assessing the home health client's environment and his or her neurologic, emotional, and cognitive status, the client's ADL and IADL should be assessed. Included in the ADL discussed here are grooming, dressing, bathing, toileting, transferring, ambulation or locomotion, and feeding/eating. The IADL include preparing meals, accessing transportation, doing laundry, housekeeping, shopping, and using the telephone.

If the patient is able to perform a particular ADL or IADL using an assistive or adaptive device, then the patient should be considered independent in this area. If the patient, however, is unable to perform ADL or IADL without the assistance of another person, then the patient should be referred to the occupational therapist or rehabilitation nurse.

Grooming

Grooming refers to the patient's ability to wash face and hands, brush hair, brush teeth, shave, apply makeup (females only), and present an overall neat, clean personal appearance. The patient is independent with grooming if these tasks can be performed alone, even with the use of assistive or adaptive devices such as a long-handled mirror, reacher, extender, or thickened handles.

Dressing Upper and Lower Body

Before assessing function with regard to dressing, it is important to think carefully about the tasks required in dressing. The patient must be able to retrieve the clothes from the closet or drawer, put them on, and remove them. It should be remembered that ability to retrieve clothes independently requires being able to get into the room that has the clothes, get next to the bureau or into the closet, open the drawer or reach the hanger, and bring out the clothes. The use of assistive or adaptive devices such as a buttonholer, shoe horn, velcro on shoes, sock aid, or pants held by elastic or velcro may help the patient to dress independently.

Bathing

The patient should be assessed for ability to wash his or her entire body in the bath tub or shower. Assistive devices that may be needed include a tub or shower seat, nonskid mat, or long-handled scrub brush. A patient that must be watched or supervised while bathing or showering cannot be regarded as independent.

Toileting

If the patient can get to and from the bathroom toilet without the assistance of another person, even though a walker, wheelchair, or other assistive device must be used, then the patient is independent with toileting. If the patient needs supervision, someone to open the door, or help from another person in any way, then the patient is not independent. This includes the incontinent patient who does not go to the bathroom in time to control urine or bowel movements unless told to do so, as well as the client who cannot perform his or her own perineal hygiene.

If the patient cannot make it to the bathroom because of incontinence, poor mobility, memory loss or any other reason, then it should be determined whether the patient can make it to the bedside commode or use a urinal or bedpan with or without the assistance of another person.

Transferring

Ability to transfer independently means that the patient can move from one place to another, including turning and repositioning in bed, without the assistance of another person. The patient may use an assistive device such as a trapeze or sliding board. Perhaps only minimal assistance from another person is required in the form of guarding or supervising, or another person is needed to hold the patient's arm or arms during the transfer. It should be determined whether the assistance of another person is required for the transfer to occur, and whether the patient can bear weight on at least one limb and pivot. The patient may be bedbound (unable to get out of bed without being carried), or the patient might not even be capable of turning in bed.

Walking

The patient should be assessed for ability to walk safely and without assistance from another person or device. It should be determined whether the patient needs a device of any kind to walk alone, or if supervision is needed for safe walking. Does the patient need any assistance from a device or a person to walk in particular areas or on particular surfaces?

The home care professional should assess whether the patient must have a wheelchair for mobility. If the patient can use a wheelchair, walker, cane, or other ambulatory device without any assistance, including supervision, then the patient has independent mobility.

Feeding or Eating

To be independent in eating, the patient must be able to bring the food to the mouth, chew it and swallow it. The patient may use assistive devices such as utensil adapters, special plates/bowls, dicem to help stick the plate to the table surface, or other devices that enable independent eating. However, if the patient needs to have the meal arranged in front of him, be assisted or supervised occasionally, be coaxed or reminded to eat the meal, or need food that has been altered in texture then the patient is not independent with this ADL. If the patient can eat using his or her mouth but must also receive food through the nose or stomach then the patient does not eat independently.

Planning and Preparing Light Meals

A light meal refers to a small meal or one that does not include a hot meat, vegetable, and starch. For home care patients, it could also mean a delivered meal reheated by the patient to be eaten later. A light meal could be a sandwich, bowl of cereal, bowl of soup or small salad. The ability to plan and prepare meals is an important part of function because if the patient cannot do these things, then help from others will be needed. The home care professional should determine whether the patient understands how to plan and prepare the meal. That is, the patient not only knows what constitutes a sandwich or a salad, how to open a can of soup, how to heat food and use utensils safely, but can actually do these things. There may be a physical, mental, or cognitive reason why this patient cannot plan or prepare meals on a regular basis.

Traveling

To be able to travel independently, the patient must have both the mental and physical ability to use transportation safely, whether assistive devices are used or not. If the patient can drive his or her own car with or without adaptations, or can use bus or van transportation without the assistance of another person, then the patient can be regarded as independent with transportation.

Doing Laundry

The ability to do laundry is an IADL. That is, it is not necessary to basic function as are feeding, toileting, or bathing. Saying that the patient can do his or her own laundry means that the patient can understand what is being done, why it is being done, and how to do it. The patient must also be physically, cognitively, and mentally able to move the dirty laundry from where it is kept to the washing machine or sink, apply soap, turn on the water, move the laundry into the dryer or hang the clothes in an appropriate place to dry (not out in the rain), and transport the laundry to the place where it belongs (i.e., drawers, closets, etc.). If the patient can perform all of these functions without the assistance of another person, then the patient is independent in doing laundry.

Housekeeping

Keeping house is another IADL category. "Light" housekeeping refers to tasks such as dusting, wiping surfaces, changing bed linens, and tidying. "Heavy" housekeeping means tasks such as vacuuming, taking out the trash, bringing in groceries, gardening, mowing the yard, and moving furniture. To function independently, the patient must be able to physically, cognitively, and mentally perform all of these tasks, which involves understanding what the task is and how it is performed, then being able to perform it safely.

Shopping

Shopping is another IADL task. To shop independently, the patient must understand the concept of shopping, know why it is done, comprehend how and where it is done, and then be able to do it without the assistance of another person. The independent patient must be able to determine what food items are lacking in the home, what food items are needed, and where and how to go to the appropriate store and bring the items home. Independence with shopping is determined by the patient's ability to get to the store, select the items, pay for them, bring them home, carry in the bags, unpack the bags, and put the items away.

Most home care patients will not be completely independent with shopping because to qualify for home care, they usually are expected to be homebound. If the patient cannot perform all the steps required to be independent with shopping, then assistance may be needed from the caregiver, neighbor, or a grocery delivery person.

Using the Telephone

The ability to use the telephone requires several steps. The patient must be able to understand the concept of making a call, know who is being called, comprehend why the call is being made, locate the correct phone number, dial the numbers, and make appropriate (socially correct) conversation. The patient may need to use a special phone or adaptive equipment on his phone.

● CONCLUSION

Function means not only mobility, but also the patient's capability to perform ADL and IADL, as well as to manage safely in, around, and outside the home. For the patient to function independently he or she must have appropriate mental, physical, and cognitive resources. A patient may use an assistive device and still be independent because independence from the assistance of another person is nevertheless maintained.

If the patient needs the assistance of another person for any reason to perform a particular function, then the patient is not performing that particular function independently. If the patient cannot think, see or hear clearly, speak and understand his/her own language, get and eat food, toilet, dress or groom self, or move, then the patient has a functional impairment. The healthcare professional must assess the extent of the functional impairments and then assist the patient to become as independent as possible despite those impairments.

REFERENCES

Narayan, M. (1997). Environmental assessment. *Home Healthcare Nurse, 15*(11), 798–805.
Neal, L. J. (1995). The rehabilitation nurse in the home care setting: Treating chronic wounds as a disability. *Rehabilitation Nursing, 20*(5), pp. 261–264.
Neal, L. (1997). Is anybody home? Basic neurological assessment of the home care client. *Home Healthcare Nurse 15*(3), 156–167.

Clients in both community and acute care settings experience problems with nutrition. However, it is much more difficult to monitor nutritional intake in community settings. The following article describes a nutrition-screening tool developed for community settings.

What type of patients could benefit from a nutritional assessment? Who does the Level I assessment? Who does the Level II assessment? What are some of the commonly recommended changes that may result from a nutrition assessment?

Lyman B., & Marquardt, P. (1997). Nutrition screening tool for Home Care Patients: Development and Utilization. *Home Healthcare Nurse*, 15(12), 835–841.

Nutrition Screening Tool for Home Care Patients: Development and Utilization

BETH LYMAN, PATRICIA MARQUARDT

Caring for individuals with nutritional problems is a part of nursing practice. Nurses often struggle with how to categorize nutrition-related maladies. Signature Home Care (now a subsidiary of Integrated Health Services) modified an existing tool to assist nurses in their assessment of nutrition status. This article describes the process of adapting the Nutrition Screening Initiative and implementing the screening tool.

● NUTRITION SCREENING TOOL DEVELOPMENT AND UTILIZATION FOR HOME PATIENTS

In response to the Joint Commission on Accreditation of Healthcare Organizations (JC-AHO) mandate requiring nutrition assessment for home patients, one home care company, Signature Home Care, elected to devise a nutrition screening tool modeled after the Nutrition Screening Initiative (JCAHO, 1995). This tool screens all types of home care patients for nutrition risks and assesses high-risk patients for specific nutritional deficiencies. The role of the nurse who collects this data for nutrition screening and assessment is not well defined in the literature and has not been a routine or in-depth part of the home

Beth Lyman, RN, MSN, CNSN, is a clinical nurse specialist, G.I. Department, The Children's Mercy Hospital, Kansas City, Missouri. Ms. Lyman served as the nurse consultant for Nutrition Support Services for Signature Home Care (now a subsidiary of Integrated Health Services).

Patricia Marquardt, RN, BSN, is Regional Director of Clinical Services, SHS-Symphony Home Care, Irving, TX. Ms. Marquardt was Vice President of Clinical Operations at the time of the Nutritional Screening Tool Development.

care nurse interviewing process. (Melnik, Helferd, Firmery, Wales, 1994; Cope, 1996). Therefore, an easy-to-use tool, training, and information flow all needed to be developed. The purpose of this article is to describe the process of Signature Home Care's development, implementation, and utilization of a nutrition screening tool adapted from the Nutrition Screening Initiative (NSI) (Wellman, 1994).

Signature Home Care, at the time of this project development and implementation, was a small national full-service home care company. With 21 branches from New Jersey to Arizona, the company provided Medicare-certified service, private duty care, home medical equipment, and respiratory therapy services, as well as infusion nursing and home care pharmacy services. Not all branches provided all services, depending on local market needs. However, all branches were Joint Commission accredited. The comprehensive nature of the services offered the opportunity for highly coordinated home care services.

Recognizing the need to evaluate the nutritional status of the patients, particularly the pediatric and geriatric populations, Signature searched the literature and found that the NSI format could be adapted to the home care population. It was decided by upper management to niche a market for nutritional services by contracting with a free-standing nutritional consultation service, Nutritional Medical Associates. Further evaluation of a patient's nutritional status revealed that subsequent appropriate alterations in the nutrition interventions could result in financial benefits related to the capitated population cared for by the company. The development of the screening tool and the use of specialty consultants created a cost-effective, clinically sound program that could be offered to the physicians of the local communities, while providing appropriate nutritional guidance to the patient.

The use of Home Parenteral and Enteral Nutrition (HPEN) doubled from 1989 to 1992, and utilization of these therapies is expected to continue to rise in the near future (Howard, Ament, Fleming, Shike, Steiger, 1995). Routine nutritional assessment of HPEN patients is imperative for early intervention and prevention of complications. These individuals and their nutritional problems are often so challenging that outside expertise is sought to assist with management of this population. The use of standardized tools to collect nutrition status-related data is essential for consultants who recommend changes for HPEN solutions. The Signature Home Care screening tools were designed in conjunction with consultants so that all needed information was included.

● NUTRITION SCREENING INITIATIVE BACKGROUND

The NSI is a tri-level screening tool developed by a multidisciplinary Blue Ribbon Advisory Committee representing over 30 national professional organizations. Nutrition screening is defined by the American Dietetic Association (1994) as the process of identifying characteristics known to be associated with nutrition problems. The impetus for developing the screening tools came from a U.S. Surgeon General mandate in 1988. This mandate was based on the belief that nutrition screening would lead to interventions promoting good nutritional status that would result in improved overall health and enhanced quality of life (Wellman, 1994).

In 1992, six intervention areas that could identify poor nutritional status were identified: social service, oral health, mental health, medications, nutrition education, and nutrition support. The tri-level screening tool is usable in several of these intervention areas (Cope, 1994). The first part of the tri-level screening tool, the Checklist, is an educational tool for lay people to raise awareness. The second part of the tool, The Level 1 Screen, is used by healthcare professionals to quantify risk factors and identify needs for further assessment, counseling, education, or nutrition support. The Level 1 Screen records height, weight, adequacy of food intake, socioeconomic issues, and functional status. On the basis of the results from the Level 1 Screen, a Level II Screen, the third part of the tool, may be initiated to diagnose the specific form of malnutrition and identify specific interventions and monitoring that are indicated. The Level II Screen looks at medication use, laboratory test results as well as cognitive, functional, and emotional status. Because this tool has proven to be valid and reliable, Signature Home Care decided to use it as the basis for its internal nutrition screening tool.

● SIGNATURE'S SCREENING TOOL DEVELOPMENT

Development of the Level I screening tool was Signature Home Care's first priority. As shown in Figure 23-1, Signature created a one-page document that collected data on an individual's height, weight, diagnosis, and diet history and evaluated pertinent psychosocial, environmental, and functional parameters. The information was then weighted for relative malnutrition risk. For example, an individual who had a greater than 10 percent unintentional weight loss in the past 6 months would immediately be progressed to a Level II assessment because such weight losses are highly predictive of nutritional deficiencies.

The Level I Screen is an effective use of staff time because it should require no more than 5–10 minutes to complete. The form should be completed within 5 days of a patient's admission to any type of home care service, except for home medical equipment, and again anytime the clinician deems it appropriate or every 120 days. Much discussion occurred regarding who should conduct the Level I screening. Because this tool is written in a simple format, it was decided that nonnursing staff, such as respiratory therapists, could complete this form after appropriate training, then give it to a registered nurse to review. Staff were advised that any individual thought to be at nutritional risk for any other reason should be referred for a Level II screening, which is done only by a nurse.

The Level II Screen was planned to evaluate all HPEN patients, as well as patients who were identified at risk through Level I. A score high enough to move a patient to a Level II Screen indicated a nutritional need that should be further evaluated and discussed with the physician and patient. In addition, Signature Home Care arranged for registered dietitians to provide staff education and consultation, as well as occasional patient home visits for each of the Signature locations. Thus, the tool met the objectives of serving the broadest patient population base with a minimum amount of staff time, while avoiding multiple forms.

Signature's policy stated that any individual who required HPEN should automatically have both Level I and Level II screens, so the two tools were designed to minimize repetition from one tool to the other. Only the initial height, weight, diagnosis, and diet information is repeated on both forms because in the case of an obtunded and completely dependent individual, the Level I screen is not done at all. A review of the Level II screen (Fig. 23-2) shows that a more detailed evaluation of weight loss, diarrhea, emesis, dietary intake, and functional status is conducted. A focused physical exam is also an integral part of this assessment. Nurses were asked to attach existing documentation of history, lab test results and other significant information.

Signature's plan called for the Level II screening tool to be incorporated into the nursing assessment, and to require no more than 15 minutes to complete. The Level II Screen is to be repeated every 120 days or sooner if the clinician deems it necessary. For example, a Level II screening should be repeated for an individual who receives an enteral tube

	LEVEL I	PATIENT		
Signature HOME CARE	NUTRITION SCREEN	PAYOR	TEAM	MR#
		DATE		TIME

BODY WEIGHT AND HEIGHT *(Measure height to the nearest inch and weight to the nearest pound)*:

PRIMARY DIAGNOSIS: _____ Weight (lbs): _____ Height (in.): _____

OTHER DIAGNOSIS: _____ Special diet. Type: _____ Calorie limitations: _____

Check any boxes that are <u>*TRUE*</u> *for the individual:*

● ☐ Has lost or gained 10 pounds (or more) in the past six (6) months without wanting to.

EATING HABITS

■ ☐ Has appetite changed?	● ☐ Has difficulty chewing or swallowing.
■ ☐ Consumes dairy or dairy products once or not at all daily (and does not take calcium supplement).	◆ ☐ Has pain in mouth, teeth or gums.
	☐ Anorexia
■ ☐ Consumes fruit or drinks fruit juice once or not at all daily.	☐ Has more than one alcoholic drink per day (woman); more than two drinks per day (man).
● ☐ Does not have adequate fluid intake (less than 4 glasses (8oz) per day).	☐ Usually eats alone.
◆ ☐ Eats vegetables two or fewer times daily.	● ☐ Does not have enough food to eat each day.
◆ ☐ Eats breads, cereals, pasta, rice, or other grains five or fewer times daily.	◆ ☐ Does not eat anything on one or more days each month.

LIVING ENVIRONMENT

◆ ☐ Lives alone.	☐ Does not have a stove and/or refrigerator.
■ ☐ Are there more than 6 people living in household?	☐ Lives in a home with inadequate heating or cooling.
■ ☐ Is housebound.	● ☐ Is unable or prefers not to spend money on food (< $25-30 per person spent on food each week).
■ ☐ Does not have significant caregiver.	

FUNCTIONAL STATUS

Usually or always needs assistance with: *(check each that apply)*	Other Problems:
◆ ☐ Walking or moving about.	● ☐ Nausea ☐ Vomiting
■ ☐ Eating.	● ☐ Diarrhea (> 3-5 per/day for > 2 days)
■ ☐ Preparing food.	● ☐ Constipation (> 2 weeks)
☐ Shopping for food or other necessities.	◆ ☐ Over 80 years of age.

INSTRUCTIONS: To be completed within 5 days from Start of Care date. Repeat Level I screen at least every 120 days (every other recertification).

HIGH RISK:
● Proceed to Level II Nutritional Screen.
◆ 5 or more "◆", proceed to Level II Nutritional Screen.
■ 8 or more "■" go to Level II Nutritional Screen.

TOTALS:

●_____

◆_____

■_____

Categories left blank should be addressed by the Signature Nutrition Screener or go to Level II.

Signature of Screener: _____   Date: _____

FIGURE 23-1. Signature Home Care Level I Nutrition Screen. (Used with permission.) Note: One or more • = Proceed to Level II Nutritional Screen.

Signature HOME CARE	LEVEL II NUTRITIONAL SCREEN	PATIENT		
		PAYOR	TEAM	MR#
		DATE		TIME

PATIENT'S REPORTED AVERAGE DAILY INTAKE:

	BREAKFAST	LUNCH	DINNER	SNACKS
Type of food:				
Serving size:				
Beverages:				

(Specify type, i.e. skim milk or soda [diet or regular])

ENTERAL FEEDING:

How long has patient been on enteral therapy: _____

Expected duration of therapy: _____ Prognosis: _____

Type of Tube: ☐ NG ☐ Gastric ☐ PEG ☐ Jejunostomy - Insertion Date: _____

Method of Feeding: ☐ Bolus ☐ Gravity ☐ Pump ☐ Amount per Feeding _____

Enteral solution: _____ Volume per day _____ Number of days per week: _____

Number of feedings per day _____ Prescribed amount received per day: ☐ Yes ☐ No

If NOT, how much _____

Why: _____

How aggressive does the patient/caregivers want therapy to be: _____

COMMENTS:

INSTRUCTIONS:

If Patient is on TPN, refer to MPSS.

If Patient is enteral patient who is tube or pump, refer to MPSS.

If Patient is oral enteral feed, refer to a dietician.

ATTACH MEDICATION PROFILE (if available)

Signature of Screener: Date:

FIGURE 23-2. Signature Home Care Level II Nutritional Screen. (Used with permission.)

feeding and develops fluid overload, diarrhea, or any other complication often associated with this therapy.

● SCREENING TOOL IMPLEMENTATION

Once the forms were completed, they were pilot tested at a selected branch. A nutrition support nurse consultant made a site visit and conducted a half day of training on nutritional assessment. This training included explaining the forms, demonstrating anthropometric measurements (arm subcutaneous fat and lean muscle), a mock screening using the forms and interviewing techniques. A video tape was made at one of the branch in-service sites so that all branch offices would have access to the same information. Part of the implementation phase involved determining the most effective flow of information. Figure 23-3 describes how the data from the screening tools were to be used to make referral and intervention decisions.

● SCREENING TOOL UTILIZATION

After completing the assessment, the nurse's role includes identification of specific nutrition problems, appropriate teaching, referral to a dietitian or community resource, and reevaluation of the nutritional status of the patient. Use of the form for admission assessment, periodic reassessments, and documentation of consultations and referrals sufficiently addresses the need for documentation of a patient's nutritional status as outlined by JCAHO.

The most common problems with the Level II screening involved the weight, height, and anthropometric measurements. It is very difficult to get an accurate weight on an ob-

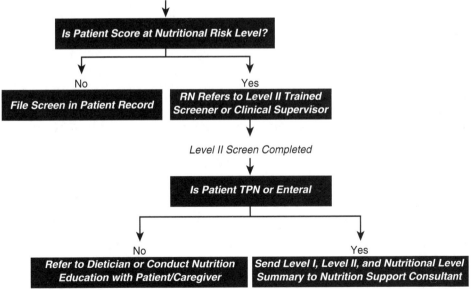

Patient Admission Nutrition Level I Screen Completed

Is Patient Score at Nutritional Risk Level?

No — File Screen in Patient Record

Yes — RN Refers to Level II Trained Screener or Clinical Supervisor

Level II Screen Completed

Is Patient TPN or Enteral

No — Refer to Dietician or Conduct Nutrition Education with Patient/Caregiver

Yes — Send Level I, Level II, and Nutritional Level Summary to Nutrition Support Consultant

FIGURE 23-3. Nutrition screening decision tree.

tunded, bedfast individual. Rarely is a height of an adult patient measured, despite the known fact that height decreases with age. Initially, anthropometric measurements were on the Level II screening tool. Nurses perceived anthropometric measurements to be difficult and unreliable, so they often omitted this section completely. In fact, anthropometric measurements are most accurately done by individuals who perform them on a regular basis. The revised Level II forms deleted anthropometric measurements with no apparent negative impact on decision making.

Standardized utilization of the results from the follow-up consultations from the Level II screens has also been difficult. Branch management staff had to determine how to introduce the home nutrition assessment concept to referring physicians so that they would not view the information as an infringement on their expertise. Informing the physician that this is now a JCAHO-mandated aspect of care, and that it is part of the nursing agency's routine assessment has proven effective. Most physicians are willing to adjust rates, utilize a more cost-effective enteral solution, or make other minor changes that improve the quality of care delivered to their patients. It is often effective to use the physician's office nurses as advocates for the program and enlist their help in presenting needed changes in the plan of care. The key factor in presenting changes to physicians or nurses is to give the rationale for the changes. Consultants must be forthcoming with their reasoning so that staff feel comfortable advocating a change in the plan of care. Table 23-1 outlines the most common recommendations made as a result of the screening tools.

Patients who received total parenteral nutrition were monitored weekly by the home healthcare nurse or nutrition support nurse consultant who assessed the patient's tolerance of the formula by a telephone call or visit to the home. That weekly contact allowed the nurse to advise the patient on diet progression, measures to prevent metabolic bone disease, and venous access complication prevention. One patient had a rare disease that was extremely painful and required high doses of morphine via pump to control the pain. The nurse consultant sent the home infusion service and local physician articles on the disease to validate that pain was indeed characteristic of this condition. The physician consultant was particularly helpful when it became evident that total parenteral nutrition was no longer in the patient's best interest.

Lessons Learned

The use of information from the nutrition screening tool benefits the local branch, the patient, and the third party payor. This value-added service made the home care branches more efficient by recommending the most cost-effective therapy for patients without compromising quality service, an issue of increasing importance in the managed care arena. This, in turn, saved payors money as patients were switched from parenteral to en-

TABLE 23-1 • Commonly Recommended Changes in Order of Frequency
1. Decrease calorie intake
2. Increase free water intake
3. Change from a specialized formula to a less-expensive enteral solution
4. Alter elixir medication schedule
5. Add some fiber-containing enteral formula to feeding regimen

teral nutrition support or a less-expensive enteral formula. The patient received a higher quality of care without being billed for consultative services.

The use of nutrition screening tools that addresses the needs of higher risk, more problem-prone individuals in a cost-effective manner is a challenge for home healthcare providers. Signature Home Care's solution was to adapt and improve an already existing and valid tool so that much of their work was in "fine tuning" a tool and developing an effective process for information flow. The result is a process that is workable for them and beneficial to the populations they serve. The following are some of the lessons learned by the Signature staff:

1. Be careful to build in a triage system so that low-risk patients do not consume the same level of time and resources as high-risk patients.
2. Make the follow-up of assessments and consultations for high-risk patients as simple as possible, so that the paperwork does not become burdensome.
3. Carefully determine how to market the program to referral sources so that the screening results are viewed as a value-added service.
4. Keep the Level I Screen to a one-page document.
5. Delete anthropometric measurements from the Level II screening form.
6. Use consultants who are active in research and are nationally known so that name recognition will help market the program to referral sources.
7. Ensure that you allow sufficient time in the initial design of the tool and in motivating staff nurses.
8. Provide ongoing education and re-education to home care branch staff to produce the most consistent and effective results possible.

REFERENCES

Cope, K. A. (1996). Nutritional status: A Basic Vital sign. *Home Healthcare Nurse, 12*(2), 29–34.

Howard, L., Ament, M., Fleming, C. R., Shike, M., Steiger, E. (1995). Current use and clinical outcome of home parenteral and enteral nutrition therapies in the United States. *Gastroenterology, 109,* 355–365.

Joint Commission on Accreditation of Healthcare Organizations. (1995). *Accreditation manual for home care* (Volume II, Scoring Guidelines Standard PE.1.3, pp. 27–28). Chicago, IL: Author.

Melnik, T. A., Helferd, S. J., Firmery, L. A., Wales, K. R. (1994). Screening elderly in the community: The relationship between dietary adequacy and nutritional risk. *JADA, 9*(12), 1425–1427.

Wellman, N. (1994). The nutrition screening initiative. *Nutr Rev, 52*(8), 44–47.

White J. V., (1996). The nutrition screening initiative: A 5-year perspective. *Nutrition in Clinical Practice, 11*(3), 89–93.

Clients in community settings often suffer from conditions that put them at risk for altered skin integrity. Those most at risk include clients with diabetes mellitus, renal failure, and malnutrition where neuropathies are common. In addition, loss of sensation may result from trauma, AIDS, a central nervous system disorder, spinal problems, or Hansen's disease. Neuropathy may also be experienced by the client as part of the normal physiologic aging process.

What are some preventive strategies to avoid developing foot ulcers? What screening and general assessments are essential to identify those at risk for foot ulcers? Identify some components of patient education for foot care.

Van Rijswijk, L. (1998). Assessing the risk of foot ulcers. Home Healthcare Nurse, 16(1), 25–32.

Assessing the Risk of Foot Ulcers

LIA VAN RIJSWIJK

Home care nurses are in an ideal position to screen clients and assess their risk of developing foot-related problems, including ulcers. An increased awareness of the potential serious consequences of foot ulcers together with agency assessment and practice guidelines, will help nurses prevent foot-related problems.

Most people can relate to the adverse effects of feet problems on mobility. At the end of a long day, the desire to take off one's shoes and give those feet a break is almost universal. During the first 3 or 4 decades of life, feet usually recuperate quickly from the tasks of standing or walking for prolonged periods. Even the occasional use of ill-fitting shoes does not appear to harm them permanently. As a result, healthcare professionals and their clients often assume that feet require minimal attention.

According to Pock, Frankel, and Shiu (1995), the foot is the most neglected part of the body in the routine physical examination. Indeed, recent guidelines on measuring the quality of healthcare for patients with diabetes include recommendations related to asking them if they recall taking their shoes and socks off during a recent physician visit (FACCT, 1996).

Traditionally, the treatment and prevention of foot ulcers is discussed in the context of their etiology (e.g., diabetic, arterial, or pressure ulcer). This approach helps healthcare professionals focus on the importance of addressing the underlying cause of these wounds. Unfortunately, using an etiology-based classification may lead one to conclude that mobile people without diabetes or arterial insufficiency will not get foot ulcers. In the United States, most patients with foot ulcers have diabetes mellitus. However, the most

Lia van Rijswijk, RN, ET, is a nurse consultant, Newtown, PA, and a RN-MSN student at La Salle University School of Nursing, Philadelphia, PA.

common underlying etiology of wounds on the feet (neuropathy, altered biomechanics, arterial insufficiency or peripheral vascular disease) is not limited to people with diabetes mellitus.

Health risk appraisals provide clients with an estimate of health threats to which they may be vulnerable because of genetic makeup, age, biologic characteristics, personal health habits, lifestyle, or environment (Pender, 1996). When conducting a nursing risk assessment, it is always important to remain oriented to the individual instead of to the disease. With respect to foot ulcers, focusing on a disease (e.g. diabetes mellitus) instead of the individual may cause one to miss the opportunity to educate or provide referral for other populations who are at risk for impaired skin or tissue integrity. Home healthcare nurses are in an ideal position to assess risk factors for the development of foot ulcers. The purpose of this paper is to review the economic and public health implications of foot ulcers, review risk factors, and screening, assessment and prevention strategies for home healthcare professionals.

● CLIENTS AT RISK

Clients with insulin-dependent or noninsulin-dependent diabetes mellitus are at high risk for developing chronic wounds on their feet (Litzelman, et al., 1993). In the United States, between 5% and 6% of the population has diabetes (FACCT, 1996). Noninsulin-dependent diabetes mellitus is the most prevalent type of metabolic disorder, affecting up to 10% of the elderly population. Many patients do not know that they have diabetes. For example, when older persons seeking care to treat their hypertension were tested, 11.6% of the 43 people evaluated had undiagnosed noninsulin-dependent diabetes mellitus (Johnson et al., 1997). One study suggests that most clients with diabetes (75%) have diabetic foot symptoms and many (44%) do not seek or obtain hospital care (Rosenquist, 1984). The most devastating consequence of nonhealing foot ulcers, amputation, has been found to occur in 7 to 8 of every 1000 people with diabetes (Kahn, Banks, Welch and Landrum, 1992; U.S. Department of Health and Human Services, Public Health Service, 1990). As a result, approximately 50,000, or half of all nontraumatic amputations in the United States, occur in people with diabetes.

Although trauma from stepping on a sharp object may precede the development of foot ulcers, most wounds are caused by moderate, repeated stress. In general, it is believed that clients with insensitive feet accept an unvarying pattern of repetitive stress long after a normal foot would have started to feel sore (Brand, 1988).

Diabetes mellitus, renal failure, and malnutrition are examples of systemic conditions that may slowly diminish sensation. Neuropathies can also be caused by trauma, AIDS, central nervous system disorder, spinal problems or Hansen's disease. The latter is caused by *Mycobacterium leprae* and causes chronic skin lesions and peripheral neuropathy. Once nerve damage has occurred, recurrent trauma, ulceration, and subsequent infection may lead to permanent tissue loss or amputation (Smith et al., 1995).

As persons age, a decrease in perception of deep pain, temperature stimuli, and vibratory sense at the ankle are commonly observed (Kozier, Erb, & Olivieri, 1991). Another aspect of the physiologic aging process, a decrease or absence of position sense in the large toes, combined with peripheral vascular disease, atherosclerosis, or inappropriate foot care, may further increase a person's risk for developing foot problems, including ulcers. The risk of different foot abnormalities increases with age (Plummer & Albert, 1996).

Because sensory loss is often a gradual process, many people in the general population do not know that they have neuropathy. When examining 125 elderly patients without diabetes who were referred to a foot care service, investigators found that 18% had peripheral neuropathy and 21% had peripheral vascular disease (Plummer & Albert, 1996). Moreover, 6% of these patients (mean age, 70.4 years) had peripheral neuropathy and peripheral vascular disease, two risk factors for developing foot ulcers.

Wounds on the heel can develop in mobile patients with neuropathy, but also in chair-bound or bed-bound individuals. Impaired mobility, sensation, or perfusion, as well as alterations in nutritional status, are some of the known risk factors for the development of pressure ulcers on the heel (Maklebust & Sieggreen, 1995). Heels are susceptible to pressure, and even relatively short periods (up to 40 minutes) of pressure in healthy individuals have been shown to cause a significant hyperemic response (Mayrovitz, Smith, Delgado, & Regan, 1997). People at risk for developing foot ulcers include patients with diabetes mellitus, the elderly, central nervous system disorders, spinal problems, Hansen's disease, those with altered biomechanics of the foot, impaired mobility or perfusion, and peripheral neuropathy (see Fig. 24-1).

● ECONOMIC AND PUBLIC HEALTH IMPLICATIONS

Little is known about the economic burden of foot problems in general, but the economic burden of diabetic foot ulcers and pressure ulcers is considerable. In one study, the cost incurred to heal diabetic foot ulcers ranged from $22,562 to $36,185 (Bentkover & Champion, 1993), and recurrence rates of between 70% and 83% have been noted after as little as 2 to 3 months (Steed, Edington, & Webster, 1996). The national cost of treat-

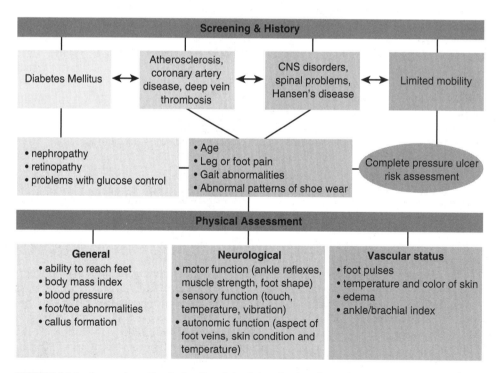

FIGURE 24-1. Assessing clients for the risk of developing foot ulcers.

ing pressure ulcers in a variety of anatomic locations has been estimated to exceed $1.355 billion per year (Miller & Delozier, 1994). In general, depending on the effectiveness of the interventions, cost of labor, and price of materials used, the cost per percentage of a wound area healed can range from $.19 to $28.40 (Bolton, van Rijswijk, & Shaffer, 1996).

Amputation, the ultimate failure of foot ulcer prevention and treatment, causes considerable morbidity, mortality, and financial burdens. In a 1988 study, hospital costs alone averaged $25,000 per amputation (Levin, 1995), and the average cost of revascularization and amputation can approach $40,000 (Cevera, Bolton, & Kerstein, in press). In 1987, amputations attributable to diabetes represented 648,570 days of hospital care (Kahn, et al, 1993). The public health implications of these findings deserve our attention, particularly because the projected 30% increase of people 85 years of age or older is certainly going to increase these costs (U.S. Department of Health and Human Services Public Health Service, 1990). Indirect costs (e.g., days lost from work or inability to work) and those of immobility or reduced quality of life have not been studied. However, based on studies of nonhospitalized patients with other chronic wounds (leg ulcers), it can be assumed that these wounds have a negative impact on patients' quality of life and limit their mobility (Phillips, Stanton, Provan, & Lew, 1994; Walshe, 1995).

Foot ulcers are expensive to treat, tend to recur, and the cost of complications is considerable in terms of dollars and reduced quality of life. Early and aggressive intervention and timely referrals can break the "causal chain to amputation" (Pecoraro, Reiber, & Burgess, 1990). Home healthcare nurses are in the ideal position to help meet the goals of *Healthy People 2000,* by

- limiting the number of people who may one day have physical activity limitations;
- preventing health problems that arise from, or are related to, disability; and
- reducing the amputation rate by 40% by ensuring that at least 80% of people with diabetes at high risk for lower extremity amputations are receiving effective clinical management and foot care (U.S. Department of Health and Human Services, Public Health Service, 1990).

● THE EFFECT OF PREVENTION EFFORTS

Controlled studies have shown that relatively simple, and noninvasive strategies, such as foot-care education and wearing appropriate shoes, reduce the likelihood of developing serious foot lesions (Litzelman et al., 1993). Similarly, teaching and follow-up programs in patients with leprosy are so successful that the U.S. Department of Health and Human Services has sponsored the Lower Extremity Amputation Prevention (LEAP) program for all patients with neuropathy (Smith et al., 1995; Gillis W. Long Hansen's Disease Center, 1994).

With respect to pressure ulcers, formal risk-based programs using valid risk-assessment scales have been shown to reduce the costs associated with prevention while reducing the incidence of these wounds (Braden & Bergstrom, 1996). When used appropriately, prevention is inexpensive. For example, in a recent study, the cost per day of ulcer-free life gained was $1.36 (Xakellis & Frantz, 1996).

It is important for home healthcare nurses to remember that, once a wound has developed, prevention efforts remain important. First, the factors that caused the wound also will delay healing and may cause wound deterioration. Second, it is not uncommon for other ulcers to develop. For example, efforts to avoid putting weight on one foot may increase pressures under the other foot.

● WHAT HOME CARE NURSES CAN DO

The first step toward reducing the incidence of foot ulcers is recognizing clients who are at risk. Fortunately, a complete, routine client assessment usually includes almost all the information needed to assess the risk of developing these wounds.

Screening and History

A complete client and family history provides the foundation for the risk assessment (see Fig. 24-1). Diabetes mellitus, increased age, a history of conditions that affect tissue perfusion (e.g. smoking, atherosclerosis, history of deep vein thrombosis), limited mobility, and signs of neuropathy (pain or numbness) all increase the client's risk for developing foot ulcers. With every additional risk factor identified (e.g., diabetes and atherosclerosis or spinal problems and coronary artery disease), the client's risk of developing these wounds increases. Complications of diabetes mellitus, such as retinopathy, nephropathy, or a history of problems with glucose control, are also reason for concern. For bed- or chair-bound clients, the above-mentioned history should be supplemented by completing a valid risk-assessment scale such as the Braden Scale for predicting pressure sore risk (Braden & Bergstrom, 1996). When using these scales, client sensory perception, exposure to moisture, activity level, mobility, nutritional status, and potential for exposure to friction and shear will be assessed.

The first step toward including the feet in the overall assessment is to always ask clients to remove their socks and shoes because it has been shown that feet are often neglected in the physical examination of outpatients simply because they keep wearing their socks or shoes (Pock, 1995). A quick glance at clients' shoes and feet can provide important information about their risk status. Foot function is complex, and minor gait abnormalities may be difficult to detect during the regular assessment process. However, gait abnormalities can often be detected by looking at the shoes. Signs of abnormal, excessive, or irregular patterns of shoe wear are often indicative of a less-than-perfect gait. Bunions, hammer toes, calluses, ingrown toenails, corns, or blisters also can negatively affect mobility and increase pressure (Saye, 1993).

General Assessment

Clients who cannot reach their feet have an increased risk of developing foot ulcers. Some clients may have been told to check their feet but are unable to do so. For example, when Enterostomal Therapy nurses evaluated home foot care practices of patients with diabetes mellitus, they found that most clients who remembered being told to check their feet were unable to visualize one or more of the sites that should be inspected (Faller & Lawrence, 1995). Obtaining an accurate body weight is important because body weight greater than normal for height/frame may affect peripheral tissue perfusion, whereas low body weight may indicate a less-than-optimal nutritional status. High blood pressure is common in clients with diabetes mellitus (Johnson et al., 1997), and foot, toe or nail abnormalities often create pressure points.

Callus formation exacerbates high plantar pressures in clients with neuropathy. The callus that forms in these clients often is firm, and extravasation of blood in the area occurs more frequently in people with, as compared to people without, diabetes mellitus

(Rosen, David, Bohanske, & Lemont, 1985). When a discolored (blue, blue/red) callus is present and the client is at risk for developing foot ulcers, a referral for callus removal and exploration of the underlying tissues is required because bacterial proliferation may extend into the joint capsule (Ennis, 1997).

Neurologic Assessment

Impaired motor function (see Fig. 24-1) can lead to one or more of the following:

- reduced or absent ankle reflexes;
- intrinsic muscle wasting;
- a flattened arch;
- prominent metatarsal heads; and
- general weakness.

Dry skin, often seen in patients with neuropathy, is caused by reduced sweating secondary to problems with autonomic function. Consequently, callus formation and increased pressure occurs. Other signs of impaired autonomic function include a warm foot and distended foot veins. Sensory function, touch, temperature, and vibration provide important information about the risk of developing foot ulcers.

To gauge sensory function, the traditional assessment methods (touch, light touch, two-point discrimination, and temperature) may be sufficient (Seidel, Ball, Dains, & Benedict, 1995). However, it is important to never use sharp or very warm objects to test sensory function, and most experts agree that when a client has other risk factors for developing foot ulcers, Semmes-Weinstein monofilaments (Gillis W. Long Hansens Disease Center, Carville, LA) should be used. Their predictive validity has been established, and they are inexpensive, easy to use, and provide quantitative data (Birke & Sims, 1986; Young & Jones, 1997; van Vliet, Novak, & Mackinnon, 1993) (see Table 24-1). Because reduced reflex responses and perception of pain, temperature stimuli, and vibratory sense may reflect the physiologic aging process, it is important to assimilate all history and physical assessment findings together when trying to determine whether the client is at risk for developing foot ulcers.

Vascular Status Assessment

The first step in assessing perfusion consists of palpating the posterior tibial and dorsalis pedis pulse. In older adults, it may be difficult to find one of these, and a Doppler Ultrasonic stethoscope may be needed. Obtaining an Ankle Brachial Index (ABI) is recom-

---

TABLE 24-1 • Using Semmes-Weinstein Monofilaments

1. Select appropriate monofilament. (Numbers 4.31 (1 g force), 5.07 (10 g force), and 6.10 (75 g) are most commonly used for diabetes screening.)
2. Select test sites. (Be consistent and always include plantar area of the foot. For example check first through fifth metatarsal head, toes, hallux, heel, and dorsum of the foot.)
3. Apply filament in random order for approximately 1.5 seconds. (Prolonged application increases cutaneous pressure threshold.)
4. Most patients with neuropathy cannot feel a 5.07 (10 g) probe.

mended for clients with existing ulcers and for clients who are at risk for developing foot or leg ulcers (Wills & Sloan, 1996). Obtaining an ABI does not require any special equipment; a regular blood pressure cuff should be applied above the ankle and the systolic pressure attained in either the posterior tibial or dorsalis pedis artery. Dividing the ankle pressure by the brachial pressure provides the ABI. An ABI of 0.9–1.0 is considered "normal" (Douglas & Simpson, 1995). A decreased ABI indicates decreased peripheral arterial blood flow. It is important to note that some conditions, including diabetes mellitus, may cause hardening of the arteries and elevated ankle pressure readings. In these instances, the ABI is not a reliable measure of arterial blood flow.

Capillary refill time can be evaluated by squeezing a toenail between your fingers. After blanching has occurred, removal of the finger normally results in immediate return of normal skin color. Elevating or dangling the legs may reveal elevational pallor or dependent rubor. In clients with darkly pigmented skin, it may be easier to assess the soles of the feet for color changes after elevating or dangling the legs. Diminished foot pulses, pale, cool skin with fissures, thickened nails, and an absence of hair growth are indicative of arterial insufficiency.

Edema can be assessed by measuring the circumference of the midcalf, ankle, and dorsum of both feet, and by pressing an index finger over the bony prominence of the tibia or medial malleolus. Edema, as well as brown/brown-red discoloration of the skin, are common signs of impaired venous return.

Skin temperature may also provide information about tissue perfusion and inflammation and is an important variable when assessing increased or reduced perfusion secondary to pressure. Checking the temperature of the skin by using the back of the hand is an excellent method for detecting problems in all clients, including those with darkly pigmented skin. For example, cellulitis or the presence of a Stage I pressure ulcer may be difficult to see but can often be felt (Bennett, 1995). Pressure ulcer risk-assessment scales (Braden & Bergstrom, 1996), home healthcare assessment forms to facilitate nursing assessment of the feet (Kelechi & Lukacs, 1996), peripheral arterial disorders (Wills & Sloan, 1996), and diabetic foot and leg ulcer risk-assessment policies and procedures (van Rijswijk, 1996) are available.

● AFTER THE ASSESSMENT

A client's risk of developing foot ulcers often can be derived from reviewing the history and physical assessment record. For example, an elderly client with a history of coronary artery disease, a low Ankle Brachial Index, and foot deformities should be considered at risk and receive appropriate interventions. Similarly, all clients with diabetes mellitus should be assessed once yearly and receive foot care instructions (Gillis W. Long Hansen's Disease Center, 1994; American Diabetes Association, 1990; FACCT, 1996).

If consistent with the overall goal of patient care, clients with signs of neuropathy, arterial or venous insufficiency, foot deformities, excess callus formation, or existing ulcers must be referred for further testing and evaluation. Foot care education, shoe accommodations, therapeutic shoes, or orthotics help these clients remain ulcer-free by reducing the deleterious effects of pressure. In addition, some may be good candidates for reconstructive vascular surgery. Finally, the conditions that predispose one to neuropathy (e.g. diabetes mellitus, atherosclerosis, etc.) also increase a client's risk of infection. Therefore, existing foot ulcers or signs of infection always require specialized care. Basic foot care instructions (see Table 24-2) should be provided for all elderly clients and for those who are otherwise at risk for developing foot ulcers.

TABLE 24-2 ● Some Components of Foot Care Patient Education Materials

Do	Do Not
Watch your diet[a]	Walk without shoes
Wash and inspect feet daily	Wear open-toed shoes or sandals
Dry feet carefully	Cut corns or calluses
Cut nails in contour with toes	Use corn plasters
Use moisturizer if skin is dry	Apply moisturizer between toes
Inspect inside of shoes	Wear shoes with heels or pointed toes
Check temperature of bath	Soak feet
water with elbow	Apply adhesive tape or antiseptic solutions to feet
Buy and wear properly fitting shoes	
Wear properly fitting/clean socks	

[a] If you have diabetes mellitus, keeping glucose levels within normal limits will help prevent some of the long-term complications of diabetes.

● CONCLUSION

Foot problems occur in various patient populations, including the elderly, people with limitations in mobility, and clients with diabetes mellitus. Fortunately, an increased awareness among providers goes a long way toward effective health promotion and disease prevention efforts. Although it may be difficult to identify high risk patients who do not seek care, provider time constraints should not be a major barrier because foot ulcer screening and risk assessment does not require a lot of extra time or equipment. Moreover, implementing relatively simple measures and reminding clients to "baby their feet," furthers efforts toward preventing the formation of foot ulcers and subsequent immobility and morbidity. For clients with impaired mobility, the use of a validated pressure ulcer risk-assessment scale can help guide ulcer prevention efforts.

● ACKNOWLEDGMENT

The author thanks Janice M. Beitz, PhD, RN, CS, CNOR, CETN, and Laura L. Bolton, PhD, for their professional support and encouragement.

REFERENCES

American Diabetes Association. (1990). *Diabetic foot care.* Alexandria, VA: Author.

Bennett, M.A. (1995). Report of the task force on the implications for darkly pigmented intact skin in the prediction and prevention of pressure ulcers. *Advances in Wound Care, 8*(6), 34–35.

Bentkover, J.D., & Champion, A.H. (1993). Economic evaluation of alternative methods of treatment for diabetic foot ulcer patients: Cost-effectiveness of platelet releasate and wound care clinics. *Wounds, 5*(4), 207–215.

Birke, J.A., & Sims, D.S. (1986). Plantar sensory threshold in the ulcerative foot. *Leprosy Review, 57,* 261–267

Bolton, L.L., van Rijswijk, L., & Shaffer, F.A. (1996). Quality wound care equals cost-effective wound care; a clinical model. *Nursing Management, 27*(7), 30,32–33,37.

Braden, B.J., Bergstrom, N. (1996). Risk assessment in pressure ulcer prevention. *Ostomy/Wound Management, 42*(10A), 6S–12S.

Brand, P.W. (1988). Repetitive stress in the development of diabetic foot ulcers. In M. E. Levin, & L. W. O'Neal (Eds.), *The diabetic foot* (4th ed.). St. Louis, MO: The C.V. Mosby Company.

Cevera, J.J., Bolton, L.L., & Kerstein, M.D. (in press). Options for diabetics with chronic heel ulcers. *Journal of Diabetics and its Complications.*

Douglas, W.S., & Simpson, N.B. (1995). Guidelines for the management of chronic venous leg ulceration. Report of a multidisciplinary workshop. *British Journal of Dermatology, 132,* 446–452.

Ennis, W. J. (1997). Personal communication.

FACCT. (1996). *Measuring healthcare quality: Diabetes.* Rockville, MD: Foundation for Accountability, Agency of Health Care Policy and Research.

Faller, N.A., & Lawrence, K.G. (1995). An assessment of diabetic foot care in a rural New England community and the nursing implications. Symposium on Advanced Wound Care, San Diego, CA.

Gillis W. Long Hansen's Disease Center Rehabilitation Branch. (1994). LEAP program, care of the foot in diabetes; the Carville approach. Carville, LA: U.S. Department of Health and Human Services.

Johnson, K.C., Graney, M.J., Applegate, W.B., Kitabchi, A.E., Runyan, J.W. & Shorre, R.I. (1997). Prevalence of undiagnosed non-insulin-dependent diabetes mellitus and impaired glucose tolerance in a cohort of older persons with hypertension. *Journal of the American Geriatrics Society, 45,* 695–700.

Kelechi, T., & Lukacs, K. (1996). Foot care in the home: Nursing and agency responsibilities. *Home Healthcare Nurse, 14*(9), 721–731.

Kahn, R., Banks, P., Welch, C., & Landrum, S. (1993). *Direct and indirect costs of diabetes in the United States in 1992.* Alexandria, VA: American Diabetes Association.

Kozier, B., Erb, G., & Olivieri, R. (1991). *Fundamentals of nursing: Concepts, process and practice* (4th ed.). Redwood City, CA: Addison-Wesley.

Levin, M.E. (1995). Diabetic foot lesions: Pathogenesis and management. In M. Kerstein, & J.V. White, (Eds.). *Alternatives to open vascular surgery* (pp. 94–126). Philadelphia: J. B. Lippincott Company.

Litzelman, D.K., Slemenda, C.W., Langefeld, C.D, Hays, L.M., Welch, M.A., Bild, D.E., Ford, E.S., & Vinicor, F. (1993). Reduction of lower extremity clinical abnormalities in patients with non-insulin-dependent diabetes mellitus. *Annals of Internal Medicine, 119*(1), 36–41.

Maklebust, J., & Sieggreen, M. (1995). *Pressure ulcers: Guidelines for prevention and nursing management.* Springhouse, PA: Springhouse Corp.

Mayrovitz, H.N., Smith, J., Delgado, M., & Regan, M.B. (1997). Heel blood perfusion responses to pressure loading and unloading women. *Ostomy/Wound Management, 43*(7), 16–26.

Miller, H., & Delozier, J. (1994). Cost implications of the pressure ulcer treatment guideline. (Contract No.282-91-0080, p.17, sponsored by the Agency for Health Care Policy and Research). Columbia, MD: Center for Health Policy Studies.

Pecoraro, R.E., Reiber, G.E., & Burgess, E.M. (1990). Pathways to diabetic limb amputation: Basis for prevention. *Diabetes Care,* 513–521.

Pender, N.J. (1996). *Health promotion in nursing practice* (3rd ed). Stamford, CT: Appleton & Lange.

Phillips, T., Stanton, B., Provan, A., & Lew, R. (1994). A study of the impact of leg ulcers on quality of life: Financial, social, and psychologic implications. *Journal of the American Academy of Dermatology, 31,* 49–53.

Pock, A., Frankel, S.L., & Shiu, W.S. (1995). Dysvascular foot care. In M.D. Kerstein & J.V. White (Eds.), *Alternatives to open vascular surgery* (pp. 127–153). Philadelphia: J.B. Lippincott Company.

Plummer, E.S., & Albert, S.G. (1996). Focused assessment of foot care in older adults. *Journal of the American Geriatrics Society, 44,* 310–133.

Rosen, R.C., Davids, M.S., Bohanske, L.M., & Lemont, H. Hemorrhage into plantar callus and diabetes mellitus. *Cutis, 35,* 339–341.

Rosenquist, U. (1984). An epidemiological survey of diabetic foot problems in the Stockholm County, 1982. *Acta Medica Scandinavia, 687,* 55–60.

Saye, D.E. (1993). The foot: Biomechanics and orthotics. *Ostomy/Wound Management, 39*(8), 46–54.

Seidel, H.M., Ball, J.W., Dains, J.E., & Benedict, G.W. (1995). *Mosby's guide to physical examination* (3rd ed.). St. Louis, MO: Mosby-Year Book, Inc.

Smith, W.C.S., Zhang, G., Zheng, T., Watson, J.M., Lehman, L.F., & Lever, P. (1995). Prevention of impairment in leprosy: Results from a collaborative project in China. *International Journal of Leprosy, 63*(4), 507–517.

Steed, D.L., Edington, H.D., Webster, M.W. (1996). Recurrence rate of diabetic neurotrophic foot ulcers healed using topical application of growth factors released from platelets. *Wound Repair Regeneration, 4,* 230–233.

U.S. Department of Health and Human Services Public Health Service. (1990). *Healthy people 2000* (DHHS Publication No. [PHS] 91-50212). Washington, DC: Author.

van Rijswijk, L. (1996). Wound care practices in the home: Signposts to effective patient outcomes. *Wound Care Policies and Procedures Manual* (2nd ed). Skillman, NJ: ConvaTec House Calls total wound management program.

van Vliet, D., Novak, C.B., & Mackinnon, S.E. (1993). Duration of contact time alters cutaneous pressure threshold measurements. *Annals Plastic Surgery, 31,* 335–339.

Walshe, C. (1995). Living with a venous leg ulcer: A descriptive study of patients' experiences. *Journal of Advanced Nursing, 22,* 1092–1100.

Wills, E.M., & Sloan, H.L. (1996). Assessing peripheral arterial disorders in the home: A multidisciplinary clinical guide. *Home Healthcare Nurse, 14*(9), 669–680.

Xakellis, G.C., & Frantz, R.A. (1996). The cost-effectiveness of interventions for preventing pressure ulcers. *Journal of the American Board of Family Practice, 9,* 79–85.

Young, M.J., & Jones, G.C. Diabetic neuropathy: Symptoms, signs and assessment. In A.J.M. Boulton (Ed.)., *Diabetic Neuropathy* (pp. 41–61). Lancashire, United Kingdom: Marius Press.

According to this article, older adults use 31% of all prescription drugs and receive prescriptions for an average of 7.5 to 17.9 medications per person. Not surprising, mismanagement of medications by the elderly is not uncommon, with subsequent unwanted side effects, loss of functional abilities, and unnecessary clinic and hospital visits.

What was the purpose of this study? How was the questionnaire developed? Who was the sample used in the pilot? What are some characteristics of this group? What were the major findings? What other information was discovered? How could you use this questionnaire in your practice?

DeBrew, J., Barba, B., & Tesh, A. (1998). Assessing medication knowledge and practices of older adults. *Home Healthcare Nurse*, 16(10), 686–692.

Assessing Medication Knowledge and Practices of Older Adults

JACQUELINE KAYLER DEBREW, BETH E. BARBA, ANITA S. TESH

An assessment instrument for home health nurses to use in assessing medication knowledge and practices of older adults was developed and tested on a convenience sample of 20 adults 65 and older admitted to a local home health agency. The tool was found usable by nurses, understood by patients, and had adequate test-retest reliability. The results emphasized the need for thorough medication assessments of all home health patients and provided a tool that home care nurses can use.

● BACKGROUND AND PROBLEM

Of all age groups, older adults are prescribed the largest number of medications. They use 31% of all prescription drugs (Cornish, 1992) and are prescribed an average of 7.5 to 17.9 medications per person every year (Ali, 1992). A physician visit results in a new prescription nearly 80% of the time for this age group (Cornish, 1992). Older adults are also the biggest consumers of over-the-counter (OTC) drugs (Cornish, 1992), the most common being aspirin, laxatives, and vitamins. Caffeine intake, alcohol consumption, nicotine use, and use of narcotics can interact with prescribed medications, and are common among older adults (Conn, 1992).

Polypharmacy, the use of multiple medications, is widespread among older people, primarily because of the multiple chronic illnesses they experience (Baker & Napthine, 1994; Wolfe & Schirm, 1992). These chronic illnesses and multiple medications, along

Jacqueline Kayler DeBrew, MSN, RN, CS, is a clinical instructor, Beth E. Barba, PhD, RN, is associate professor, and Anita S. Tesh, EdD, RN(c), is associate professor at the UNC-Greensboro School of Nursing, NC.

with normal changes of aging, place older adults at great risk for side effects from drug therapy. In addition, older adults frequently have difficulty managing their complicated medication regimens, which poses a great challenge to healthcare providers, particularly those in home health.

Mismanagement of medications, intentional or unintentional, may cause unwanted side effects, loss of functional abilities, unnecessary hospital admissions, and even death. Voluntary misuse includes not having prescriptions filled or refilled, stopping medications too soon, and not taking medications because of side effects. Involuntary misuse includes administering medications incorrectly, often because of cognitive or sensory changes (Mullen, 1993), the complexity of the medication regimen (Conn, Taylor, & Kelly, 1991), or the lack of financial resources (Kluckowski, 1992).

These risks point to the necessity of thoroughly assessing the medication practices of each elder so as to provide individualized teaching and care. The home care nurse will witness firsthand any problems that might be occurring, and can assist the patients in developing solutions. Home care nurses also have a responsibility for reviewing all medications and contacting prescribers about potential problems, because they may be the patients' primary contact with the healthcare system.

Many authors advocate the use of a standardized assessment tool to evaluate medication practices accurately (Benzon, 1991; Hahn & Wietor, 1992; Messner & Gardner, 1993; Sidel et al., 1990; Simpson, 1993). There are several medication assessment tools in existence, but none have been tested for use in the home care setting. The purpose of this study was to develop and test an assessment instrument for use by home health nurses in evaluating the medication knowledge and practices of older adults.

● METHODS

Instrument Development

Construction of items in the instrument was based on a literature review concerning instrument development and medication practices of older adults. Items were written as complete sentences and placed in logical order to improve respondents' recall. According to Flesch-Kincaid's measurement of reading level, items were written on a fifth grade level, which was consistent with the literature on instrument development (Lewis, 1993).

The instrument consists of three sections. The first section asks about basic patient demographics: date of birth, race, gender, physicians, current health problems, and allergies. This demographic section also requests data that might influence a patient's ability to complete an interview such as highest level of education completed, ability to read and write, and orientation.

The second section focuses on the patient's overall medication practices. The areas addressed are medication administration and storage; medication purchasing habits; attitudes toward medications and health; lifestyle habits including use of nicotine, caffeine, alcohol, and street drugs; and home environment (Fig. 25-1).

The final section is designed to determine the patient's knowledge of each medication currently used. The patient is asked about the action, administration, and side effects, both potential and actual, of each medication.

The content validity of the tool was established by a panel of experts consisting of faculty from a local school of nursing and nurses employed in community health nursing. Data were collected using semistructured interviews. This allowed the test administrators to tailor the order and phrasing of questions to respondents' needs. The administrators were given the freedom to explain or restate items so the instrument would be easier to

Medication Assessment

Note to administrator: The sequence of the interview, along with the instructional statements are merely suggestions, and should be considered guidelines when using the interview. It is acceptable to reword statements or change the format to better meet the needs of the individual, yet all topics must be included in the assessment.

Start Time: _____ Who is the respondent? ☐ Patient ☐ Spouse ☐ Other (list) _____

Please Check The Appropriate Response.

Administrator: *"I need to see all of your medications. Please show me those you take every day, and those you take occasionally. Don't forget to show me eyedrops, insulin, laxatives, vitamins, antacids, ointments or any over-the-counter drugs you sometimes use. Are there any other medications that you regularly take that are not here today?"* (Attach copies of medication profiles to document drugs.)

I. Medication Administration and Storage

☐ Yes ☐ No   Can patient open a pill bottle? (Have patient demonstrate.)

☐ Yes ☐ No   Can patient break a pill in half? (Have patient demonstrate. Omit if not applicable)

☐ Yes ☐ No   Does someone help you take your medicine?

☐ Yes ☐ No   Do you use any type of system to help you take your pills, such as a pill box, or a calendar?

List: _____

☐ Yes ☐ No   Do you have problems swallowing your pills?

Where do you store your medicines? _____

II. Medication Purchasing Habits

What drug store do you use?

☐ Yes ☐ No   Does the drug store you use deliver the medications to your home? _____

If no, then how do you get your medications? _____

_____

☐ Yes ☐ No   Do you always use the same drug store? If no, explain: _____

☐ Yes ☐ No   Do financial difficulties ever prevent you from buying your medications?

III. Attitudes

☐ Excellent   How would you describe your health? _____

☐ Good   What do you see as your health needs? _____

☐ Fair   _____

☐ Poor   _____

☐ Yes ☐ No   Does taking your medications upset your daily routine? If yes, explain: _____

☐ Yes ☐ No   Do side effects from your medications upset your daily routine?

☐ Yes ☐ No   Do your medications help you?

☐ Don't Know

☐ Yes ☐ No   Do you ever share your medications with anyone else?

FIGURE 25-1. Medication assessment tool that was administered during research study.

(continued)

IV. Lifestyle Habits
TIMES PER WEEK

_____ How often do you drink coffee, tea, colas or eat chocolate?

_____ How often do you use cigarettes, snuff, or tobacco products?

_____ How often do you consume beer, wine or liquor?

_____ How often do you use recreational drugs such as marijuana?

V. Home/Environment

Who else stays at your residence? (List relationship and age) _____

_____

If someone else lives in home, does that person participate in your healthcare? _____

VI. Medication Profile

Record each medication separately on the form below: (Attach additional sheets as necessary.)

_____

(MEDICINE NAME, DOSAGE, ROUTE, EXPIRATION DATE EXACTLY AS PRINTED ON LABEL)

☐ Yes ☐ No Can you read the name, dosage, and expiration date of this medicine?

Why do you take the medication? _____

_____

How long have you taken this dosage? _____

When do you take the medicine and how many do you take? _____

_____

Do you know what the side effects are? List: _____

_____

☐ Yes ☐ No Does the medicine cause you any problems or side effects? _____

What do you do if you experience side effects? (stop the pills, call the doctor, etc.)

_____

FIGURE 25-1. _(Continued)_

administer to older adults who have varying educational levels, sensory changes, and memory deficits.

Five volunteer registered nurses enrolled in the baccalaureate nursing program at a local university were trained by the researcher to administer the instrument. Training included information on administration of the tool and on the procedures for making a home visit.

Interrater reliability, determined by percentage of agreement on items, was established by role-playing among the test administrators. Interrater reliability was established at 82% during the training session by the use of two videotaped scenarios. These videotaped scenarios gave the raters an opportunity to observe the tool being administered and to practice using it.

Test-retest reliability was determined by administering the tool to the same subjects on two occasions, one week apart, and correlating scores. Usability was established by determining how long it took to administer the tool. Administrators assessed clarity by noting on the instrument any items that seemed difficult for subjects to understand, or that had to be paraphrased. Any problems the test administrators encountered were also included in these comments.

Sample

The instrument was tested with a sample of elders who were currently being served by a southeastern home health agency. All were older than 65 years, had been admitted to a home health agency for nursing care, and met the criteria for home health services under Medicare (i.e., homebound, needing skilled care, and possessing a physician's order for treatment). The sample consisted of 20 patients newly admitted over a 7-day period. The only subjects excluded were those who did not speak English. Potential subjects were telephoned before the interview to obtain their consent to participate and to establish a convenient time for a visit. Written consent was obtained before data collection.

● RESULTS

Sample Characteristics

Data were collected from 20 elders, and test-retest reliability was determined for 14 of these subjects. A second interview was not conducted with the remaining six subjects because two were not found, two refused, one had been admitted to a skilled nursing facility, and one had discontinued all medications.

The primary respondents were the elders, but family members and spouses often took part in the interviews. Subjects had a mean age of 72. They used an average of 6.7 different prescription and nonprescription medications. The number of medications sometimes varied from the first visit to the second. Housing varied among subjects from single family homes to senior housing facilities. Most subjects had recently been discharged from a hospital. Education levels ranged from completion of fourth grade to completion of a doctoral degree, and all subjects were able to read and write English. Only one subject was disoriented.

Major Findings

Content validity of the instrument was endorsed by the panel of 10 experts, who agreed that the tool was logical and contained the necessary information. Interrater reliability was 82%, and test-retest reliability was 92%. Data collection took an average of 25 minutes on the first visit and 22.5 minutes on the second.

Administrators reported few difficulties in using the tool. Some expressed concern that the instrument did not prompt the administrator to indicate whether a person had answered a question correctly. For example, when the administrator asked about the purpose of a medication, the person's response was recorded, but there was no space for the nurse to note whether that response was correct. When the person was asked to read the prescription label, there was no way to indicate whether the person could read the entire label or just parts of it. Respondents had difficulty answering questions about managing side effects if they had not experienced any side effects from a medication. Some people had difficulty calculating lifestyle habits on a weekly basis, and felt more comfortable addressing them on a daily basis.

● DISCUSSION

Subjects used an average of 6.7 different medications. The most common OTC medications were aspirin, laxatives, and vitamins. Caffeine use was reported by all but one subject. Most used it as many as seven times per week. Nicotine was used by only one subject. Alcohol was used weekly or more by three subjects. Multiple physicians and multiple pharmacies were common among subjects.

The use of an unstructured interview to collect data worked well because nurses were able to paraphrase questions, leading subjects to give them more detailed responses. Some subjects wanted to talk about individual medicines immediately, before answering other questions, and the unstructured interview made this possible. When questioned about personal topics such as lifestyle, subjects appeared to give socially acceptable answers initially, but the unstructured format allowed for in-depth questioning to reveal more reliable answers.

Questioning subjects about each medication revealed valuable information. The greatest knowledge deficits concerning drug action, administration, and side effects were found for medications that had been prescribed during a recent hospitalization. Subjects lacked knowledge of side effects for almost all medications, even those taken for years. This section of the tool should revised to include the name of the prescriber of each medication, particularly for OTC medications.

Two items pertaining to time were unclear. On the demographic section, the item "recent hospitalization?" should be clarified to say, for example, "hospitalization within 3 months?" When questioning respondents about each individual medication, "How long have you taken this dosage?" was answered differently by several subjects on retesting. Providing choices such as "new," "less than 6 months," or "longer than 6 months" would probably reduce this discrepancy.

These results supported the usefulness of a formal instrument to assess the medication knowledge and practices of older adults. A clear and logical instrument can be used easily by home health nurses. The tool took an average of 23 minutes to administer, which could seem overwhelming to both patient and nurse when other forms also must be completed and signed. In a more appropriate use of the tool, the assessment nurse, who makes the initial patient visit, could obtain a list of current medications and verify it with the physician or family. The primary nurse could then complete the tool on the next visit and use the results as a blueprint for providing teaching and care.

Improved medication teaching is needed in the hospital when new medications are prescribed. It was noted that older adults kept teaching leaflets given to them by pharmacists. In the acute care setting, these teaching tools may prove valuable in preparing patients for discharge. Also, home health nurses must complete a thorough assessment of clients' and caregivers' medication knowledge. It cannot be assumed that because a caregiver administers the medications, he or she is knowledgeable of them. For example, one of the elders had been a patient in the same agency three times, yet the caregiver lacked knowledge about most of his medications.

REFERENCES

Ali, N. (1992). Promoting safe use of multiple medications by elderly persons. *Geriatric Nursing, 13*(3), 157–159.

Baker, H., & Napthine, R. (1994). Polypharmacy and older people: What can nurses do? *Australian Nursing Journal, 2*(1), 28–30.

Benzon, J. (1991). Approaching drug regimens with a therapeutic dose of suspicion. *Geriatric Nursing, 12*(4), 180–183.

Conn, V. (1992). Self-management of over-the-counter medications by older adults. *Public Health Nursing, 9*(1), 29–35.

Conn, V., Taylor, S., & Kelley, S. (1991). Medication regimen complexity and adherence among older adults. *Image: Journal of Nursing Scholarship, 23*(4), 231–235.

Cornish, J. (1992). Color coding patient medications. *Caring, XI* (11), 46–51.

Hahn, K., & Wietor, G. (1992). Helpful tools for medication screenings. *Geriatric Nursing, 13*(3), 160–166.

Kluckowski, J. (1992). Solving medication noncompliance in home care. *Caring, XI* (11), 34–41.

Lewis, P. (1993). Guidelines for developing questionnaires for older respondents. *Perspectives, 17*(2), 2–6.

Messner, R., & Gardner, S. (1993). Start with the medicine cabinet. *RN, 12*(1), 51–53.

Mullen, R. (1993). Noncompliance: The homecare provider's critical role. *Homecare Provider's Buyer's Guide,* Fall(11), 19–21.

Sidel, V., Beizer, J., Lisi-Fazio, D., Kleinmann, K., Wenston, J., Thomas, C., & Kelman, H. (1990). Controlled study of the impact of educational home visits by pharmacists to high-risk older patients. *Journal of Community Health, 15*(3), 163–174.

Simpson, J. (1993). Assessing elderly people: Should we all use the same scales? *Physiotherapy, 79*(12), 836–838.

Wolfe, S., & Schirm, V. (1992). Medication counseling for the elderly: Effects on knowledge and compliance after hospital discharge. *Geriatric Nursing, 13*(3), 134–138.

This article presents a cultural assessment that is concise but comprehensive. Both a cultural assessment and a documentation tool demonstrate ways to elicit a client's health care beliefs. This creates a foundation from which culturally sensitive care can be provided.

What areas should be assessed in a cultural assessment? What follow-up questions can be used to elicit additional information about cultural beliefs? How should a cultural assessment be documented? What characteristics describe effective transcultural nursing?

Narayan, M. (1996). Cultural assessment in home healthcare. *Home Healthcare Nurse*, 15(10), 664–671.

Cultural Assessment in Home Healthcare

MARY CURRY NARAYAN

Performing cultural assessment is the starting point for providing culturally competent care to patients of diverse cultures. In this article, instruction for performing a concise cultural assessment is given, and ways to elicit a client's culturally determined healthcare beliefs, values, and practices are explored. A cultural assessment documentation tool is also included.

Although influenced by education, life experience, and creative thought, culture is the lens through which we see everything. Whether patient or nurse, our views, decisions, and actions are seen through our own particular cultural lens. Our reactions to pain and illness, health-seeking behaviors, and healthcare decisions are culturally determined. "Culture is the fabric of meaning through which humans interpret their experiences and guide their actions" (Juliá, 1994, p. 2). Leininger (1995) describes culture as the learned and shared beliefs, values, and practices that are transmitted intergenerationally and influence one's thinking and action. Because culture plays such a crucial role in how a client feels about and manages a health problem, it is vital that home care nurses assess the client's cultural beliefs, values, and practices (Andrews & Boyle, 1995). To provide holistic care, the home care nurse must assess the patient physically, psychosocially, spiritually, and culturally.

Nurses used to be told to "treat all patients alike." Color, creed, or socioeconomic status were not to affect the assessment or interventions. This "culture blindness" led to congruent care that "felt right" to those who shared a similar cultural background with the nurse. However, patients who came from a different cultural background frequently felt misunderstood, "out of sync," alienated, and in conflict with the healthcare provider (Leininger, 1991; Germain, 1992). This cultural dissonance frequently leaves patients

Mary Narayan, MSN, CNS, RN, is a specialty nurse and nurse coordinator with Inova VNA Home Health, Springfield, VA.

without the benefit of a therapeutic relationship and without an understanding of why they were supposed to do what they were told to do.

Nurses may erroneously label these patients as "noncompliant," not realizing the patients were complying with their valued cultural beliefs. Campinha-Bacote (1994) states that when the patient is noncompliant, the problem is not so much with the client as with the provider. It is the provider who is responsible for developing a mutually agreeable plan based on an understanding of the problem from the client's culturally determined perspective. In this way, culturally competent care can facilitate adherence to the therapeutic regime.

Culturally competent care is an important and critical standard of care. The Joint Commission on Accreditation of Health Care Organizations has stated that "the impact of the person's culture is an important component of the assessment process . . ." (JCAHO, 1994, p. 88). In *Position Statement on Cultural Diversity in Nursing Practice,* the American Nurses Association (1991) stated:

> Ethnocentric (see footnote 1 on p. 204) approaches to nursing practice are ineffective in meeting the health and nursing needs of diverse cultural groups of clients. Knowledge about cultures and their impact on interactions with healthcare is essential. . . . (p. 1).

As Meleis (1995), a nursing theorist and leader, has said

> Providing care that is culturally competent care is no longer a luxury; it is a necessity that is being demanded by patients and by those who act as advocates for patients in both hospital and community settings (Meleis, 1996, p. 1).

As we enter the 21st Century, American nurses (see footnote 2 on p. 204) will care for more and more patients who have different cultural values and norms. According to the U.S. Census Bureau, minority populations are growing. We are truly a multicultural nation. Although diversity is America's strength, this diversity presents a challenge for nurses in providing care to meet the cultural needs of all clients.

● CULTURAL ASSESSMENT

The cultural assessment is the point at which the home healthcare nurse can begin to meet the challenge of providing care to meet the clients' diverse cultural needs.

> Cultural assessments elicit beliefs, values, and practices that are relevant to health behaviors. They are performed to identify patterns that may assist or interfere with a nursing intervention or planned treatment regimen (Tripp-Reimer, Brink, & Saunders, 1984, p. 78).

Multiple cultural assessment tools have been developed by nurse-anthropologists and nurses interested in transcultural nursing care. Andrews and Boyle's (1995) *Transcultural Nursing Assessment Guide,* Bloch's (1983) *Assessment Guide for Ethnic/Cultural Variations,* Fong's (1985) *CONFHER Model for Cultural Assessment,* Giger and Davidhizar's (1991) *Six Cultural Variables Assessment,* Leininger's (1991) *Acculturation Health Care Assessment Tool for Cultural Patterns in Traditional and Non-Traditional Lifeways,* Spector's (1996) *Heritage Assessment Tool,* and Tripp-Reimer's (1985) *Cultural Assessment* are among the cultural assessment tools available in the nursing literature.

Sidebar Footnotes

[1]Ethnocentrism is the belief that one's own culture is superior to others and is the norm against which other cultures should be measured. Conversely, ethnorelativism is the belief that all cultures are equally valid and equally deserving of respect (Eliason, 1993). When providing patient care cultural relativism is considered "best practice."

[2]American nurses are primarily of European heritage and have been socialized through their nursing education to the Western biomedical perspective on health and illness (Andrews & Boyle 1995).

[3]Kleinman's Exlanatory Model Interview is grounded on the medical model. It seeks to understand the patient's explanation of the diagnosis, etiology, course, treatment, and prognosis of the health problem. Because it is based on the medical model, some nurses have criticized it as being "illness-oriented with limited value in chronic illness, health promotion and illness prevention, or with patients whose health cultural orientation leads to the expectation they will be told by, rather than tell, the healthcare provider what is wrong with them" (DeSantis 1994, p. 710). Yet, according to Dougherty & Tripp-Reimer (1990), although disease (the biomedical understanding of the problem and the purview of physicians) is not the domain of nursing, nurses are concerned with illness (the patient's lived experience of and response to the disease). Furthermore, by changing the word "illness" to "health problem," the questions lend themselves to addressing chronic illness, health promotion, and illness prevention. The Explanatory Model Interview assists nursing in discovering the patient's illness experience and response to health problems. Many nurses find the Explanatory Model Interview to be among the easiest ways of obtaining the most culturally relevant assessment data in the shortest amount of time.

[4]"Cold" and "hot" foods do not refer to temperature. Instead, this is a culturally defined food characteristic. There may be variations from one culture to another in how this food characteristic is defined. The same foods that are considered to be hot in one culture can be considered to be cold in another culture.

However, the busy home healthcare nurse rarely has the time to go into the depth these tools require. As Lipson and Meleis (1985) state, "Although most assessment guides are quite comprehensive, there may be neither time nor need to gather data on all the suggested topics" (p. 50). Other nurse-anthropologists agree (Tripp-Reimer, Brink, and Saunders, 1984; DeSantis, 1994).

Figure 26-1 presents a concise, yet comprehensive, assessment checklist of cultural variables that often influence the perspective of home care patients. By spending some extra time performing the cultural assessment initially, the nurse is likely to develop a culturally congruent plan that is agreeable to the client. This care plan can reach desired outcomes more efficiently and effectively than one that is not.

To complete a cultural assessment using the guide in Figure 26-1, the nurse needs two resources and several extra minutes during the assessment process. The first resource is the client and the client's family, who are the experts on how their culture affects their health beliefs, values, and practices (Lipson & Meleis, 1985). The second resource is a reference guide to various cultures. One excellent resource is Lipson, Dibble, and Minarik's (1996) *Culture & Nursing Care: A Pocket Guide,* which contains information about 24 different ethnic cultures frequently encountered by American nurses in their practice.

Patient Identified Cultural/Ethnic Group

Religion

Etiquette and Social Customs

- ✔ **Typical greeting.** Form of address? Handshake appropriate? Shoes worn in home?
- ✔ **Social customs before "business."** Social exchanges? Refreshment?
- ✔ **Direct or indirect communication patterns**

Nonverbal Patterns of Communication

- ✔ **Eye contact.** Is eye contact considered polite or rude?
- ✔ **Tone of voice.** What does a soft voice or a loud voice mean in this culture?
- ✔ **Personal space.** Is personal space wider or narrower than in the American culture?
- ✔ **Facial expressions, gestures.** What do smiles, nods and hand gestures mean?
- ✔ **Touch.** When, where and by whom can a patient be touched?

Client's Explanation of Problem

- ✔ **Diagnosis.** What do you call this illness? How would you describe this problem?
- ✔ **Onset.** When did the problem start? Why then? What started the problem?
- ✔ **Cause.** What caused the problem? What might other people think is wrong with you?
- ✔ **Course.** How does the illness work? What does it do to you?
  What do you fear most about this problem?
- ✔ **Treatment.** How have you treated the illness? What treatment should you receive?
  Who in your family or community can help you? Traditional practitioners?
- ✔ **Prognosis.** How long will the problem last? Is it serious?
- ✔ **Expectations.** What are you hoping the nurses will do for you when we come?

Nutrition Assessment

- ✔ **Pattern of meals:** What is eaten? When are meals eaten?
- ✔ **Sick foods**
- ✔ **Food intolerance and taboos**

Pain Assessment

- ✔ **Cultural patterns to pain**
- ✔ **Patient's perception of pain response**

Medication Assessment

- ✔ **Patient's perception of "western" medications**
- ✔ **Possible pharmacogenetic variations**

Psychosocial Assessment

- ✔ **Decision maker**
- ✔ **Sick role**
- ✔ **Language barriers, translators**
- ✔ **Cultural/ethnic community resources**

FIGURE 26-1. Cultural assessment checklist.

Social Etiquette and Nonverbal Patterns of Communication

The cultural resource guide can be used to gain background information about the culture's etiquette rules and can assist in establishing rapport even before the first visit. What are the social customs usually practiced when visiting a person of this culture? (Are shoes typically removed before entering the home? Should a small amount of "refreshment" be accepted?) What are the nonverbal communication patterns? (Is eye contact considered polite or rude behavior? Is touch valued? Are there taboos about where or by whom a person can be touched? Is personal space wider or narrower than that typically used by Americans?)

Client's Understanding of Problem

Cultural resource guides can sensitize a nurse to the many cultural beliefs, values, and practices that may influence a client's health behaviors. However, these guides cannot indicate what we need to know: how culture affects this particular client's healthcare decisions and practices. Each individual is a unique blend of multiple subcultures (ethnic, religious, socioeconomic, occupational, geographic, age and sex), education, acculturation, and creative thinking. Although focusing on the client's ethnic group and its beliefs, values, and practices is helpful, understanding the client's unique perception of the health problem is paramount. Kleinman, Eisenberg, & Good (1978) recommend the use of an Explanatory Model Interview (see footnote 3 on page 204). The Explanatory Interview elicits the client's explanation and understanding of the health problem from the patient's cultural perspective and experience. In its simplest form, the assessment questions are:

- What do you call this illness?
- When did it start? Why then?
- What do you think caused it?
- How does the illness work? What does it do to you?
- How have you treated the illness? How should it be treated? By whom?
- How long will it last? Is it serious?

According to Buchwald et al. (1994), approaching these questions with a conversational approach can be more effective than a direct approach. One nondirect technique is to ask the client what another family member thinks is causing the problem or how the client's mother would treat the problem. Often, the client is more likely to reveal the cultural perspective of the problem when the explanation can be ascribed to another, especially when it is feared that the nurse may be scornful of the client's cultural beliefs and practices. Another piece of valuable information is to determine what the client expects of the nurse and the nursing visits.

The client feels "heard" and that his or her perceptions are valued by the nurse when these questions are asked. Because the client believes that the nurse truly understands the problem, the client is able to place trust in the nurse's recommendations. With this information, the nurse can develop a mutually agreeable care plan, congruent with the client's culturally determined understanding of and goals for the health problems.

However, there is still other cultural information that is essential to a good nursing assessment. According to Campinha-Bacote (1995), much of the cultural assessment should be embedded in assessment and history taking. Biologic, psychologic, and sociologic variations that are based on ethnicity should be incorporated into the systems and psychosocial assessments. Parts of the cultural assessment that can be embedded in the traditional nursing history include cultural aspects related to the nutrition, pain, medication, and psychosocial assessments.

Nutrition Assessment

When and what is eaten is culturally determined. A 2-day dietary recall, as part of the nutrition assessment, may be helpful in determining the cultural aspects of the patient's diet. The American pattern of three meals daily may not be shared by clients of diverse cultures. The types of foods Americans eat for breakfast, lunch, and dinner may vary from those that our patients eat. Many patients of Asian, African, and Middle Eastern origin are prone to lactose intolerance.

Certain foods are taboo to some cultures. Pork, beef, and meat are some of the foods that are not eaten by some cultural groups. The nurse can determine whether there are any food taboos or intolerance by asking, "Are there any foods you cannot eat?" In some cultures, it is important to balance foods with the type of condition—a cold food is paired with a hot condition (see footnote 4 on p. 204). Foods that are eaten when a person is sick, such as chicken soup, also vary from culture to culture. Therefore, the nurse might also ask, "Are there any foods that should be eaten by a person with your health problem?" With this information, the nurse can provide culturally acceptable diet education.

Pain Assessment

When a patient seeks pain treatment, how pain is expressed and what types of treatments the patient believes one should receive also are culturally determined. Unfortunately, because cultural information about appropriate pain response is transmitted through a cultural group implicitly, rather than explicitly, the client is not able to verbalize the answers to questions such as, "Do you prefer to cope with pain stoically or expressively?" It is here that the cultural resource guide can also be helpful. For instance, Lipson, Dibble, and Minarik's (1996) *Culture & Nursing Care: A Pocket Guide* describes pain response patterns for the 24 ethnic cultures frequently seen by American nurses. By consulting such a reference, the nurse can be aware of how the client might respond and can intervene appropriately and quickly. To gain insight into the patient's pain response, the nurse may also ask questions such as, "When was the last time you had severe pain? What caused it? What did you do to relieve the pain?"

Medication Assessment

Because of genetic variations in drug metabolic pathways and protein-binding capacities, different racial/ethnic groups may react differently to medications than the reactions depicted in our drug reference books. In the relatively new field of ethnopharmacology, discoveries have been made that require the nurse's attention. "Pharmacogenetic research in the last 15 years has uncovered significant differences among racial and ethnic groups in the metabolism, clinical effectiveness and side effects of important medicines" (Levy, 1993). In the initial medication assessment, the nurse should ask questions about the client's medication history. "Do the medications the physician prescribes work well for you? Are they too strong? Do they seem to cause problems?" Answers to these questions may indicate important genetic variations. Similarly, with each follow-up medication assessment, the nurse should be vigilant in identifying indications of pharmacogenetic variation.

Psychosocial Assessment

In addition to the standard psychosocial questions, there are four important topics nurses should consider when assessing clients from diverse cultures:

1. Who is the "decision maker" in the family?
2. What are the characteristics of the "sick role" in the client's culture?
3. Are there language barriers?
4. What are the resources available from the client's cultural community?

Decision Maker. In the American and Western biomedical cultures, the person who usually makes the decisions about the patient's healthcare is the patient. Most Americans would say that they value independence and autonomy. However, many other cultures value interdependence, which is characterized by hierarchical or cooperative decision making. In hierarchical decision making, decisions are made by the head of the household, usually the eldest male in a patriarchal household and the eldest female in a matriarchal household. Other cultural groups may make health decisions consensually as a family or a group. It is important to include the decision maker in any health teaching or intervention. Background information about family structure and decision making is usually included in cultural reference guides. Still, the best source for this information is the client and the client's family. Frequently, this information can be obtained by asking questions such as, "Who will help you decide what to do about this problem? Who will help you with this problem?"

Sick Role Behavior. In the American culture, self-reliance, self-care, and achievement are highly valued. However, people from other cultures often expect that the sick person will be "cared for" by other members of the family for much longer periods than we might believe, from our cultural perspective, is appropriate. When sick or disabled, it may be culturally appropriate for the patient to rest while other family members meet the patient's needs. Self-care and rehabilitation may be foreign concepts (Hoeman, 1989). Therefore, it may be appropriate to ask the patient questions such as, "How will this problem affect your ability to do your usual activities? Who will help you? How will they help you?"

Language Barriers. When the client does not speak English, the nurse should determine whether the patient speaks any other languages. Perhaps the client and the nurse share a second language. For instance, a Vietnamese patient may speak French, a language the nurse might speak or for which an interpreter may more easily be found. Are there family members who can serve as translators? When are they available? How can they be contacted? When English is a second language, the nurse should assess the client's ability to speak and read English. Printed materials may be at a level that is too challenging for the client.

Community Resources. In areas where there is a sizable population of a particular ethnic or religious group, there may be community or religious organizations that provide helpful services. These services may include the assistance of interpreters or community liaisons who might provide help when needed.

● PLANNING NURSING CARE

To remember the multiple variables that may influence a client's healthcare, the nurse can use the cultural assessment outline presented in Figure 26-1 as a guide for completing a cultural assessment documentation form as presented in Figure 26-2. The Cultural

Cultural Assessment

Patient _____ Patient Number _____ Team _____

Cultural/Ethnic Identity _____ Religion _____

Etiquette and Social Customs _____
_____

Nonverbal Communication Patterns _____
_____

Client's Explanation of Health Problem _____
_____
_____
_____

Traditional Treatments/Healers _____
_____

Expectations of Nurse/Care Providers _____
_____

Pain Assessment

Cultural Patterns/Patient's Perception of Pain Response _____
_____

Nutrition Assessment

Meal patterns _____
_____

Sick foods _____
_____

Food Intolerances/Taboos _____
_____

Medication Assessment

Patient's Perceptions of Medications _____
_____

Possible Pharmacogenetic Variations _____
_____

Psychosocial Assessment

Family Structure and Decision-making Patterns _____
_____

Sick Role Behavior _____
_____

Language Barriers and Resources _____
_____

Cultural/Ethnic/Religious Resources/Supportive Systems _____

FIGURE 26-2. Cultural assessment form.

Assessment documentation form can become part of the client's permanent record. Once cultural information is assessed and documented, the home care nurse can develop a nursing care plan that is mutually agreeable, culturally acceptable, and potentially capable of producing positive outcomes. "Only when a nurse recognizes and respects a client's cultural values can the basic rapport necessary for successful teaching occur" (Spruhan, 1996, p. 449). The nurse can involve the client in identifying sources of potential conflict between cultural practices and the biomedical treatment plan.

Leininger (1988) suggests that decisions about planning care can be made using a maintain-preserve, accommodate-negotiate, and restructure-repattern framework. Using this framework, the nurse structures the cultural assessment data (beliefs, values, and practices) into three categories:

1. those that are helpful to the treatment plan and should be preserved;
2. those that are neither helpful nor harmful, but can be incorporated in the nursing care plan; and
3. those practices that are harmful and should be repatterned to a health-enhancing, but culturally acceptable, practice.

By incorporating helpful or neutral cultural practices into the care plan, the nurse gains the client's trust and increases the likelihood that the patient will adhere to the treatment plan. However, it is the nurse's role to provide to the client information and options from which the client can choose the beliefs, values, and practices with which he or she is comfortable.

● SUMMARY

As the nurse becomes adept at performing cultural assessments and culturally competent care, it will become clear that "although it is critical to conduct a cultural assessment with culturally and ethnically diverse groups, it is also important to realize that every client needs a cultural assessment. Every client has values, beliefs, and practices that must be considered when a clinician renders healthcare services. Therefore, cultural assessments are not limited to specific ethnic groups, but rather should be conducted on each individual" (Campinha-Bacote, 1995, p. 148).

Nurses who have been identified as good transcultural nurses have been found to be empathetic, caring, open, and flexible. They have a positive attitude toward cultural differences and have a genuine interest in learning from the client about the client's culture (Emerson, 1995). Talabere (1996) states that openness, appreciation of another's perspective, holistic communication, genuine interest, and a nonjudgmental attitude are central to cultural sensitivity. When a culturally sensitive nurse develops mutually agreeable goals with a patient from another culture, a kind of cultural synergy occurs, resulting in care that is "meaningful, satisfying and beneficial to clients" (Leininger, 1988, p.155).

● ACKNOWLEDGMENT

The author thanks Rita L. Ailinger, PhD, RN, College of Nursing and Health Science of George Mason University, Fairfax, Virginia, for reviewing this manuscript.

REFERENCES

American Nurses Association. (1991). *Position statement on cultural diversity in nursing practice.* Washington, DC: Author.

Andrews M., & Boyle, J. (1995). *Transcultural concepts in nursing care.* Philadelphia: Lippincott-Raven Publishers.

Bloch, B. (1983). Bloch's assessment guide for ethnic/culture variations. In M. S. Orque & B. Bloch (Eds.), *Ethnic nursing care: A multi-cultural approach* (pp. 49–75). St. Louis: Mosby.

Buchwald, D., Caralis, P., Gany, F., Hardt, E., Johnson, T., Mueche, M., & Putsch, R. (1994). Caring for patients in a multicultural society. *Patient Care, 28*(11), 105–123.

Campinha-Bacote, J. (1994). *The process of cultural competence in health care: A culturally competent model of care.* Wyoming, OH: Transcultural C.A.R.E. Associates.

Campinha-Bacote, J. (1995). The quest for cultural competence in nursing care. *Nursing Forum, 30*(4), 147–153.

Desantis, L. (1994). Making anthropology clinically relevant to nursing care. *Journal of Advanced Nursing, 20,* 707–715.

Dougherty, M., & Tripp-Reimer, T. (1990). Nursing and anthropology. In T. M. Johnson & C. F. Sargent (Eds), *Medical anthropology: A handbook of theory and method* (pp. 174–186).

Eliason, M.J. (1993). Ethics and transcultural nursing care. *Nursing Outlook, 41,* 225–228.

Emerson, J. (1995). *Intercultural communication between community health nurses and ethnic-minority clients.* (Doctoral Dissertation). Fairfax, VA: George Mason University.

Fong, C.M. (1985). Ethnicity and nursing practice. *Topics in Clinical Nursing, 7*(3), 1–10.

Germain, C. P. (1992). Cultural care: A bridge between sickness, illness, and disease. *Holistic Nursing Practice, 6*(3), 1–9.

Giger, J.N., & Davidhizar, R.E. (1991). *Transcultural nursing: Assessment and intervention.* St. Louis: Mosby.

Hoeman, S.P. (1989). Cultural assessment in rehabilitation nursing practice. *Nursing Clinics of North America, 24*(1), 277–289.

Joint Commission on Accreditation of Healthcare Organizations (1994). *1995 Comprehensive accreditation manual for hospitals.* Oakbrook Terrace, IL: Author.

Juliá, M.C. (1994). *Multicultural awareness in the health care professions.* Needham Heights, MA: Allyn & Bacon.

Kleinman, A., Eisenberg, L., & Good, B. (1978). Culture, illness and care: Clinical lessons from anthropologic and cross-cultural research. *Annals of Internal Medicine, 88,* 251–258.

Leininger, M.M. (1988). Leininger's theory of nursing: Cultural care diversity and universality. *Nursing Science Quarterly, 1*(4), 152–160.

Leininger, M. (1991). Leininger's acculturation health care assessment tool for cultural patterns in traditional and non-traditional lifeways. *Journal of Transcultural Nursing, 2*(2), 40–42.

Leininger, M. (1995). *Transcultural nursing: Concepts, theories, research & practices.* New York: McGraw-Hill.

Levy, R.A. (1993). Ethnic and racial differences in response to medicines: Preserving individualized therapy in managed pharmaceutical programmes. *Pharmaceutical Medicine, 7,* 139–165.

Lipson, J.G., Dibble, S.L., & Minarik, P.A. (Eds.). (1996). *Culture & nursing care: A pocket guide.* San Francisco: UCSF Nursing Press.

Lipson, J. & Meleis, A. (1985). Culturally appropriate care: the case of immigrants. *Topics in Clinical Nursing, 7*(3), 48–46.

Meleis, A. I. (1996). Culturally competent scholarship: Substance and rigor. *Advances in Nursing Science, 19*(2), 1–16.

Spector, R.E. (1996). *Cultural diversity in health and illness.* Stamford, CT: Appleton & Lange.

Spruhan, J.B. (1996). Beyond traditional nursing care: Cultural awareness and successful home healthcare nursing. *Home Healthcare Nurse, 14*(6), 445–449.

Talabere, L.R. (1996). Meeting the challenge of culture care in nursing: Diversity, sensitivity, competence, and congruence. *Journal of Cultural Diversity, 3*(2), 53–61.

Tripp-Reimer, T., Brink, P.J., Saunders, J.M. (1984). Cultural assessment: Content and process. *Nursing Outlook, 32*(2), 72–82.

Tripp-Reimer, T. (1985). Cultural assessment. In J. Bellack & P. Bamford (Eds.), *Nursing assessment.* North Scituate, MA: Duxbury Press.

This environmental assessment uses Maslow's Hierarchy of Needs as a framework. Assessment of the client's surroundings is essential to make care safe and therapeutic.

Why do an environmental assessment? What are the standard elements? How is the information from the assessment used to plan care?

Narayan, M., & Tennant, J. (1997). Environmental assessment. *Home Healthcare Nurse*, 15(11), 799–805.

Environmental Assessment

MARY CURRY NARAYAN, JULIE TENNANT

The significance, standard elements, components, and documentation of an environmental assessment in home care are discussed. This assessment is delineated within Maslow's Hierarchy of Needs and from a functional perspective. An Environmental Assessment Form that can be used as a documentation tool is included.

● SIGNIFICANCE OF ENVIRONMENTAL ASSESSMENT

Madeleine Mazar is a 72-year-old insulin-dependent diabetic who lives alone in an apartment building. While hurrying to answer the phone yesterday, she tripped when her cane became caught on the edge of the carpet. She fell, breaking her right arm. When sending her home, the emergency room physician, worried about her ability to manage her diabetes with her new disability, made a referral to a home care agency.

John Murphy, 84 years old, had a stroke 2 months ago. After 2 weeks in the hospital and several weeks at an extended care facility, he has just arrived home. Although his wife was very anxious to have him home, she is now in tears as she opens the door for the home care admissions nurse. Mr. Murphy has just been incontinent while trying to negotiate his walker up a step and into the bathroom.

The home care nurses seeing Ms. Mazar and Mr. Murphy need a broad range of assessment skills. One of these skills, with limited use in an institutional setting but of utmost importance when nursing in the community, is the ability to assess the environment. Most new home care patients on being discharged from the hospital find that their homes are not as comfortable or "easy" as they remember. Illness, disability, fatigue, and weakness place new demands on the patient in the home. That home, which had always offered comfort and security, is now filled with obstacles and hazards. Yet, as home care nurses we believe that the patient's home, surrounded by people, things, and routines that give life meaning, is the most therapeutic environment. The challenge then is to adapt this environment, making it safe and therapeutic for the patient.

Mary Curry Narayan, MSN, CNS, RN, is a member of The Extended Hours Team, Inova VNA Home Health, Springfield, VA.

Julie Tennant, MEd, RN, is the manager of The Extended Hours Team, Inova VNA Home Health, Springfield, VA.

Home care nurses assist patients in meeting their optimal health goals. These goals can be either enhanced or inhibited by the patient's home environment. There should be a match between the patient's abilities and the demands placed on the individual by the environment (Letts, 1994). Assessment of the patient's surroundings is crucial in determining a care plan to meet the patient's health goals. As the nurse makes the assessment, she asks: Does this environment meet the patient's needs? Does it keep the patient safe? Does it promote a sense of well-being in the patient? After assessing the patient's surroundings, the nurse can implement teaching and interventions that will create a safe home environment meeting the patient's needs and maximizing the quality of the patient's life.

Lange (1996) reported that environments that appear safe for fully functioning individuals can be filled with hazards for the frail and the old. Aging decreases visual acuity, sensory awareness, and muscle strength. Side effects of medications are dizziness and confusion putting patients at high risk for accidents and falls. Accidents are the fifth leading cause of death in individuals 65 years of age and older (Lange, 1996). Sadly, the fear of falling causes many older individuals to restrict their activities, decreasing their quality of life.

Environmental assessment takes on added urgency when a patient such as Ms. Mazar is living alone. Without a caregiver, there must be an appropriate fit between the environment and the patient's abilities. Homes with stairs and bathrooms on different levels pose challenges to patients such as Mr. Murphy.

● IMPORTANCE OF ENVIRONMENTAL ASSESSMENT DOCUMENTATION

Standards guiding home healthcare are clearly stated by such accrediting agencies as the Joint Commission on Accreditation of Healthcare Organizations (JCAHO) and by such regulatory bodies as the Health Care Financing Administration (HCFA) in the text of the *Federal Register* (1991). JCAHO requires any organization it accredits to have policies and procedures for initial and ongoing assessments of safety in the home setting. The safety assessment must include a home assessment consisting of attention to fire response, electrical safety, environmental and mobility safety, bathroom safety and medication safety (JCAHO, 1997). It also requires a safety review of medical equipment in the home, a safety evaluation of the storage and handling of supplies and medications, and a review of identification, handling, and disposal of hazardous materials and wastes in a manner consistent with law and regulation.

In its *Interpretative Guidelines for the Conditions of Participation,* The Department of Health & Human Services, Health Care Financing Administration (1996) requires attention to client safety in more than one area. It calls for the plan of treatment to include safety measures to protect against injury. HCFA also requires the home care nurse to document information about the patient's living environment that might detract from the home healthcare agency's ability to implement or complete the plan of care.

● STANDARD ELEMENTS OF ENVIRONMENTAL ASSESSMENT

The Nurse Is a Guest

The nurse–client relationship is built on respect, and this respect must extend to the patient's environment if the nurse is to establish a therapeutic relationship. The nurse must be very aware that she is a guest in the patient's home. Homes and belongings are cherished. The nurse is a consultant, assessing the locations of shortcomings in the environment and offering suggestions for adaptation.

Patient's Hierarchy of Needs

There are many guides and recommendations for performing a comprehensive environmental assessment (Humphrey, 1994; Hyer, 1996; McClelland, Thompson, Pretz, & Hatcher, 1996). One helpful way to assess the patient's environment involves looking at the home in terms of Maslow's Hierarchy of Needs (Maslow, 1954; Hogstel, 1985). Does the patient's environment meet the patient's physiologic and survival needs? Does it meet the patient's needs for safety and security? For love and belonging? For self-esteem and self-actualization? As the pyramid of needs is ascended, the patient's needs move into the psychosocial realm and are less in the strictly physical environment. Yet the physical environment can either promote or inhibit the patient's psychosocial well-being.

The patient's activities of daily living (ADL) and instrumental activities of daily living (IADL) are components of the pyramid that assist in assuring that the environment meets the patient's needs (see Fig. 27-1). During the initial assessment, have the patient "walk through" the ADL either physically or through visualization to see the physical barriers

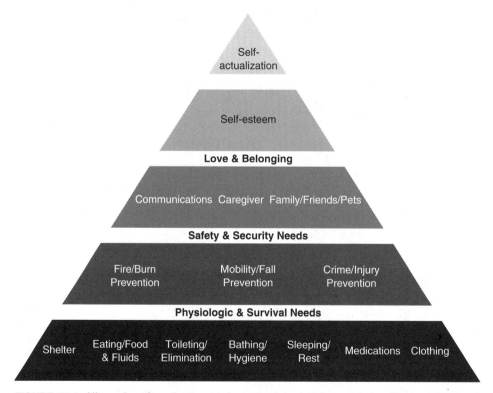

FIGURE 27-1. Hierarchy of environmental needs. Adapted from *Motivation and Personality,* by A.H. Maslow, 1954, New York: Harper & Row.

and hazards the patient will encounter (Robbins, Armstrong, York, Brown, & Swank, 1991).

Nurse Safety

Unfortunately, in today's world, nurses must also assess the environment for their own safety and the safety of all visiting staff. JCAHO (1997) standards and Occupational Safety and Health Administration (1996) regulations demand safe environments for employees. Thobaben (1996) stated, "It is the agency's responsibility to ensure that potentially dangerous environmental conditions are noticed during the initial screening process." In the initial assessment, the nurse considers the neighborhood and the patient's home, attempting to measure the presence of risks to the agency's home care personnel. Is this a high crime area? Is parking far from the door? What is this neighborhood like at night and in the early morning hours? Are there aggressive and dangerous pets? Do firearms and weapons exist in the home of a patient with a history of violent behavior or mental illness with aggressive and irrational tendencies? Can a plan be created to offset the dangers of the environment? Hunter (1997) provided an excellent tool to assist the nurse in determining the potential for violence. Despite the nursing tradition of providing care to all, nurses have an obligation to themselves and their colleagues to determine if this environment is too dangerous for the provision of home care services.

● COMPONENTS OF ENVIRONMENTAL ASSESSMENT

As the nurse "walks through" the patient's environment, a complete assessment is assured by using an environmental assessment documentation form. The checklist in Figure 27-2 addresses each of the ADL as a brick within Maslow's Hierarchy of Needs. Such a checklist of questions pertaining to each of the "bricks" can guide the new home care nurse until the environmental assessment becomes easy and natural (see Fig. 27-3).

Conclusion of Case Studies

When the nurse assessed Ms. Mazar's home, she discovered many shortcomings in the patient's home environment. There were safety concerns about uneven floor surfaces, a torn and frayed carpet, a single telephone at the farthest corner of the patient's apartment, and the burned-out light bulbs in the hallway leaving it very dark. Ms. Mazar is right-handed and therefore had trouble drawing up her insulin, using her cane to ambulate steadily, and preparing her meals. The nurse discovered that the patient had little food in the home and did not have a plan for obtaining groceries. Referrals were made for occupational therapy, social work, and a home health aide. While awaiting professional intervention, Ms. Mazar was assisted by a neighbor who agreed to help.

Mr. Murphy had gone straight to his study on returning to his home. The nurse discovered that the study was removed from the main part of the house. She suggested that Mr. Murphy's family set up a space for Mr. Murphy in the sunny family room right off the kitchen and downstairs bathroom. Mr. Murphy's son then brought the books and papers his father needed from the study to the family room. On the Environmental Assessment Checklist, the nurse also noted that the commode seat was quite low and recommended a raised seat and a pullbar. The nurse showed the family how Mr. Murphy's energy could be conserved by having items within easy reach.

Environmental Assessment Checklist

Patient _____ Patient Number _____ Team/Person Completing Form _____

Date and initial as each assessment area is addressed. Describe unsafe/unmet needs. Suggest modifications.

Assessment Areas	Safe/Meets Client's Needs	Unsafe/Needs Adaptation	Recommended Modifications and Possible Referral
Physiologic and Survival Needs Food/Fluids/Eating			
Elimination/Toileting			
Hygiene/Bathing/Grooming			
Clothing/Dressing			
Rest/Sleeping			
Medications			
Shelter			
Safety and Security Mobility and Fall Prevention			
Fire/Burn Prevention			
Crime/Injury Prevention			
Love and Belonging Caregiver			
Communication			
Family/Friends/Pets			
Self-Esteem, Self-Actualization Enjoyable/Meaningful Activities			

FIGURE 27-2. Environmental assessment checklist (see Figure 27-3 for questions for each category).

Questions To Complete: Environmental Assessment Checklist

Physiologic and Survival Needs
Food and Fluids/Eating
What does the patient plan to eat? Drink? Who will prepare the food?
Is there food in the home? Who will do the grocery shopping?
Is the food properly stored? Does the refrigerator work?
Is there drinkable water?
Does the kitchen have barriers to the patients actually preparing the food?
Are the pathways clear? Can the items be reached? Are there clean dishes?

Elimination/Toileting
Can the patient get to the bathroom? Is the pathway clear? Is a bedside commode indicated?
Do assistive devices (wheelchairs, walkers) fit through the doorways and can the patient turn?
Will the patient have a hard time getting up and down from the commode? Would a raised toilet seat help? Grab bars? (Towel racks, if used for steadying, can pull away from the wall.)
Will the patient be able to wash hands? Able to turn water off and on?

Hygiene/Bathing/Grooming
What is the plan for bathing? Bathtub? Shower? Shower chair? At the sink? Requires help?
Is there hot and cold running water? Is the water temperature 120° or less?
Are there grab bars next to the tub and shower?
Are there nonskid tiles/strips/appliques/rubber mats on tub bottom and shower floor?
Are the bathroom and fixtures clean?
What provisions are there for mouth care? Hair care?

Clothing/Dressing
Does the patient have shoes or slippers which are easy to put on, fit properly with nonskid soles?
Will the patient be able to change clothes?
Are the clothes so baggy that they could trip the patient?
Are there clean clothes? How will the laundry be washed?

Rest/Sleeping
Where will the patient sleep? Would the patient benefit from a hospital bed? A trapeze?
How far is the bed from the floor? Can the patient get in and out of the bed?
How much time will the patient spend in bed? Does the patient need a special mattress?
How far is the bed from the bathroom? From other family members?

Medications
Does the patient have a plan for taking the right medications at the right time?
Is there a secure place to store the medications? Are they safe from children and the cognitively impaired?
Can the patient reach the medications needed? Open the container? Read the label?
Is there adequate lighting where the patient will be preparing medications?
Is there a safe way to dispose of syringes? Medical supplies?

Shelter
Is the house clean and comfortable for the patient? Who will do the housework?
Are the plumbing and sewage systems working?
Is there a safe heat source? Are space heaters safe? Are the electrical cords in good condition?
Is there adequate ventilation?
Is the house infested with roaches, other insects, or rodents?

Safety and Security
Mobility/Fall Prevention
Is the patient able to get around the home? Does the patient have good balance? Steady gait?
Is the caregiver thinking of using restraints? What sort of restraints? Are they necessary?

Figure 27-3. Environmental assessment questions to complete.

(continued)

Does the patient use assistive devices (walkers, canes) correctly? Are they the right height?
Do the devices fit through the pathways without catching on furnishings?
Are the pathways, hallways and stairways clear? Are there throw rugs?
Are there sturdy handrails on the stairs? Are the first and last steps clearly marked?
Is there adequate lighting in hallways and stairways? Is the path to the bathroom
well-lighted at night?
Are the floors slippery? (Floors should not have a high gloss or be highly waxed.)
Are there uneven floor surfaces?
Are the carpets in good repair without buckles or tears that could cause tripping?
Can the patient walk steadily on the carpets? (Thick pile carpets can cause tripping if the patient
has a shuffling gait.)
Are the chairs the patient uses sturdy? Are they stable if the patient uses them to prevent a fall?
Does the patient use furniture or counters for balance when walking? Are these sturdy enough
to withstand the pressure?
Are there cords or wires that could cause the patient to trip?

Fire/Burn Prevention
Is there a smoke detector on each level of the home? Is there a fire extinguisher?
Is there an escape plan for the patient to get out of the house in case of fire?
Is the patient using heating pads and space heaters safely?
Are wires and plugs in good repair?
If the patient smokes, are there plans to make sure the patient smokes safely?
Are there signs of cigarette burns? Burns in the kitchen?
Are oxygen tanks stored away from flames and heat sources?

Crime/Injury Prevention
Are there locks on the doors and the windows?
Can the patient make an emergency call? Is the telephone handy? Are emergency numbers
clearly marked?
Are firearms securely stored in a locked box? Is the ammunition stored and locked away
separately?
Is there evidence of criminal activity?

Love and Belonging
Caregiver
Is there a caregiver? Is the caregiver competent? Willing? Supportive?
Does the caregiver need support?
Can the caregiver hear the patient? Should there be an intercom? "Baby Monitor?" Handbell?

Communication
Is the telephone within easy reach of the patient?
Should the telephone have an illuminated dial? Oversized numbers? Memory feature? Audio
enhancer?
Are needed numbers clearly marked? Police? Fire? Ambulance? Nurse? Doctor? Relatives?
Neighbors?
Is there a daily safety check system? Should there be an alert system like Lifeline?
How will the patient obtain mail?

Family/Friends/Pets
Are the neighbors supportive?
Does the patient have family, friends, church/synagogue members to help and visit?
Is the patient able to take proper care of any pets? Are pets well-behaved?

Self-Esteem and Self-Actualization
Are there meaningful activities the patient can do? Listening to music/book tapes? Interactive
activities?
What kind of activities does the patient enjoy? Are there creative ways that these activities can
be brought to the patient?

Figure 27-3. *(Continued)*

From these cases, the importance of environmental assessment for the success of the care plan can be seen. A commonsense tool that serves as both a reminder and a form of documentation provides the nurse with structure for this assessment.

REFERENCES

Department of Health and Human Services, Health Care Financing Administration. (1996). Interpretative Guidelines for the conditions of participation. Rockville, MD: Author.

Hogstel, M.O. (1985). *Home nursing care for the elderly.* Bowie, MD: Brady Communications.

Humphrey, C.J. (1994). *Home care nursing handbook.* Gaithersburg, MD: Aspen.

Hunter, E. (1997). Violence prevention in the home health setting. *Home Healthcare Nurse, 15*(6), 403–409.

Hyer, K. (1996). Home safety assessment. *Home Health Focus, 2*(9), 70–71.

Joint Commission on Accreditation of Healthcare Organizations. (1997). *Comprehensive accreditation manual for home care.* Oakbrook, IL: Author.

Lange, M. (1996). The challenge of fall prevention in home care: A review of the literature. *Home Healthcare Nurse, 14*(3), 198–206.

Letts, L., & Marshall, L. (1995). Evaluating the validity and consistency of the SAFER tool. *Physical & Occupational Therapy in Geriatrics, 13*(4), 49–66.

Maslow, A.H. (1954). *Motivation and personality.* New York: Harper & Row.

McClelland, C., Thompson, P.A., Pretz, S.M., & Hatcher, P.A. (1996). Assessing firearm safety in inner-city homes. *N&HC: Perspectives on Community, 17*(4), 174–178.

Occupational Safety and Health Administration. (1996, March). *Violence prevention guidelines in the workplace.* Washington, DC: OSHA Publications.

Robbins, D., Armstrong, C., York, R., Brown, L., & Swank, A. (1991). Home visits for pregnant diabetic women: Environmental assessment as a basis for nursing intervention. *Clinical Nurse Specialist, 5*(1), 12–16.

Thobaben, M. (1996). A safe and healthy work environment. *Home Care Provider, 1*(2), 91–96.

Community assessment is used to determine the health status, resources, and/or needs of a group. This article provides an introduction to community assessment that may be used by all community-based practitioners.

What is community assessment? What are the advantages of community assessment? How does the nurse perform a community assessment? What are some strategies for using community assessment data to improve the quality of life and productivity in community-based settings?

Lindell, D. F. (1997). Community assessment for the home healthcare nurse. *Home Healthcare Nurse*, 15(9), 618–627.

28

Community Assessment for the Home Healthcare Nurse

DEBORAH F. LINDELL

Home health clients and their families live within the context of a community. To deliver effective care, home health nurses must understand how the community influences the health of their clients and families. This article describes a community assessment, how to incorporate it into daily practice, and suggests strategies for using the data to enhance the quality and efficiency of home healthcare.

Which agency would you call in your area to arrange home-delivered meals for a client? Which pharmacy in your area has the best price on insulin and syringes? Where is the nearest location a family can take its infant for low-cost or free immunizations? A home health nurse who seeks this type of information is performing a community assessment.

The purpose of this article is to share with the home health nurse: 1) what a community assessment is; 2) its advantages; 3) how to perform a basic community assessment; and 4) strategies for using community assessment data to improve the quality of and productivity in home healthcare.

● WHAT IS COMMUNITY ASSESSMENT?

In nursing, community assessment is a technique used to determine the health status, resources, and/or needs of a group of individuals. The approach is similar to basic nursing assessment in that the nurse collects data about the physiologic, psychologic, sociocultural, developmental, and spiritual health of the client. However, in the case of commu-

Deborah F. Lindell, MSN, RNC, is a lecturer, BSN Program, Frances Payne Bolton School of Nursing, Case Western Reserve University, Cleveland, OH.

nity assessment, the client is a group of individuals rather than a single person or family. It is noteworthy that the technique of community assessment is not unique to nursing: rather, it used by several health and social service-related professions.

● THE HOME HEALTH NURSE AND COMMUNITY ASSESSMENT

Historical Perspective

Community assessment has been a strategy of nursing intervention since the late 1800s. Lillian Wald (1915), in writing of her work at The Henry Street Settlement in New York, noted that the visiting nurses and members of the community should work together to identify ways to improve social and physical living conditions.

During the middle to latter part of this century, community health nursing as a specialty diverged along two paths: public health nurses, who practice health promotion and illness prevention in settings such as health departments and schools, and visiting nurses, who practice illness-oriented home care. The advent of Medicare-funded home health services, diagnosis-related groups, and other changes in the healthcare system led to a dramatic growth in home health nursing, whereas that of public health nursing lagged behind (Clark, 1996).

Home Health Nursing and Community Health Nursing

Today, the relationship between home health nursing and community health nursing is frequently discussed. Clark (1996) sees community health nursing as an umbrella under which several subspecialties practice, including public health, school health, occupational health, and home health nursing. Green & Driggers (1989) identified distinct differences between the roles of the home health nurse and those of community health nurse, yet stated that home health nurses should address the needs of the larger community.

The 21st century will see dramatic changes in the United States' approach to healthcare. To provide cost-effective, comprehensive, high-quality care, the healthcare system of the future will increasingly emphasize health promotion of groups rather than sick care of individuals. A modified community health nursing role is likely to emerge, reflecting a blend of the public health, home health, and acute-care nursing roles. This hybrid nurse will care for clients with all levels of health needs in various community-based settings. These settings could include private and group residences; shelters; hospice facilities; schools of all levels; senior centers; wellness facilities; and even shopping malls (personal communication, C. Lamade, 1996).

For the purposes of this article, home health nurses will be considered to be a subgroup of community health nurses. Home health nurses can use the information gained from community assessment in the care of individual clients and groups of clients with similar problems. Use of community assessment techniques will allow care to be more efficient, enhance the quality of care, and improve the level of client outcomes. Let's consider clients with ostomies. The client may know how to manage the ostomy, but does he or she know where to purchase ostomy supplies, the types of insurance the suppliers accept, the product lines carried, the timeliness of delivery, etc? Does the client know how to contact the nearest ostomy support group? Knowing this information will certainly improve care outcomes. However, productivity will also be enhanced if the information is available to all nurses at the agency to avoid duplication of effort.

Improving the Health of Individual and Family Clients

Home care clients do not exist in a vacuum. Many homebound clients, particularly the frail elderly, are highly dependent on community agencies to supply services that they are unable to provide for themselves. Often, a scenario such as that described below, develops.

A client experiences an acute illness and, on discharge from the hospital, has multiple needs related to activities of daily living (personal care activities) and instrumental activities of daily living (home maintenance activities). A referral is made to a home care agency whose staff members assist the client in meeting those needs. With excellent skilled nursing and other home health services, the client's medical condition stabilizes and he or she is ready for discharge. The client wishes to remain in his home, but the need for support will be indefinite.

Will discharge from home care be abrupt and stressful, leaving the client without resources for continuing support? Or, will the discharge from home care be smooth and coordinated, because the nurse has thorough, advance knowledge of community resources and is able to make appropriate, timely referrals?

Improving the Health of Population or Community Clients

Community assessment also has a second, broader purpose. The data collected can be analyzed to determine the overall health status of a particular population or community. A population is a group of individuals who have one or more characteristics in common. Examples of populations are listed in Column A of Table 28-1.

A community is a type of population. Clark (1996, p. 6) defines a community as a group of individuals who share some common characteristic, interact with each other, and function collectively regarding common concerns. To many people, the word community might mean a group of individuals whose boundaries are defined in geographical or political terms (e.g., a county, town, or neighborhood). However, a community can also be defined by other characteristics such as a common social or health concern or social characteristic. An excellent, yet basic example of the difference between a population and a community, emerges from school athletics. In this context, a population would be a group of students who like to play a particular sport. A community would be that group of students working together as a team to play the same game. See Column B of Table 28-1 also for types of communities that parallel the examples of populations.

TABLE 28-1 ● Examples of Populations and Communities the Home Health Nurse Might See	
A. Populations	**B. Communities**
1. Clients who live in the same area	1. Local governmental unit (i.e., city, county) Local community development group
2. Clients in the same age group	2. Senior citizens center, women's club Boy or Girl Scouts, athletic teams
3. Clients who need assistance with meals	3. Meals on Wheels Program
4. Students who attend a nursing program	4. The Student Nurses Association
5. Home health clients with diabetes	5. American Diabetes Association

The health of a group of individuals is more than the sum of the health of its members. Each community has its own personality, and each has a different health level. Just as with individual clients, the health of communities can be assessed using a hierarchy of needs. The health concerns of residents of an affluent suburb differ from those of residents of a Native American reservation, which differ from those of residents of an inner-city neighborhood. This article will later examine in detail how to use community assessment data to improve the health of various types of clients.

● TECHNIQUES OF COMMUNITY ASSESSMENT

The easiest starting point for the home health nurse performing a community assessment for the first time is the community in which the nurse's clients live. The nurse may know much about the community already, and the information acquired can be easily used to enhance the care of those clients.

Although the community assessment process can be incorporated into a home care nurse's daily practice and doesn't take much additional time, it is critically important. Just as with assessment of an individual, there are several tools available that provide a list of factors for assessment; most are organized according to particular theoretical model of nursing or public health practice (Christensen & Kenney, 1995; Clark, 1996; Smith & Maurer, 1995; Stanhope & Knollmueller, 1997). Figure 28-1 illustrates eight characteristics of communities that should be investigated during a community assessment; they are derived from a systems approach to nursing care of the community.

Assessment tools are guides. The amount and type of data to be collected should be adjusted according to the type of clients served and the time available for the assessment process. For example, if the home care clients are predominantly elders, the nurse would seek information pertaining to elder day care services, home-delivered meals, assisted-living facilities, and transportation for those with impaired mobility. If the clients are children, the nurse might seek information on programs such as lead screening, immunizations, or support for children with chronic health problems. Four techniques of data collection will be discussed in this article: the windshield survey, networking, analysis of existing data, and interviews.

Windshield Survey

The ideal approach to community assessment is to live in the community in which one practices. However, the windshield survey, a systematic assessment that is performed while the nurse travels through the community, is an excellent alternative.

It is important to put aside any prior impressions or opinions of the community and view it as a clean slate. Table 28-2 lists some points to consider when performing a windshield survey. All of the senses should be used to look closely at the community and note its sounds, smells, and tastes. Are the noises pleasant (e.g., children playing in a park or waves lapping on a shore), or are they noxious (e.g., industrial, vehicular, or overly loud music)? Are there various ethnic restaurants or generic fast food restaurants? Is there a sense of a community that is open and warm or closed and cold? What types of buildings are visible: residential, retail, light, or heavy industry? What is the condition of the roads, side-walks, and buildings? What is the developmental stage of the community?

Just as individuals and families move through various levels of maturity, so do communities. For example, is the community mature and stable, or is it young and growing? Are the residents predominantly families with young children, elders, or a mix? Is the

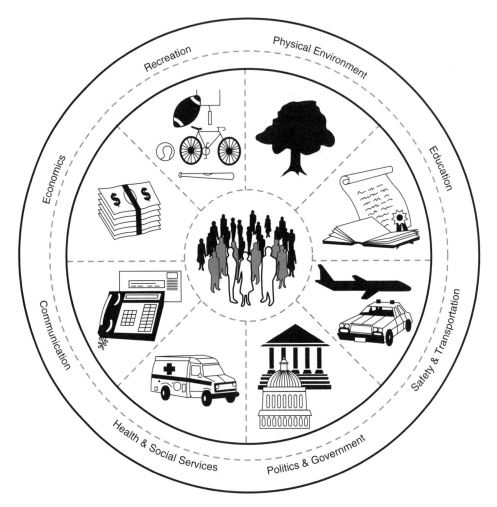

FIGURE 28-1. Categories of information for community assessment source. From "Community as partner: Theory and practice in nursing," by E. Anderson & J. McFarlane, 1996. 2nd. ed. Philadelphia: Lippincott-Raven Publishers, p. 178. Adapted with permission.

community in a transition phase as elders sell their homes and young families move in? What housing resources are available for elders or other individuals who need assistance in planning new living arrangements?

A windshield survey can reveal much about the personality and character of a community. It is a continuous process because communities are dynamic—always changing and evolving.

Networking

Another way to learn about a community is by networking with other professionals. For example, colleagues may be familiar with the community from working or living in it. Per-

TABLE 28-2 • Community Windshield Survey

Housing

Age? Construction, condition, repair? Separate? Connected? Yards?

Environmental

Green space? How used? Public or private? Terrain? Safety hazards? Sounds and odors? Pleasant, noxious? Source? Air and water quality? Sources of pollution? Type of boundaries (natural, physical, or economic)? Are there distinct neighborhoods? Name or identity?

Transportation

Types (plane, car, train, bus, walk)? Availability and condition of streets and roads? Major highway near? Is public transportation available? Transport for those with special needs? How access? Cost?

Shopping/Common Areas

What types of stores are there? How do residents get to the stores? How do the prices compare with other areas? Where do people gather? Do they form groups? Who are they? What times of day?

On the Street

What people do you see on the streets during the day? Homeless? Animals—strays, watchdogs, pets, wild animals (i.e., deer)? Is the community young and growing? Mature? Is it "alive"?

Race, Ethnicity

What evidence do you see of various ethnic groups, races, cultures?

Culture, Spiritual

Eating places, languages, private schools? Places of worship? Types?

Safety Services

What safety services (fire, police, EMS) are available? What is their location? Response time? Lost cost smoke alarms?

Health

Healthcare facilities? Type or level of care? Cost? Nearest emergency room? Nearest public health facilities? Services? Cost? Mental health resources? AA? Social services? Cost? Recreation services? Cost?

Community Development

Any political posters? What parties? Evidence of community groups? Nearest public offices? Public services are available?

Communication

What TV and radio stations are available? What print media is read? Is there a community newsletter? Community event signs? Signs of community pride? Industry? Type?

Education

Public? Private? Cost? Transportation? Adult education?

Note. Adapted from *"Community as partner: Theory and practice in nursing,"* by E. Anderson & J. McFarlane, 1996, 2nd. ed. Philadelphia: Lippincott-Raven Publishers, p. 186. Previously adapted from Terry Mizrahi, School of Social Work, Virginia Commonwealth University. Adapted with permission.

haps a colleague knows about a the values, goals, beliefs, and practices of a cultural group that lives in the community. The knowledge and experience of social workers at the agency, local hospital, or governmental human services office should be used. Discharge planning coordinators also can be helpful. Some communities have community resource guides that may be found at city halls, community development offices, and libraries. Other communities have a phone number that may be used to access a central clearing-house of community services.

Assembling a community resource notebook or card file for the agency is also a consideration. This can save time, prevent duplication of effort, and facilitate continuity of care. It is particularly useful for agencies whose districts have frequent turnover of case managers. Does more than one staff member work in the community? Anderson and Mc-Farlane (1994, p. 179) suggest that the group work as an interdisciplinary team by dividing the community assessment process and having each staff member be responsible for a portion of the data collection. This allows those who are new to the process to ease into it and avoid feeling overwhelmed.

Analysis of Existing Data

The community assessor can also learn about the health of a community by analysis of data that is already available (Christensen & Kenney, 1995, p. 104). The most common types of data include demographic and health status statistics. Demographic data relates to social characteristics including age, sex, employment, housing, ethnicity, education, and income. Information in census surveys consists of demographic statistics. From a community's demographic data, one can learn about the distribution of age groups, proportion of people receiving food stamps, poverty rate, average educational level, average age of homes, median income, and proportion of one- or two-parent homes.

Health status statistics can be used to divulge information about births, deaths (mortality), illnesses (morbidity), communicable diseases, and injuries. Two terms related to illnesses are incidence and prevalence. According to Clark (1996), incidence is the number of new cases of a particular health problem during a period of time and prevalence is the number of people affected by a particular health problem at a specified point in time.

Some common health status statistics are listed in Column A of Table 28-3. The statistical data kept for each community may vary; however, by using available data, the community assessor can form an overall impression of the community's health.

Sources for demographic and health status statistics include state, county, or local health departments; city halls; community development organizations; and libraries. Often, the desired data can be requested by phone and delivered by mail or information can be provided to the nurse about how to access an on-line database. Indicators of morbidity (illness) may be more difficult to find than those of mortality (death). However, if the nurse has an interest in a particular social or health problem, such as teen pregnancy, data may be found through governmental agencies and/or voluntary associations that specialize in the problem. Another data source is the local environmental protection office, which often can provide the community assessor with information on sites of environmental concern and those being actively managed.

Once the community assessor has collected various statistics, the data must be interpreted. Three aspects of data interpretation will be discussed:

1. Many health statistics are reported as rates. A rate is a calculation that converts raw data, such as how many deaths occurred in a particular area, to a common population base of 1000 or 100,000. Raw data from two communities of different popu-

TABLE 28-3 ● Comparison of Public Health Statistics

A. Statistic	B. Healthy People 2000 Objective	C. U.S. Statistics
Infant mortality rate	7 per 1000 live births	8.5 per 1000 live births (1992)
Low birth weight	No more than 5% of live births	7.1% of live births (1992)
Pregnancy in females ages 15–17 yr	50 per 1000	74.3 per 1000 (1990)
Deaths due to coronary artery disease	100 per 100,000 people	114 per 100,000 (1992)
Deaths due to cancer	130 per 100,000 people	134 per 100,000 (1992)
Immunization levels in children younger than 2 yrs	At least 90%	67%—19–35 mos. (1993)

Note. Adapted from "Healthy People 2000: Midcourse Review," by the U.S. Department of Health and Human Services, U.S. Public Health Service, 1995. Washington, DC: Gov't Printing Office. Adapted with permission.

lations are difficult to compare. However, with a common base, the data can be compared and interpreted. Some examples of rates and how to calculate them are noted in Table 28-4. "Age-adjusted" rates are those that take into consideration the differences in death rates of various age groups.

2. One item of data is not significant. For example, to know that 85% of the preschoolers of City A had received all their required immunizations to date in 1995 is not significant. The statistic must be compared with that of another community or the same community over time. An entirely different picture is presented, for example, when it is learned that in 1990, only 60% of the preschool children in City A had received all their required immunizations to date or that in 1995 for the county in which City A was located, 95% of the preschoolers had received all their required immunizations to date.

3. Always compare "apples to apples"; make sure two pieces of data have the same labels.

TABLE 28-4 ● Formulas for Common Public Health Rates

Crude Birth Rate	No. of live births during the year × 1000
	Average population at midyear
Crude Death Rate	No. of deaths during the year × 1000
	Average population at midyear
Cause-Specific Death Rate	No. of deaths from stated cause in 1 year × 100,000
	Average (midyear) population
Infant Mortality Rate	No. of deaths in 1 year of children aged < 1 year × 1000
	No. of live births in the same year
Neonatal Mortality Rate	No. of deaths in 1 yr. of children < 28 days × 1000
	No. of live births in the same year

Note. Adapted from "Community health nursing: Promoting the health of aggregates," by J. Swanson, & M. Albrecht, 1993. Philadelphia: W.B. Saunders, p. 90. Adapted with permission.

An important source of comparison data is *Healthy People 2000* (DHHS, 1995). Developed by a group of national health experts in 1990, this document specifies objectives for the health of the people of the United States by the year 2000. *Healthy People 2000* focuses on prevention, and the objectives have important implications for health promotion. An example of a health objective of *Healthy People 2000* objective is to reduce coronary heart disease deaths to no more than 100 per 100,000 people (age-adjusted baseline, 135 per 100,000 in 1987 [DHHS, 1995, p. 232]). By comparing community data with the *Healthy People 2000* objectives, areas requiring improvement can be identified. The National Health Objectives may be purchased from the U.S. Government Printing Office and may be found in textbooks of community health nursing. Many states have year 2000 health objectives that integrate the national objectives with state priorities (DHHS, Foreword) (see Columns A, B, & C of Table 28–3 for examples of comparisons of common health statistics).

Interviews

The fourth means of community data collection is interviewing residents or health professionals in the community. Through interviews, the nurse can learn the community's history, perceived assets and deficits, and details of various community and government services (i.e., lead testing and abatement programs), voluntary agencies, or community businesses (e.g., which pharmacy delivers or accepts Medicaid, etc.). Services may be provided from within or outside of the community.

Local voluntary agencies such The American Heart Association, The American Cancer Society, or The March of Dimes are invaluable resources to home health nurses and their clients. A voluntary agency is a private, non-profit organization. Voluntary agencies may provide services such as educational programs and materials, supplies, financial assistance, direct care, and research support. Information on voluntary agencies may be obtained by phone or in writing. To facilitate referrals, the agency's phone number, address, name of contact person, target clients, types of services, fee schedule, eligibility criteria, and desired referral process should be noted.

Information about the community can also be obtained by talking with clients; many are long-time residents and can offer insights into the community's history, changes over time, community resources, strengths, and weaknesses. Such interviews allow the nurse to implement a basic principle of involving the client in the assessment process.

Pastors of churches are often helpful resources and are knowledgeable as to the social, cultural, and spiritual life of the community. Depending on the type of information the nurse is seeking, other possible sources include police officers, firefighters, paramedics, and other local and state services. Their perspectives and statistics often can lead to implications for health promotion interventions by the nurse. For example, families with children can be educated by home health nurses on the importance of bicycle helmets and informed as to whether local law requires their use.

Two points to consider about interviews are that: 1) employees of some agencies must obtain permission, or are not permitted, to give an interview; and 2) information gained in interviews often represents personal opinions and should be considered in light of other data.

● USING COMMUNITY ASSESSMENT DATA

How can the home health nurse use the information acquired during community assessment to improve the quality of client care? It is helpful to look at this question from three points of view: 1) the individual or family client; and 2) the client group; and 3) the community client.

The Individual or Family Client

The information gained from a community assessment can be used to enhance the care of the individual or family client. In making referrals, the nurse's goal is to promote client independence so that the client will contact the agency directly. However, the nurse may choose to perform a direct referral when a crisis situation exists, the client is unable to contact the agency, or the nurse intends to role model the process for the client or caregiver.

Assessment data may also be used to identify health promotion activities geared specifically to the community in which the client lives. For example, the fact that a community has high levels of air pollution has implications for clients with chronic respiratory problems; or residents of communities with a high number of older homes should be educated as to the problem of lead toxicity and available abatement programs.

Community assessment can also facilitate the home health nurse's progress toward culturally competent practice. Through community assessment, the home health nurse can learn about the beliefs, practices, and community resources for clients whose cultural background differ from that of the nurse (Stanhope & Lancaster, 1996, p. 121). This knowledge can be used to provide a background for assessment of the individual client's cultural perspective.

Groups or Populations of Clients

The home health nurse can also look at individual clients as members of groups (or populations). Home health nurses work with many groups of clients. Examples include elderly clients with chronic wounds or clients who speak a particular language. Once aware of the various populations nurses serve, they can identify health needs common to the group, develop nursing strategies, and identify community resources that may apply to group members. For example, the nurse can locate local merchants who will accept Medicare for dressing supplies and who will ship or deliver the supplies. This information will likely be relevant to a number of home care clients at the nurse's agency and could be noted in the agency's resource file. Duplication of effort will be avoided, and the quality of care for all clients in the population will improve.

In some cases, the individual clients may be assisted to become members of a group with interests similar to their own. For example, the parents of a child with diabetes might join the Juvenile Diabetes Association to locate a parent's support group or a summer camp for their child.

The Community as Client

An important role of the community health nurse and often the home care nurse, involves efforts to improve the health of various communities. Often, these activities are interdisciplinary, and the community health nurse functions as a member, or leader, of a committee or task force.

The information gained during a community assessment, whether broad-based or specific, can be the first step in the nursing process applied to the community client. In collaboration with the community, the nurse can use community assessment data to identify strengths and deficits of the community, define health-related needs, and develop a plan for intervention. Nurse-managed foot clinics, mobile women's health vans, community-based nursing clinics, and on-site nurse-managed primary health clinics are examples of such programs.

As with individual clients, community health nursing interventions are not always directed toward a problem; the goal may be to maintain or improve an aspect of the community's health. For example, a particular community may currently have a successful program of services geared to its elderly citizens but may be concerned about the ability to continue these services with decreasing state subsidies and the anticipated increased proportion of elderly in the 21st century.

Clark (1996) sees the clinical nurse specialist in community health nursing as having a leading role in the nursing process at the population and community level. However, the home health nurse can contribute significantly to that process by acting as a key informant, sharing existing community assessment data, and assisting in all phases of the nursing process. In doing so, the home health nurse will be able to explore a broader scope of nursing practice and participate in improving the health of the community.

● SUMMARY

The home health nurse can enhance the quality of care of clients at all levels—individual, family, and populations—through the use of the community assessment process, which may be integrated into the nurse's daily practice. Through a windshield survey, networking, interviews, and secondary data analysis, the nurse can acquire in-depth knowledge of the community from several perspectives: physiologic, psychologic, sociocultural, developmental, and spiritual.

With the information gained during community assessment, the home health nurse will have a prospective, comprehensive bank of resources to use in planning nursing interventions. The home health nurse, as part of a interdisciplinary team of health providers, can also explore a broader scope of practice through identification of and intervention for health concerns at the population or community level.

REFERENCES

Anderson, E., & McFarlane, J. (1996). *Community as partner: Theory and practice in nursing* (2nd. ed.). Philadelphia: Lippincott-Raven Publishers.

Christensen, P., & Kenney, J. (1994). *Nursing process: Application of conceptual models* (4th ed.). St. Louis: Mosby.

Clark, M.J. (1996). *Nursing in the community* (2nd ed.). Stamford, CT: Appleton and Lange.

Green, J., & Driggers, B. (1989). All visiting nurses are not alike: Home health and community health nursing. *Journal of Community Health Nursing, 6*(2), 83–93.

Department of Health and Human Services, Public Health Service. (1995). *Healthy People 2000: Midcourse Review and 1995 Revisions.* (1995). Washington, DC: Gov't Printing Office.

Smith, C., & Maurer, F. (1995). *Community health nursing:* Theory and practice. Philadelphia: W.B. Saunders.

Stanhope, M. & Knollmueller, R. (1997). *Public and community health nurse's consultant.* St. Louis: Mosby.

Stanhope, M. & Lancaster, J. (1996). *Community health nursing: Promoting the health of aggregates, families, and individuals.* (4th ed.) St. Louis: Mosby.

Swanson, J., & Albrecht, M. *Community health nursing: Promoting the health of aggregates.* (1993) Philadelphia: W.B. Saunders.

Wald, L. (1915) *The house on Henry Street.* New York: Henry Holt and Company.

With the renewed emphasis on holistic care, nursing is truly returning to its professional roots. Defined as care considering the relationships among the biologic, psychological, social, and spiritual dimension of a person, holistic nursing attempts to understand the individual as an integrated whole interacting with both internal and external environments. This article outlines the basic tenets of holistic nursing.

What is holistic nursing? How can holistic nursing be applied to community-based practice? What does research tell us about the relationship between spirituality and health and longevity? What are some resources for providing holistic nursing in community-based settings?

Dossey, B., & Dossey, L. (1998). Attending to holistic care. *American Journal of Nursing*, 98(8), 35–38.

Attending to Holistic Care

BARBARA M. DOSSEY, LARRY DOSSEY

It's time we listened to our patients' concerns about soul and spirit.

Why are we justified as clinicians in speaking about soul and spirit in an age of science? Why not concentrate exclusively on the body, the sick organs, and the deranged biochemistry of our patients, as we've done for most of this century?

Our majestic predecessors in nursing, such as Florence Nightingale, spoke boldly about the need to honor the psychological and spiritual aspects of our patients. For her and many others, it was unthinkable to consider sick humans as mere bodies who could be treated in isolation from their minds and spirits. In Nightingale's holistic approach, the role of love and empathy was considered paramount. Early physicians agreed. As Paracelsus, the sixteenth-century Swiss physician and alchemist who discovered mercury as a treatment for syphilis, put it, "The main reason for healing is love." But with the rise of scientific, materialistic medicine in the nineteenth and twentieth centuries, these lessons in love, which had seemed obvious throughout the history of healing, were set aside and virtually lost. Nurses and physicians set their sights almost exclusively on objective, physically based approaches. Emotional involvement, we learned, might get in the way and contaminate our clinical objectivity. We went to unbelievable lengths to sanitize health care, to rid it of the "subjective." For example, for most of this century, when one spoke of "the mind," what one really referred to was the chemistry and physiology of the brain. As a result, mental illness has increasingly been considered a biochemical or genetic derangement, which can best be treated pharmacologically. And one spoke about "love," "soul," and "spirit" almost apologetically, if at all. Such talk was considered unscientific and antiquated; it did little to enhance one's professional advancement; it wasn't "modern."

Barbara M. Dossey is director, Holistic Nursing Consultants, Santa Fe, NM, and author of *Holistic Nursing: A Handbook for Practice* (Aspen Publishers, 1995), and *Florence Nightingale: Mystic, Visionary, Reformer* (Springhouse Corporation, 1999).

Larry Dossey is executive editor, *Alternative Therapies in Health and Medicine*, Santa Fe, NM, and author of *Healing Words* (Harper San Francisco, 1997). This series on holistic nursing care has been coordinated by Barbara D'Alessio, RN, C, MPA, and J. Brent Foward, MD, FACP, of the Institute of Complementary Medicine, Randolph, NJ.

Yet, the more things change, the more they stay the same. This is nowhere truer than in nursing and medicine, in which the time-honored concepts of soul and spirit are making a comeback after sitting on the sidelines for more than a century. The transition taking place is profound. We're approaching the point where, if clinicians do not honor the concepts of mind, soul, and spirit in our approaches to patient care, we will be considered unscientific.

● 'SOUL LEVELS' AND NURSING PRACTICE

It's true that we don't have "spirit meters" or lab tests for a "serum soul level." But we are developing powerful tools that help us assess the spiritual welfare of our patients, and the impact of the meanings, values, goals, and purposes in their lives. And powerful data show that if these are deranged, patient health will suffer. The lesson is plain: Any comprehensive approach to nursing and medical care must focus acutely on these issues. We must learn to pay as much attention to them as we would our patients' blood pressure, cholesterol level, or diet. The reason is straightforward: This focus makes the difference between health and illness, life and death.

Consider the fact that more patients under 50 years of age experience fatal heart attacks on Monday morning, around 9:00 am, than at any other time of the week, and that one of the best predictors of heart attack has been found to be job dissatisfaction. This has given rise to what's been called Black Monday syndrome. What is the significance of one's occupation? What value does one place on work? What fulfillment does one sense on returning to the workplace on Monday mornings? If our patients give negative responses to these questions, we must tackle them as aggressively as we would a cardiac arrhythmia, because they, too, are a matter of life or death.

When Dr. Thomas Oxman and his colleagues at Dartmouth Medical School examined the factors that correlated with successful coronary artery bypass surgery, they discovered that the degree of religious faith and spiritual meaning in patients' lives was the single best predictor of survival of surgery. The same results have been found in assessing the postoperative course of elderly patients undergoing hip surgery.

It's time we listened to our patients. They want us to be concerned about their souls and spirits. A recent survey of hospitalized patients found that 75% believed their physicians should be concerned about their spiritual welfare; 50% said they wanted their doctors to pray not just for them but with them.

● SPIRITUALITY IS GOOD SCIENCE

In study after study, social contact—the richness of one's interactions with others—is correlated with positive health outcomes. Over 250 studies now show that religious practice—the specific religion doesn't seem to matter—is correlated with greater health and increased longevity. Intercessory prayer in a hospital coronary care unit, in a double-blind study, was effective in promoting a lower incidence of cardiac arrest, need for cardiopulmonary resuscitation, and intubation; decreased need for potent medications; and a lower incidence of pneumonia and pulmonary edema.

These are touchy issues, and some say that clinicians have no business taking on the role of spiritual guide; that's what pastoral counselors, hospital chaplains, ministers, priests, and rabbis are for. But we are not being asked to become spiritual counselors. We're being asked to integrate a holistic approach and extend love, compassion, and empathy (which are the bedrock on which nursing and medicine have always rested); to en-

Applying Holistic Nursing

Dorothy Lavigne is a 45-year-old woman with end-stage breast cancer with metastases to the bone and liver. Pain management has been difficult for her, and she's been reluctant to discuss end-of-life issues, even when you have approached her. You wonder how she might respond to holistic nursing interventions. The following questions and answers define holistic nursing and its potential implications for your practice—and for patients like Ms. Lavigne.

Q*What is the difference between "healing" and "curing"?*

ACuring has been described by Mary McGlone as the alleviation of symptoms or the termination or suppression of a disease process through surgical, chemical, or mechanical intervention. Cure doesn't take into account causal or contributing factors, It's not uncommon for an ill person to continue developing a new set of symptoms until the underlying causes are addressed.

Healing may be spontaneous, but more often it's a gradual awakening to a deeper sense of self (and of the self in relation to others) in a way that effects profound change. McGlone has noted that there are clear distinctions between the kind of relationships and interactions that lead to healing and those that lead to cure. For example, a health care provider who cures focuses on the disease and its symptoms, while one who heals (or, rather, facilitates healing), focuses on the person with the disease. It's important to note that a patient may be cured without being healed, or healed without being cured. Coming to accept emotional or physical limitations—and eventual death—has tremendous healing power. And healing is transformation.

Margaret A. Newman describes this transformation as a move away from treating symptoms and diseases and toward a search for "patterns" which she characterizes as the constantly moving or changing interpenetration of human energy as transformation takes place. There is also a shift from seeing pain and disease as wholly negative to a view that pain and disease are information, along with a perspective of the body as a "dynamic field of energy," at one with a larger field. Martha Rogers views each person as a unitary being, eliminating the dichotomy between health (healing) and disease (cure). She sees illness and health as equal expressions of being, and that the meaning of these phenomena is derived from an understanding of the larger processes of life.

McGlone has described healing as coming from within, and that the rate of healing is consistent with a person's own readiness to grow and to change. The rate of healing cannot be determined by the care provider, no matter how much she would like to see a patient relieved of his symptoms. Healing is a matter of honoring who the patient is, rather than who we think he should be.

McGlone has also described a healing attitude as "a belief system that recognizes that all of life's experiences, including injury, illness, and other setbacks, provide us with opportunities to learn and to grow toward that which we are meant to be. Seen in this light, disease is not an enemy but a teacher and motivation. Disease is manifesting, in a physical way, the desire or need of the psyche to reestablish balance and integration through a change of direction in one's lifestyle, behavior, or attitudes."

Q*What is holistic nursing?*

AThe American Holistic Nurses Association defines holistic nursing as "all nursing practice that has healing the whole person as its goal." Holistic nursing recognizes that there are two components of holism: first, that holism involves understanding the relationships among the biologic, psychological, social, and spiritual dimensions of a person—and that the whole is greater than the sum of its parts, and second, that holism involves understanding the individual as an integrated whole interacting with internal and external environments.

(continued)

Applying Holistic Nursing (*Continued*)

Holistic practice draws on nursing knowledge, theories, expertise, and intuition to guide nurses in becoming therapeutic partners in strengthening clients' responses to the healing process. Practicing holistic nursing requires practitioners to integrate self-care into their own lives. Self-responsibility can lead us to a greater awareness of the interconnectedness of all individuals and permits us to use this awareness of a global community to facilitate patients' healing.

Q *What are the differences between the terms "holistic modalities," "complementary and alternative medicine," and "preventive therapies"?*

A The National Institutes of Health's Office of Alternative Medicine defines these terms as follows: "Complementary and alternative medicine . . . [are] those treatments and health care practices not taught widely in medical [or nursing] schools, not generally used in hospitals, and not usually reimbursed by medical insurance companies. Many therapies are termed 'holistic,' which generally means that the health care practitioner considers the whole person, including physical, mental, emotional, and spiritual aspects. Many therapies also are known as 'preventive,' which means that the practitioner educates and treats the person to prevent health problems from arising, rather than treating symptoms after problems have occurred."

Q *Why is it important to develop this type of practice when I am already a practicing nurse?*

A Recent research has been able to assist clinicians in understanding the interconnectedness of the body and the mind. Barbara Dossey has noted that treating an illness solely through the body doesn't take into account the profound influence of the mind on disease states, and that treating illness exclusively from a physical perspective may be only a partial solution. The growing popularity, efficacy, and legitimacy of many holistic therapies could be just what our ailing health care system needs.

Holistic nurses are integrating complementary therapies into clinical practice to treat physiologic, psychological, and spiritual patient needs. Doing so doesn't negate the validity of conventional medical therapies but serves to complement them and broaden and enrich the scope of nursing practice, and helps the patient access his greatest healing potential.

Ms. Lavigne's anxiety and pain have responded to your holistic interventions. The nursing staff have taught her guided imagery and relaxation techniques, which have decreased her anxiety. She's also received therapeutic touch treatments to augment her pain medication. Her decreased anxiety and pain levels have allowed her to more openly express her feelings and needs regarding her illness.—Anna M. Acee, EdD, RN,C, holistic nursing consultant, New York, NY, and a member of AJN's editorial advisory board.

SELECTED REFERENCES

Achterberg, J., et al. *Rituals of Healing: Using Imagery for Health and Wellness*. New York, Bantam Books, 1994.

Burkhardt, M.A., and Nagai-Jacobson, M.G. Reawakening spirit in clinical practice. *J. Holist. Nurs.* 12:9–21, Mar. 1994.

Dossey B.M., et al. *Holistic Nursing: A Handbook for Practice,* 2nd ed. Gaithersburg, MD, Aspen Publishers, 1995.

McGlone, M.E. Healing the spirit. *Holist. Nurs. Pract.* 4(4):77–84, July 1990.

National Institutes of Health, Office of Alternative Medicine. What is complementary and alternative medicine? Available online < http://altmed.od.nih.gov/oam/what-is-cam/faq.shtml>, accessed June 18, 1998.

Newman M.A. *Health as Expanding Consciousness,* 2nd ed. (Pub. No. 14–2626). New York, National League for Nursing, 1994.

courage patients themselves to address these issues and to suggest how they might do so. We don't expect ministers to perform appendectomies, and we shouldn't expect clinicians to be expert spiritual guides. But we can be mediators of spiritual resources for those we serve. This is not an outrageous mandate; it is merely a return to the core values implicit in nursing's history, and it is good science.

But let's not be naive; this expanded role for nursing presents immense challenges. Just when we thought it was sufficient to "be scientific" and focus on the physical, nursing science is becoming richer, fuller, and more complex than we ever imagined. It will be tempting to ignore the data pushing us in these new directions. It is far easier to take refuge in the body and its infinitely complex physiology than to entertain an expanded nursing role that includes soul and spirit. It will be tempting to say, "Let the psychiatric

Resources for Holistic Nursing and Complementary Therapies

Following are resources for nurses wishing to expand their understanding of holistic modalities.

American Holistic Nurses Association
P.O. Box 2130
Flagstaff, AZ 86003-2130
(520) 526-2196
<http://www.ahna.org>

Nurse Healers-Professional Associates, Inc.
1211 Locust Street
Philadelphia, PA 19107
(215) 545-8079
<http://www.therapeutic-touch.org>

Stress Reduction Clinic
University of Massachusetts
    Medical Center
58 Lake Avenue North
Worcester, MA 01655
(508) 856-2656

Dean Ornish's Opening Your Heart Program
Preventive Medicine Research Institute
900 Bridgeway. Suite 2
Sausalito, CA 94965
(415) 332-2525

Academy for Guided Imagery
P.O. Box 2070
Mill Valley, CA 94942
(800) 726-2070

American Yoga Association
P.O. Box 19986
Sarasota, FL 34276
(914) 927-4977

Acupressure Institute
1533 Shattuck Avenue
Berkeley, CA 94709
(610) 845-1059

American Chiropractic Association
1701 Clarendon Blvd.
Arlington, VA 22209
(703) 276-8800
<http://www.amerchiro.org>

American Massage Therapy Association
820 Davis Street, Suite 100
Evanston, IL 60201
(847) 864-0123
<http://www.amtamassage.org>

American Reflexology Certification
    Board and Information Service
P.O. Box 246654
Sacramento, CA 95824
(916) 455-5381

American Association of
    Oriental Medicine
433 Front Street
Catasauqua, PA 18032
(610) 266-1433
<http://www.aaom.org>

—*Compiled by Anna M. Acee, EdD, RN, C, holistic nursing consultant, New York, NY, and a member of AJN's editorial advisory board* nurses do it; that's not my role. Call the chaplain; I'm not trained to be that kind of nurse."

We may specialize or subspecialize, but our patients don't. They come to us as a whole, not as a body cut off from their soul and spirit. And it is the whole to which a nurse responds, if she deserves to be called a nurse instead of a technician.

Are nurses up to it? Yes! We have talked with thousands of nurses around the country who are hungry and eager for these changes. They deeply desire a greater sense of professional, personal, and spiritual fulfillment, which comes about, they say, when they honor the psychospiritual needs of those they serve.

Modern science, including nursing and medicine, has evolved into one of the most spiritually malnourished endeavors in recent history. It's paradoxical that it's science that is now showing that soul and spirit are essential to health. Science, long the enemy of spirituality, is pointing the way back. As these developments proceed, it is not just our patients who will benefit, but nurses as well. What a glorious prospect with which nursing can phase out one millennium and enter a new one.

SELECTED REFERENCES

Byrd, R.B. Positive therapeutic effects of intercessory prayer in a coronary care unit population. *South. Med. J.* 81:826–829, 1988.

Dossey, B., et al. *Holistic Nursing: A Handbook for Practice.* Gaithersberg, MD, Aspen Publishers, 1995.

Dossey, B., ed. *AHNA Core Curriculum for Holistic Nursing.* Gaithersberg, MD, Aspen Publishers, 1997.

Dossey, L. The return of prayer. *Alternative Therapies.* 1997:3(6)10–17, 113–120.

King, D.E., et al. Beliefs and attitudes of hospital inpatients about faith healing and prayer. *J. Fam. Pract.* 49:349–352, 1994.

Levin, J.S. Investigating the epidemiologic effects of religious experience: Findings, explanations, and barriers. In *Religion in Aging and Health: Theoretical Foundations and Methodological Frontiers,* edited by J.S. Levin. Thousand Oaks, CA, Sage Publications, 1994, pp. 3–17.

Nightingale, F. *Suggestions for Thought to the Searchers after Truth among the Artizans of England.* London, Eyre & Spottiswoode, 1860, 3 vols. Cited in Calabria, M.D., and Macrae, J.A. *Suggestions for Thought by Florence Nightingale: Selections and Commentaries.* Philadelphia, University of Pennsylvania Press, 1994, p. 121.

Oxman, T.E., et al. Lack of social participation or religious strength or comfort as risk factors for death after cardiac surgery in the elderly. *Psychosom. Med.* 57:5–15, 1995.

Pressman, P., et al. Religious belief, depression, and ambulation status in elderly women with broken hips. *Am. J. Psychiatry* 147:758–60, 1990.

Rabkin, S.W., et al. Chronobiology of cardiac sudden death in men. *JAMA* 244:1357–1358, 1980.

Special Task Force to the Secretary of Health, Education, and Welfare. *Work in America.* Cambridge, MA, MIT Press, 1973.

This article discusses basic spiritual assessment and intervention useful for families and clients in all settings. Recently, the Joint Commission on Accreditation of Healthcare Organizations added as a standard the right to receive care that respects individual spiritual values of the client. This further expands the nurse's professional responsibility to address spirituality as an important aspect of care.

How might spiritual distress manifest itself in clients? Define spirituality. Define religion. How does spirituality differ from religion? What barriers are common to spiritual care? Discuss some interventions that provide spiritual support to clients and families.

Sumner, C. H. (1998). Recognizing and responding. *American Journal of Nursing*, 98 (1), 26–30.

Recognizing and Responding

CONSTANCE HARRIS SUMNER

The right to receive care that respects individual spiritual values was recently added to the Joint Commission standards. Here are some points to consider as you strive for maximum effectiveness in this aspect of patient care.

Nia sits quietly in a yoga position in the middle of her hospital bed. The nagging pain in her right breast continues to draw her attention and she cannot focus her mind. Although Nia receives pain medication, she prefers to use guided imagery, deep breathing, and meditation to assist with pain control. Nia tries desperately to center herself by meditating to make her pain go away. As the level of pain intensifies, she begins to question the meaning of her suffering and, ultimately, her life.

As you enter Nia's room you notice that she's grimacing and touching her lumpectomy site. You ask, "Would you like something for pain?" "No!" Nia replies. She pauses for a few seconds and continues. "Why is this awful thing happening to me? Why have I developed cancer?" You hesitate for a moment, searching for the appropriate response, and reply, "Shall I call the chaplain?" The young woman repositions herself, stares at you with a puzzled look, and says, "No, I'll be okay. I just need to meditate and connect with my Higher Power so I can push the pain out!"

Nia is experiencing spiritual distress—and the intervention of first resort, calling on the clergy, is of no use in her case. When that happens, we aren't always prepared.

Constance Harris Sumner is an oncology nurse and data manager at Allegheny University Hospital Medical College of Pennsylvania and Graduate Hospital and a graduate student at LaSalle University, both in Philadelphia, PA.

● THE TRUE SCOPE OF SPIRITUAL DISTRESS

Spiritual distress sometimes takes the obvious form of anger toward God or inner conflict about one's religious faith. But concerns about "meaning"—of pain, suffering, life, and death—are equally important indicators of spiritual distress. Nia's spiritual concerns arise during her encounter with the psychological experience of breast cancer and the physical experience of an unfamiliar pain. She wonders, "Why me?" and attempts to find meaning in the experience.

Viktor Frankl, founder of a form of existential therapy called logotherapy, articulated the link between meaning and spirituality. He declared that "to live is to suffer, to survive is to find meaning in the suffering," a perspective born of his own personal tragedies while confined to a concentration camp.

What Frankl and others have recognized is that spirituality includes religion but doesn't equate with it. It's a broader concept, a phenomenon not confined to churches, temples, and synagogues, although it tends to be viewed that way in Western cultures.

If you believe, as many theorists do, that spirituality is humanity's single unifying and transcendent dimension, it follows that a life-threatening diagnosis such as cancer or AIDS—by challenging every aspect of a person's being—can trigger a spiritual crisis. The onset of serious illness brings the nonphysical aspects of life into the conscious mind.

The demands of caring for patients faced with a life-threatening disease, intense by nature, have grown more difficult to meet as the restructuring and downsizing trends in health care erode nurse-patient ratios. At the same time, new standards from the Joint Commission for Accreditation of Health Care Organizations are explicit about the patient's right to care that considers his personal dignity and respects his spiritual values (August 1994). We may sometimes wonder, "How can we possibly do any more than we are doing now?" I believe the answer lies in a combination of intuition, creativity, and a broader view of spirituality.

● WHAT IS SPIRITUALITY?

The definition of spirituality is broad and varies depending on whom you ask. And in today's multicultural environment, its implications for both patient and nurse differ from case to case. There is, however, general agreement that spirituality is a basic human phenomenon that helps create meaning in the world. In presenting their humanistic interpretation of spirituality, David Elkins and colleagues have described it as "a way of being and experiencing that comes about through awareness of a transcendent dimension and that is characterized by certain identifiable values in regard to self, other, nature, life, and whatever one considers to be the Ultimate." They note that it is quite different from religion and is experienced long before one is aware of religion.

A useful way of viewing spirituality was expressed by David Moberg. He sees it as composed of a horizontal and a vertical aspect. One's sense of well-being in relation to God evolves from the vertical aspect. Within the horizontal aspect is our sense of life purpose and life satisfaction, independent of religious context. It encompasses the search for transcendence, purpose, hardiness, serenity, peace, connection, and hope. The vertical aspect concerns our eternal being; the horizontal, our earthly existence.

Religion is a specific manifestation of spirituality's drive to create meaning in the world. It can be thought of as part of spirituality, although spirituality is not necessarily related to religion. Religion is both a concept and a social system that supports group expression and devotional activity. It's a formal medium for expressing belief in God or gods. In recent times, however, religious practice has shifted away from formal structure toward greater individuality, contributing to the diversity of spiritual expression that nurses encounter in practice.

● BARRIERS TO SPIRITUAL CARE

In everyday nursing practice, we're sometimes prompted to engage in prayer with patients or read to them from scriptures, but spiritual care isn't usually planned. Often, too many tasks and not enough time discourage us from even thinking about this aspect of care. Beyond that, many of us are uncomfortable in interacting with patients regarding matters of the spirit. Some observers blame inadequate training for that discomfort, but it can also be rooted in failure to fully address one's own spiritual issues.

In 1990 Karen Boutell and Frederick Bozett surveyed 238 practicing nurses and found that the majority didn't assess for spiritual needs. Another survey by Elizabeth Taylor and colleagues revealed that oncology nurses provided spiritual care sparingly and were uncomfortable doing so. Fifty-three percent rarely or never prayed with patients, and 66% rarely or never read religious or spiritual passages with a patient. The majority rarely or never addressed components of the horizontal aspect of spirituality when interacting with patients.

You can see inadequate attention to spirituality reflected in almost any nursing admission assessment form. The section that refers to spiritual matters typically asks, "What is your religion?" If the patient answers "none," there's no further pursuit of spiritual concerns. We need to revise assessment forms to reflect spiritual values if we are to effectively meet patient needs and JCAHO requirements.

● REAFFIRMING A NURSING TRADITION

You might be wondering whether it's ultimately appropriate for nurses to address patients' spiritual needs. I believe it is. We can't and shouldn't replace religious leaders, and there will always be times when spiritual care is best referred to other members of the health team—chaplain, minister, rabbi, psychologist, or a family member. But we can provide spiritual care that is meaningful and effective because it's patient-centered.

If the goal of our work is to help people reach optimal levels of functioning of mind, body, and spirit, then spirit must be restored to its rightful place. When the nursing profession was first establishing itself as a science, words like biophysical and psychosocial were dominant. We avoided subjective terms like spirit, spirituality, and spiritual needs that were viewed as unscientific. In fact, however, nursing has a strong tradition in the spiritual dimension of health care. Prayer, a component of spirituality, and the "laying on of hands" have long been used in healing the sick. Janet Macrae's recent article about Florence Nightingale reveals a global approach to spirituality and a strong interest in mysticism that went beyond her religious faith.

In modern times, nurse scholars like Virginia Henderson and Martha Rogers have spoken about achieving maximum health potential and advocated a holistic approach to the patient. Joyce Travelbee included the spiritual element in her writings, defining alterations in health as spiritual, emotional, and physical experiences. To her, nursing's role is to assist patients in finding meaning in these experiences. The classic *AJN* article by Ruth Stoll, "Guidelines for Spiritual Assessment," addressed both existential and religious components of spirituality.

In the '80s and '90s, "New Age" nursing literature has placed an even stronger emphasis on spiritual care. Outstanding contributions include those of Jean Watson, with her

Transpersonal Caring Theory; Julia A. Lane, with her detailed spiritual interventions and comprehensive discussion of the nurse's role, and Margaret A. Burkhardt, with an analysis that gives thorough attention to the horizontal as well as the vertical aspect of spirituality.

● PUTTING SPIRITUALITY INTO PRACTICE

We provide care for patients and families from diverse religious backgrounds, ranging from Christianity to Taoism, as well as some who practice no formal religion at all. Incorporating inclusive spiritual care into your clinical practice is not only possible but necessary.

To succeed, though, you have to expand your knowledge base—beginning with your own spiritual self. There are several guides available to help you with this task. For example, Reed's Spiritual Perspective Scale is a 10-item questionnaire that uses a six-point scale to measure spiritual perspective to the extent that it permeates one's life and spiritually-related interaction. Ellison's Spiritual Well-Being Scale measures vertical and horizontal aspects of spirituality. Elkins' Spiritual Orientation Inventory measures spirituality based on the humanistic model.

Review your own beliefs, opinions, and biases. You may identify a need to learn the inherent difference between religion and spirituality. Take a look at some of the articles listed in *Selected References*. Keep in mind that we enter life as spiritual beings, while religions are something we acquire as we grow, develop, and become part of our communities.

As you become more receptive to your patients' spiritual orientation and mindful that it may or may not be associated with religion, your interactions can be more purposeful. Remember Nia? She was in need of spiritual—not religious—care. A more receptive response to Nia's spiritual needs would have been to encourage her to elaborate on what she was thinking and feeling, assist her in identifying the causes of her sense of disconnectedness, and help her articulate the impact of her illness on her life.

You can provide enhanced, inclusive spiritual support to your patients in the following ways [Fig. 30-1]:

- Facilitate the process of finding meaning and purpose in life. Attempt to understand the patient's unique way of experiencing and expressing spirituality. Encourage a life review process and listen attentively.
- Be fully present and open to issues as they arise when interacting with the patient.
- Support the faith needs of your patients and safely provide time for ritual and devotional practices. Be knowledgeable about different religious and nonreligious practices.
- Ask the patient questions like, "What gives your life meaning and hope? What are you searching for spiritually? To whom do you turn when you're distressed?" The answers will assist you in the planning and intervention phases of care. Share this information with the other members of the health care team.
- Establish trust and unconditional acceptance.
- Help the patient to get in touch with her spiritual self. This is accomplished in part by linking, connecting, and associating the numerous events occurring during illness.
- Know the other members of the health care team to whom you might refer your patient if spiritual distress develops, such as chaplain, psychologist, social worker, or colleague.

A SPIRITUAL NEEDS PROTOCOL

Illness often triggers spiritual wrestling in addition to emotional, mental, and physical pain. Spiritual care is an integral part of holistic care. The health care team must be comfortable with and receptive to these needs in order for them to emerge and be addressed. The concept of presence implies self-giving by the health care provider to the patient. It means being available and listening in a meaningful way. It also means having an awareness that it is a privilege to be invited into a person's life in this way, as well as an ethical responsibility.

ASSESSMENT

Assess spiritual/religious preference and request to see chaplain using database on admission.
Listen for verbal cues regarding spiritual/religious orientation:
• patient refers to God or Higher Power
• patient talks about prayer, church, synagogue, spiritual/religious leader
Look for visual cues on patient's person and in room regarding spiritual/religious orientation:
• Bible, Torah, Koran, or other spiritual books
• symbols such as the cross or Star of David
• articles such as prayer beads, medals, or pins
Listen for significant comments, e.g., "It's all in God's hands now" or "Why is this happening to me?"
Assess for signs of spiritual concerns:
• discouragement
• mild anxiety
• expressions of anticipatory grief
• inability to participate in usual spiritual practice
• expressions of concern about relationship with God or Higher Power

• inability to obtain foods required by beliefs
Assess for signs of spiritual distress:
• crying
• expressions of guilt
• disturbances in sleep patterns
• disrupted spiritual trust
• feeling remote from God or Higher Power
• moderate to severe anxiety
• anger toward staff, family, God, or Higher Power
• challenged belief or value system
• loss of meaning and purpose in life
Assess for signs of spiritual despair:
• loss of hope
• refusal to communicate with loved ones
• loss of spiritual belief
• death wish
• severe depression
• flat affect
• refusal to participate in treatment regimen
Assess for special religious concerns such as diet, refusal of blood.

INTERVENTIONS

Convey a caring and accepting attitude.
Provide support, encouragement, and respect.

Provide presence.
Listen actively.
Use therapeutic communication techniques such as restatement, clarification, or silence.
Join in prayer or reading scripture if comfortable.
Use therapeutic touch with the patient's permission.
Include family/significant other in spiritual care.
Consult physician for medications as needed for anxiety or depression.

REPORTABLE CONDITIONS

Notify physician of severe anxiety, or depression that may require pharmacologic or psychiatric intervention.
Notify chaplain, priest, rabbi, pastor or spiritual leader of spiritual concerns, distress or despair with patient's permission.

DOCUMENTATION

Document assessment on database and flow sheet.
Document significant comments, behaviors of patient/family/significant other, interventions, physician notification, and referrals to chaplain or other religious leader on nurse's notes.
Document initiation of protocol on plan of care.

FIGURE 30-1. Spiritual needs protocol.

REFERENCES: Pettigrew, J. *Intensive Nursing Care—The Ministry of Presence,* Critical Care Nursing Clinics of North America, Volume 2, #3, pg. 503–508, September 1990. *Adapted with permission from a protocol developed by Beth Villines, BS, RN, CCRN, Jean Harrington, chaplain, and the Interdisciplinary Plan of Care Team at Saint Luke's Northland Hospital, Kansas City, MO. Saint Luke's Northland Hospital is a member of the Saint Luke's/Shawnee Mission Health System.*

- Be prepared to cooperate or collaborate with the patient's spiritual official, be it high priestess, shaman, minister, or guru.
- Speak up about issues of spirituality in the health care organization where you practice. Participate on standards committees and practice guideline committees. Facilitate the development of nursing admission forms that include spiritual orientation.

● RESPECT FOR THE INDIVIDUAL

The ANA Code of Ethics specifies that "the nurse, in providing care, promotes an environment in which the values, customs, and beliefs of individuals are respected." The International Code of Nursing Ethics makes the same statement with specific reference to "spiritual beliefs." Helping patients maintain their individuality without conflicting with the dominant culture demonstrates personal respect and conforms to JCAHO standards. When you interpret the meaning of spirituality from the patient's perspective with an awareness that spirituality is a global concept, your responses may be more therapeutic to your patient's immediate needs.

Often when patients are coping with life-threatening diseases, the most consistent aspect of their experience is contact with a nurse. We're present 24 hours a day, seven days a week, regardless of physical settings. When patients are at their lowest physical, mental, and spiritual level, and when their support systems weaken or fade away, we are there. This presence gives us an opportunity to promote spiritual health and integrity by being open to and accepting the horizontal aspect of spirituality.

SELECTED REFERENCES

Boutell, K.A. and Bozett, F.W. Nurses' assessment of patients' spirituality: Continuing education implications. *J. Contin. Educ. Nurs.* 21:172–176, July–Aug. 1990.

Engebretson, J. Considerations in diagnosing in the spiritual domain. *Nurs. Diagn.* 7:100–107, July–Sept. 1996.

Frankl, V.E. *Man's Search for Meaning: An Introduction to Logotherapy,* 4th ed. Boston, Beacon Press, 1992.

Heliker, D. Reevaluation of a nursing diagnosis: Spiritual distress. *Nurs. Forum* 27(4):15–20, Oct.–Dec. 1992.

Mansen, T.J. The spiritual dimension of individuals: Conceptual development. *Nurs. Diagn.* 4:140–147, Oct.–Dec. 1993.

Redfield, J. *The Celestine Prophecy: An Adventure.* Hoover, AL, Satori Publishing, 1993.

Stoll, R.I. Guidelines for spiritual assessment. *Am. J. Nurs.* 79:1574–1577, Sept. 1979.

Taylor, E.J., et al. Spiritual care practices of oncology nurses. *Oncol. Nurs. Forum* 22:31–39, Jan.–Feb. 1995.

Teaching is an essential aspect of community-based care. Assessment of the learner is the first step to effective teaching. This article outlines a comprehensive assessment process to analyze the characteristics of the learner.

How does effective teaching lead to cost savings? How is teaching in the community setting different from teaching in the acute care setting? What are the four questions fundamental to the instructional process?

Duffy, B. (1998). Get ready—Get set—Go Teach! Analyzing patients as learners in home healthcare. *Home Healthcare Nurse*, 16(9), 597–602.

31

Get Ready—Get Set— Go Teach! Analyzing Patients as Learners in Home Healthcare

BARBARA DUFFY

Teaching is an integral part of the home care nursing role and has assumed increasing importance as a cost-saving intervention. This article gives the home health nurse insight into the importance of thoroughly assessing the patient's learning style before developing and implementing the teaching plan.

Patients come to home healthcare from all walks of life. It seems that every life challenge eventually shows up in home care. Nurses are increasingly being asked to teach this diverse population about complex and expanding healthcare issues. Quite often, referrals offer little in the way of information other than patient name, address, and diagnosis. With this information, nurses are expected to teach patients with a myriad of needs and abilities in a nontraditional, unstructured setting—the patient's home. The "student" may or may not be able to read, walk, or speak. The only prerequisite for attending this "class" is a need for assistance. It is a situation that would challenge even the most seasoned teacher.

With shorter and fewer hospital admissions and limited resources becoming realities in the transforming of the American healthcare system today, the bulk of patient education and training is occurring in the home. Home care nurses are expected to provide efficient and effective instruction for "sicker" patients. This occurs at a time when payer sources are insisting that patients become and remain independent in a shorter time.

Unlike the controlled environment of the typical classroom, home healthcare instruction takes place in the unpredictable confines of the patient's home. There is no desk;

Barbara Duffy, RN, LHRM, BS, is Director of Health Care Services, Interim HealthCare, South Daytona, FL.

there is no blackboard. Noise, low light, uncomfortable temperatures, pets, family members, and a million other interruptions and distractions are an everyday part of this "classroom." Our student is the ill or injured as well as maybe another caregiver or two. Traditional classroom educational and training methods must be adjusted to accommodate the needs, abilities, resources, and environments of this special population of students. To meet these needs best in the most effective and cost-efficient manner, the Patient Learner Analysis and Planning Tool will be discussed in this article.

● WHY IS THE PATIENT LEARNER ANALYSIS AND PLANNING TOOL NEEDED?

There are four questions fundamental to the instructional process (Kemp, 1985):

1. What are the characteristics of the learner?
2. What must the learner be able to do or learn? (objectives)
3. How is the subject content or skill best learned? (teaching methods)
4. How is the learning evaluated?

This article focuses mostly on analyzing the characteristics of the learner (question 1). However, in doing so, it also suggests the best methods for teaching those characteristics (question 3). What the learner must learn or be able to do is also addressed in this analysis/teaching plan (question 2), which in turn describes how the learner will be evaluated (question 4). The Patient Learner Analysis and Planning Tool (see Fig. 31-1) is offered as a method for obtaining pertinent information and developing an appropriate teaching plan for patients in the home.

Characteristics of the Learner

Patient education and training cannot be accomplished with a "cookbook" approach (Rankin & Stallings, 1996). Most of the literature available today dealing with patient education and training pertains to materials developed for teaching the patient about a specific illness, treatment, or procedure. Very little has been researched about analyzing patients as learners.

Patients, like all other students, have varying learning styles, motivations, and rates of learning and retention. An early and comprehensive analysis of the learner helps in targeting instruction to the needs and learning styles of the patient (or caregiver) and in developing an effective teaching plan. This analysis should answer the following questions:

Is there a problem worth solving?
Is instruction a relevant part of the solution?
If so, what should the instruction accomplish (Mager, 1984)?

The analysis should include environmental, ethnic, cultural, religious, psychomotor, cognitive, affective, and psychosocial considerations as well as the patient's communication, sensory, and motor functional abilities (Rankin & Stallings, 1996; Spector, 1996). Learning styles also must be explored with the patient, caregiver, or both. This analysis for patient education and training need not be separate from other assessment activities. Information about the learning needs of the patient, caregiver, or both is gathered with other data about the patient's condition (Rankin & Stallings, 1996).

Each patient has unique physical and cognitive limitations and requires special consideration. As a result, some patients find certain methods of learning more appealing and

Patient Learner Analysis and Planning Tool

Learner Name (Patient/Caregiver) _____ Date _____

Psychomotor Abilities of the Learner

Sensory limitations (sight, hearing, smell, taste, touch) _____
Color blind or experience of night blindness? _____
Motor/functional limitations (walking, ROM, manual dexterity, etc.) _____
What does (did) learner do to exercise? _____
Occupation/hobbies _____

Communication

How does learner communicate? _____
What is learner's primary language? Is learner able to read that language? _____
Is learner able to read/write/speak English? _____

Environment

Does learner have a working VCR and TV? _____ Cassette tape player? _____
Potential distractions (pets, poor lighting, noise, temperature) _____
Time of day and days of the week best for teaching (meds, therapy, planned/routine activity) ____
_____
Primary caregiver(s) _____ When are they able to be present? _____
Safety concerns _____

Cognitive Abilities

Current learner knowledge of illness/injury _____
Education level _____ Any learning disabilities? _____

Affective Abilities

What does the learner most value? _____
What is the healthcare goal? _____

Learning Styles
Which best describes the learner? (brain dominance)

_____ 1. Likes words, numbers, parts, sequential order, linear thought, detail-oriented, punctual, organized, language. (left-brain analytical learner)
OR
_____ 2. Likes images, patterns, wholes, simultaneous actions, nonverbal, creative, intuitive, spontaneous, graphics-oriented, music. (right-brain, global learner)

Which best describes the learner? (learning modalities)

_____ 1. Prefers verbal instruction; remember names, not faces; distracted by noise, enjoys music; likes answering machines. (auditory learner)
OR
_____ 2. Remembers faces; forgets names; vivid imagination; thinks in pictures; uses color; likes post cards. (visual Learner)
OR
_____ 3. Learns by doing; remembers what was done; touch is important; impulsive; loves games. (kinesthetic learner)

Circle the activities listed below that the learner enjoys doing:

(Visual)	(Auditory)	(Kinesthetic)
watching TV	tapes	games
reading	music	simulations
videos	radio	group activities
handouts	conversation	return demonstration
flip charts	listening to instruction	role playing

FIGURE 31-1. Patient learner analysis and planning tool.

Ethnic/Religion

In what country were the learner's parents born? _____

What foods and drinks are special to the ethnic background? _____

What is the learner's religion? _____

Psychosocial

Role of learner before this illness/injury _____

What chief problem has this illness/injury caused for learner? _____

Emotional/stress/coping level _____ Learner lives with _____

What does the learner feel he or she needs to know or must know how to do? _____

_____

_____

_____

Teaching/Lesson Plan Development

Information to be taught (number in order to be taught):

_____ diet   _____ s/s of disease   _____ infection control   _____ disease process

_____ FBS   _____ dsg change   _____ IV therapy   _____ injections

_____ ROM   _____ equipment use   _____ personal care   _____ cath care

_____ cath insertion   _____ tube feeding   _____ safety   _____ medications

_____ trach care   _____ other

other _____

Need for another discipline? _____ Which ones and why? _____

Write at least one OBSERVABLE objective for each preceding numbered item. Use back of sheet for additional space. Keep in mind knowledge, skill, attitude. **After instruction, the patient/caregiver will be able to:**

1. _____

2. _____

3. _____

Teaching method. (Place corresponding objective number before appropriate teaching method. You may use a method more than once.)

_____ handouts _____ simulation   _____ practice   _____ games _____ role play

_____ video   _____ community class _____ flip charts   _____ lecture

_____ reading   _____ problem solving _____ cassette tapes _____ other

other _____

Equipment/materials needed for preceding activities _____

_____

Evaluate (Place corresponding objective number and date met before appropriate evaluation method.)

_____ recitation _____ return demonstration _____ verbal/written test _____ correct response verbally

_____ observation _____ problem solving _____ other

other _____

Notes/opportunities for improvement:

Certificate of completion to patient _____ Date _____

Nurse signature _____ Date _____

FIGURE 31-1. *(Continued)*

effective than others. It has long been known that in preference to hearing verbal lectures (auditory learners), or reading handout material (visual learners), some individuals learn better from physical activities and the manipulation of objects (kinesthetic learners). Determining the patient's preferred learning style can be beneficial during the instructional planning (Nitko, 1996). Teaching methods can be better selected as appropriate to the learning style of the patient.

Additionally, a general understanding of how the patient routinely processes information can be beneficial to the teaching plan. Determining whether the patient is right- or left-brain dominant can assist in developing instruction. The human brain is divided into right and left hemispheres. It has been found that the two hemispheres contribute differently to the way an individual perceives and organizes information during the process of learning.

The *left hemisphere* is more efficient in handling information in a logical, sequential, and analytical manner. This side is especially well-suited to the functions of language such as reading, speaking, and interpreting written symbols.

The *right hemisphere* interprets information in a more holistic or all-inclusive manner. This side gives attention to the synthesis of information, visual–spatial relationships, and problem solving. The right hemisphere is regarded as the side of the brain used for creative thinking that results, for example, in writing music, designing a work of art, or engineering a structure. People with right brain dominance may have delayed language development or reading and spelling problems (Kemp, 1985).

The characteristics of the learner must also extend to include his or her environment. Many environmental factors can affect a person's ability to concentrate and to absorb and retain information. Consideration must be given to the physical environment (sound, light, temperature, choice of furniture) and the emotional environment (in relation to motivation, taking responsibility, and being persistent in completing a task) (Kemp, 1985). The basic human needs of the patient must also be remembered. If learning is to take place, Abraham Maslow's hierarchy of needs must be met:

- physiologic and survival needs;
- safety and security needs;
- love, affection and belonging needs;
- esteem needs; and
- self-actualization (Rankin & Stallings, 1996).

What Are the Objectives?

An objective is a description of performance the learner must be able to exhibit before being considered competent. An objective describes an intended result of instruction, not the process of the instruction (Mager, 1984).

Objectives are useful in providing a sound basis for the following:

1. selecting or designing of instructional content and procedures
2. evaluating or assessing the success of the instruction
3. organizing the student's efforts and activities for the accomplishment of the important instructional intents.

"If you know where you are going, you have a better chance of getting there" (Mager, 1984).

Successful learning is more likely when the objectives are clearly stated and the learner, at the start of a topic, is informed of the specific objectives to be achieved (Kemp, 1985).

Patients can acquire more information and retain it longer when objectives are carefully written, organized, and constructed with them. Learning is improved when the content or procedures to be learned are organized into meaningful sequences.

The material should be presented to the learner in segments, the size of which depends on logical divisions, complexity, type of learning, and associated activities such as practice and time (Dick & Carey, 1990). Using activities and feedback during instruction sessions can extend the learner's attention span and interest (Dick & Carey, 1990). This organization and procedure can assist the learner in synthesizing and integrating the knowledge or process personally (Kemp, 1985).

The Teaching/Lesson Plan Development Section of the Patient Learner Analysis and Planning Tool allows for development of objectives with the patient to meet his or her learning needs.

How Is the Information Best Learned?

After determining the characteristics of the learner and developing the objectives, many cues to effective instructional methods can be indicated. From the Patient Learner Analysis and Planning Tool, the nurse can determine the type of instruction that will likely be the most effective for the patient, the times to present the information, who needs to be present, what materials are required, and what objectives are being taught. Other motivational and personal information is provided, which also can be used as appropriate during the instructional experience.

For instance, suppose a patient indicates a visual learning preference and has a functioning video cassette recorder/player (VCR) and television. If no illness or injury is currently affecting the patient's eyesight, the patient may benefit from written handout materials, video tapes pertaining to their care, flip charts, and observation of the nurse performing the procedure. The teaching session may be scheduled at times when the patient is not receiving physical therapy, taking pain medications, or napping, and when the primary caregiver can be present. Because this patient is also a "right-brainer," he or she may enjoy applying newly acquired skills and knowledge to given scenarios and problems.

How Is the Learning Evaluated?

Did the patient and/or caregiver meet the objectives? Evaluation is done to assess patient performance and competence. It also is an opportunity to improve teacher and instructional effectiveness (Scott, 1993). The instructional program should be modified as necessary to accommodate patient needs in achieving the objectives. Documentation should be done as changes are made in the teaching plan and as the patient meets objectives. Knowledge and skill of the objectives should be demonstrated through observable means (e.g., the patient does a proper return demonstration of a sterile dressing change or the patient states the signs and symptoms of hypoglycemia).

● CONCLUSION

For centuries, the "technology" for transferring skills and knowledge has changed little: one human being teaching another (Bassi, Cheney, & Van Buren, 1997). Until the teaching of patients becomes automated, home healthcare nurses will be relied on to impart a vast amount of information to an incredibly diverse population of patients. Currently, this occurs at a time when budgets are tighter; resources are limited; and accountability is increasing.

To make the best use of the time allotted for teaching, nurses must become better acquainted with instructional processes and learner needs. One way to accomplish this is through the use of Patient Learner Analysis and Planning Tool. Targeting instruction to the learning styles and knowledge deficits of the patient makes the most efficient use of time for both the patient and the nurse while giving the patient the best opportunity to succeed.

REFERENCES

Bassi, L.J., Cheney, S., & Van Buren, M. (1997). Training industry trends in 1997. *Training and Development, 51,* 46–59.

Dick, W., & Carey, L. (1990). *The systematic design of instruction* (3rd ed.). New York: Harper-Collins.

Kemp, J.E. (1985). *The instructional design process.* New York: Harper & Row.

Mager, R.F. (1984). *Preparing instructional objectives.* Belmont, CA: Lake Publishing Company.

Nitko, A.J. (1996). *Educational assessment of students.* Englewood Cliffs, NJ: Prentice-Hall.

Rankin, S.H., & Stallings, K.D. (1996). *Patient education.* Philadelphia: Lippincott.

Scott, J.L. (1993). Cognitive achievement evaluation. In L.G. Duenk (Ed.), *Improving vocational curriculum.* (pp. 145–171). South Holland, IL: Goodheart-Wilcox.

Spector, R.E. (1996). *Cultural diversity in health and illness.* Stamford, CT: Appleton & Lange.

INTERNET RESOURCES

Calgary Conjoint Nursing Program. Available at: http://www2.mtroyal.ab.ca/mmontgon/week2.htm.

Teaching: individual. Available at: http://neurosun.medsch.ucla.edu/BMML/Stitt/new.htdocs/NIC HTML/intrv_275.html.

Wound and Skin Care Patient Education in Home Care. Available at: http://www.convatec.com/wshca4.htm.

This article presents a simple teaching process specifically geared toward adult learners. It discusses learners, objectives, and methods of instruction and evaluation using adult learning principles. Strategies for documentation of client learning are presented.

How and why do adults learn? How does the nurse decide what to teach? How does the nurse determine what method and what materials to use? What are some tips to remember when teaching? How does the nurse evaluate the effectiveness of his or her teaching?

Duffy, B. (1997). Using a creative teaching process with adult patients. *Home Healthcare Nurse*, 15(2), 102–108.

32

Using a Creative Teaching Process With Adult Patients

BARBARA DUFFY

Teaching is an integral component of the home care nurse's role in every visit. Even though many teaching materials are at the nurse's disposal, not everyone feels comfortable teaching in the home setting. A simple teaching process specifically geared toward adult learners is presented as well as strategies and games that the home care nurse can use to make the teaching process effective and efficient.

Home health nursing provides a unique and wonderful opportunity for patient education and training. Working one on one with the patient and caregivers in a familiar environment offers opportunities not found in medical facilities such as hospitals or physicians' offices. Unlike traditional scheduled classrooms of many "unrelated" students, the home health nurse is able to use the home environment as an individualized learning experience, thereby potentially increasing patient acceptance and compliance with the instruction.

Hospital staff members are frequently unable to spend the time needed to teach patients and caregivers adequately before discharge from the facility. Home health nurses must assess what the patient has retained of the hospital teaching and continue instruction from there. When appropriate and taught by a skilled nurse or therapist, teaching is a service reimbursed by many payment sources including Medicare.

Teaching patients in the home is much like any other skilled nursing intervention in that someone cannot be forced to learn any more than someone can be forced to get well. The nurse instructor's challenge is to instill in patients the desire to learn and provide every opportunity for them to participate in the learning process. Getting well and learning are determined largely by the acceptance and consequential change in behavior.

This article discusses the learners, objectives, methods of instruction, and evaluation

Barbara Duffy, RN, BS, LHRM, is Director of Health Care Services, Interim Healthcare, South Daytona, FL.

using adult learning principles and the Analyze, Design, Develop, Implement and Evaluate (ADDIE) method of instructional design (Kemp, 1985). It also demonstrates various teaching and learning concepts dealing with adult learners and makes suggestions as to how these can be applied to patient learning opportunities in the home.

● WHAT IS ADDIE?

How do you go about developing patient instruction? Is there a system that puts you in control of the content, methods, organization, and materials while allowing for individuality and flexibility? By applying an instructional design process, a reliance on intuition or trial-and-error planning can be reduced (Kemp, 1985).

ADDIE is a simple but effective model to use for instructional design. Through proper use, ADDIE answers the who, what, where, when, how, and why of instruction.

● HOW AND WHY ADULTS LEARN

The two distinguishing characteristics of adult learning most frequently advanced by androgogy theorists are the adult's autonomy of direction in the act of learning and the use of personal experience as a learning resource (Brookfield, 1986). Average adults spent years as children in educational systems, learning concepts to help them in the working world. As adults, their learning focus generally shifts to concerns closer to home and to themselves. For the purposes of home health instruction, this is ideal.

Adults learn best when they feel the need to learn and when they have a sense of responsibility for what, why, and how they learn (Brookfield, 1986). They often become ready to learn after they identify the need to know through life experience. They then want specific information relevant to their needs (Brookfield, 1986). Conversely, adults do not bother with information they cannot directly apply to a personal situation or concern. Experience has taught them the world is full of information, and out of necessity, they must limit their time and energy to relevant interests.

Like all students, adults learn at different rates, with differing comprehension and retention. Some adult patients learn best through visual means (such as watching the nurse perform a task) or auditory means (such as listening to instructions or lecture). Others learn the most through hands-on experience. Effective instruction must consider all of these strategies. Through these means of instruction, the goal is for the patient to be able to:

1. Have the **knowledge** or cognition (i.e., This is the syringe and needle filled with the proper amount of insulin required to lower my blood sugar that's now 265) (Kemp, 1985).
2. Have the **skill** or psychomotor ability (This is the proper method of injecting my abdomen) (Kemp, 1985).
3. Have the **desire, attitude,** or value (I want to do what is needed to control my blood sugar and enhance my long-range health) (Kemp, 1985).

Adult patients want to have control over their own destiny (Brookfield, 1986). Ask patients what they expect to learn or what their goals are at the beginning of the teaching process. Then, effective nursing instruction facilitates learning by helping adult patients find their level of knowledge and skill, and determines which means of instruction are most effective (visual, auditory, or hands on), and provides new learning experiences within a nonthreatening and supportive home environment.

A big part of learning is the motivation to learn or perform a task. Much of what nurses teach involves changing the patient's major long-standing actions and attitudes. Although the long-term effect may be desired by the patient, the day-to-day lifestyle changes involved are not always embraced. Reinforcing motivating factors, therefore, should be integrated into the teaching plan (Humphrey & Milone-Nuzzo, 1996).

Adults often underestimate their ability to learn new things and therefore need a lot of encouragement to cope with change in their lives. They want to fully understand *why* something must be done before they alter years of a lifestyle or practice. Nurses must give such patients a sense of accomplishment through timely reinforcement and numerous opportunities to practice new skills throughout the instructional period. Positive feedback regarding patient progress enhances motivation and encourages continued learning (Kemp, 1985). The nurse must be a patient, compassionate role model, mindful of the patient's often fragile self-esteem. Demonstrating a strong desire to teach and showing them you are interested in their welfare will greatly enhance patients' attitude toward learning.

● THE INSTRUCTIONAL DESIGN PROCESS OF ADDIE

Analysis: Who to Teach, Where, When, and Why

In preparing to teach, take a different look at the home and patient. Barking dogs, effects of pain medications, and the patient's watching a favorite soap opera on TV are things that may not significantly impede a visit for a dressing change but might make teaching more difficult.

Without denying the importance of "impromptu" mini-teaching sessions at appropriate moments, times and places for patient instruction should be planned in advance. Where and when can the nurse have the patient's full attention with the fewest distractions? Who else should be present? Why must the patient be taught and how do you anticipate the instruction will impact his or her health? The instruction must be scheduled at times other than those designated for activities such as therapy, naps, physician's appointments, and times for household construction or repairs. Depending on the situation, the instruction might occur outside on the patio away from interruptions (weather and noise permitting) or with the family gathered around a kitchen table.

Keep the patient's considerations in mind. Assess the patient's readiness, willingness, and ability to learn (Mason & Hansen, 1991). According to Abraham Maslow's theory, basic physiologic needs for food, water, oxygen, elimination, etc., take precedence over other needs. These needs must be satisfied before effective learning can occur (Rice, 1996). Pain, fatigue, medication side effects, language barriers, educational level, age, and physical, emotional, or intellectual impairments also may influence instruction time, endurance, and the ability to cope with illness and instruction (Hudson et al., 1992). Sensory loss of hearing or vision impacts the selection of the method of instruction. For example, the inability to identify color may result in the patient's taking the wrong medication; a patient with a hearing impairment may accept instruction better when the nurse's face and use of nonverbal communication are easily seen (Pollock & Altholz, 1993).

Family, social, and cultural dynamics can influence who else are involved in the teaching process, what task they will perform, and when they will do it. A caregiver may also have physical or emotional limitations. Among multiple caregivers, the nurse becomes a facilitator, encouraging the members to express their concerns, experiences, and ideas of coping and caring for the patient. Allow for the physical, emotional, and mental comfort of the patient and caregivers. Check the physician's orders for what is to be taught, make a note of your analysis of the environmental and patient considerations anticipated to affect the teaching process, and get ready to make a plan.

Design: What to Teach

Specifically what does the patient need and want to learn? Just planning for the patient to learn about tube feedings is not enough. What is the objective?

An objective is a small goal or outcome of intended patient-centered learning that is measurable and observable. It is a description of a performance you want patients (or caregivers) to exhibit before you consider them to be competent (Mager, 1984). An objective also describes the result of instruction, not the process (Mager, 1984). The objective has three components (Mager 1984):

1. **The condition:** given materials or a specific situation (e.g., a blood sugar level of 50 mg/dL, sterile supplies, low urine output due to a clogged foley catheter, etc.)
2. **The performance:** for example, the learner will be able to list four symptoms of hypoglycemia, change a sterile dressing, properly irrigate a catheter, etc.
3. **How well:** as measured by scoring, for example, 100% on a written or verbal test, a return demonstration, a free-flowing catheter, etc.

Make sure the objectives are within the physical, emotional, and intellectual abilities of the patient and that each one addresses the knowledge, skill, or attitude aspects of learning. For example:

The patient will demonstrate comprehension of how diabetes affects the importance of good foot care as evidenced by:

1. Verbal response regarding slow wound healing of feet with diabetes (knowledge)
2. Demonstration of proper washing and drying of feet (skill)
3. Always wearing shoes and socks at appropriate times (attitude)

Analyze and organize the order of information to be presented. Build one unit of instruction on top of existing knowledge or skills, as illustrated in the following dialogue:

Remember yesterday when you learned about how digoxin lowers your heart rate and how that helps your condition? Today we will discuss how to measure your heart rate and what is normal for you when you are taking digoxin.

Adult learners like to know what to expect and to have a sense of being in control. Frequently discuss the objectives with the patient and ask for agreement and inclusion of what they want to learn. This gives them a sense of shared direction with the nurse, preserves dignity, and encourages participation. For example:

Tomorrow, please have your medications ready so we can administer them together. The goal we set is to have you comfortably performing your tube feedings by Friday. How do you feel things are progressing so far?

After designing the objectives, including what needs to be taught, in what order, and identifying where, with whom, why, and when (analysis); teaching materials must be selected and collected in accordance to the patient needs.

Development: How to Teach and What to Use

Development is planning how to teach the patient objectives and what items or methods to use. This includes getting everything together and ready for the actual instruction.

At every opportunity, plan to involve the patient and caregiver in the instruction. Research has shown that a learner remembers 10% of what is read, 20% of what is heard, 30% of what is seen, 50% of what is heard and seen, and 80% of what the learner says and does (Humphrey & Milone-Nuzzo, 1996). The learner must internalize the information and not simply be told it (Kemp, 1985).

Gather and inspect patient teaching materials. Make sure the teaching materials are current, pertinent, and appropriate for the patient according to reading grade level, primary language, and ability. Look for more than printed handouts. What resources for items and supplies do you have available that would make a simulation more realistic? Do you have a video on a topic that you can lend to a patient with a video cassette player? Organize the materials according to the individualized patient teaching plan.

Provide simulations when appropriate (such as washing and diapering a baby doll before the child is born). Keep in mind the closer the simulation is to the actual environment, the better the learner will do in the real situation (Campbell 1993). Use the same furniture, tub, washcloth, etc., the learner anticipates using in "real life."

Making instruction interactive through games and role playing adds another dimension to learning in the home. Some patients enjoy playing **Medication Jeopardy!** To play, the nurse states the actions, side effects, dosage, or time to be taken for a particular drug, and the patient must respond with the name of the proper medication.

"Armchair Grocery Shopping" is another activity in which the nurse provides a list of common foods from which the patient chooses those allowed on his or her diet.

Adults learn by solving *relevant* problems. Instruction that provides scenarios challenge patients in caring for themselves in various situations. This gets the patient involved, thinking, and ready for life after discharge. For example, consider asking patients the following problem-solving questions:

- Provide a menu from a favorite restaurant, asking the patient, "How do you choose a meal you enjoy that is on your diet?"
- "How would you transport your insulin on an overnight trip to your sister's home?"
- "Since our talk about skin care, what would you need to consider if you went to the beach with your leg prosthesis?"
- "From what you have learned, how would you transfer your dad with right hemiplegia into and out of a car?"
- "In case of a disaster, how would you wash your hands if only bottled water were available?"
- "How would you change your husband's diapers using a public rest room?"
- "How would you navigate your wheelchair in the snow?"

The patient's homework assignment for the next visit may be create questions to **"Stump the Nurse."** After providing the patient with resource material about vitamin B-12 deficiency, the patient can quiz the nurse during the next visit, asking "Tell me nurse, what is intrinsic factor and where is it produced?"

Integrating the home living environment with the task the nurse is teaching increases the likelihood of long-term compliance by the patient. The nurse can make convenient suggestions that adapt the newly learned behaviors into daily activities. Look to caregivers and patients for clues of daily routines.

It isn't easy for quadriplegics to remember to shift to relieve pressure on their buttocks every hour. How can it be consistently incorporated into their daily activities? Would a wristwatch set to beep hourly during waking times help? Where can medications be placed in the home to ensure the patient remembers to take them? Can the morning dose be placed next to favorite breakfast foods and the evening dose be placed near the pajama drawer? Would a sheet of paper and pencil taped on the bathroom mirror remind patients with congestive heart failure of the importance of writing down and monitoring their weight every morning?

How can helpful tools and reminders be used in the daily environment to encourage proper health maintenance without getting into the way or announcing to the world that this person needs help? Incorporating health maintenance activities into these routines helps them to become automatic and less cumbersome.

Consider these ideas and others when developing your teaching plan.

Implementation

Prepared with the analysis, design, and development of the teaching plan, the nurse now is ready to provide learning experiences for the patient in the home. Some tips to remember during the instruction:

- Involve patients. Ask them to tell you what they know about the topic. Let them "experiment" with real equipment during practice.
- Tell them, show them, let them practice, and then let them tell you, and you can coach them through it.
- Use language patients can understand. Be careful with abbreviations and medical jargon.
- When possible, teach the task where it will occur in the home. For example, colostomy care taught in the bathroom; learning about a low-sodium diet while going through the kitchen cabinets and planning dinner.
- Put yourself at eye level with the patient. Talk slowly, allowing for breaks as needed.
- Build teaching on prior patient knowledge, skills, and experience. "Yes, this does have a lot in common with when you gave your dog insulin shots."
- Give the patient plenty of opportunities to give correct responses. Give immediate feedback to incorrect actions or responses, but never criticize. Never rush.
- Involve as many of the senses as possible. "Notice how the alcohol swab smells and feels cool on your skin."
- Relax! The use of friendly humor contributes to an effective learning environment.
- Tell the patient, "Let's find out together what works the best for you."

Research has found that precision and clarity of information presented along with teacher excitement, animation, and humor are the qualities that contribute most to high learner evaluations (Brookfield, 1986). Good organization, willingness to experiment, and encouragement of learners to think for themselves also receives high marks (Hudson, Holt, Benda, & Ebrite, 1992).

Be flexible in your teaching plan. Listen to the patient. Adjust the goals, methods of instruction, and materials to meet the needs of the patient. Remember, the nurse is there to instruct and be a helpful resource, not to inspire old memories of school teachers wielding rulers. Let the patient learn by solving problems. Lead them to the proper solution and discovery of what is going to work for them.

Evaluate

At each point, evaluate how effective the teaching plan has been. Is the patient competent in the task the nurse has taught? Does the patient have the knowledge, skill, and desire to perform the task? Was the objective met? Has there been an observable change in behavior? Routinely evaluate your patients' comprehension and skills to avoid frustrating them (Mason & Hansen, 1991).

Use checklists and performance rating scales on return demonstrations to score and document observable and measurable patient performance. Praise success, and reemphasize those areas needing further instruction, practice, or coaching. Consider providing certificates of accomplishment at discharge "graduation," having the patient and nurse date and sign the certificate as each task or objective is mastered. Leave information about where the patient can get more help from support groups, books, etc.

Always document the teaching that was was done along with listing the materials used and patient outcome. In addition to meeting requirements for various payer sources and serving as a legal safeguard, documentation of patient teaching can provide valuable information regarding competency and outcomes for quality improvement programs (Mason & Hansen, 1991).

This documentation should include a statement of the patient's health problem, any barriers affecting the ability to learn, learning outcomes or objectives agreed upon by the nurse and the patient, teaching methods, an objective statement regarding the patient's response to the teaching, and an evaluation of the patient's progress in meeting the outcomes or objectives (Mason & Hansen, 1991). Make sure the discharge summary includes a listing of the patient educational materials provided to the patient and caregiver.

Also evaluate your teaching plan and yourself. What worked well and what needs some help? Do you have the skill, knowledge, and ability to teach this subject? Update your materials and knowledge frequently. Take a good look at the teaching plan. Save the materials and methods that worked well, but constantly ask yourself, "How can I do this better next time?" What does the patient need to be taught, and what outcomes can you expect? Share your findings and suggestions with coworkers. Build resources of materials, methods, and experts in various fields. Find new ways to answer who, what, where, when, how, and why through the ADDIE process of instructional design.

● SUMMARY

Because the patient or caregiver must manage healthcare needs after the nurse has left the home, patient education is an important component to home health nursing (Rice, 1996). Fortunately, patient teaching is ideal for home healthcare. To make the most of the home learning environment with adult patients, the nurse must assess, design, develop, implement, and evaluate an individualized patient teaching plan. Throughout the ADDIE process, the nurse manipulates and integrates the home environment to maximize the possibility that the patient will accept, remember, and apply the information presented. Taking into account how adults learn, the nurse provides relevant problems and situations for the patient to practice newly acquired knowledge and skills. The instruction presents learners with alternatives to their current ways of thinking, behaving, and living (Brookfield, 1986). Given the information and the tools needed to regain a sense of control and experience life safely, within their abilities of medical illness or injury, informed adult patients are likely to experience fewer complications and enhanced self-esteem.

For pertinent, timely, and personal healthcare instruction, there is no place quite like home.

REFERENCES

Brookfield, S.D. (1986). *Understanding and facilitating adult learning*. San Francisco, CA: Jossey-Bass Publishers.

Campbell, C.P. (1993). *Manipulative performance tests. Improving vocational curriculum* (pp. 173–196). South Holland, IL: Goodheart- Willcox Company, Inc.

Hudson, L., Holt, L., Benda, B., Ebrite, L., & Hudson, L. (1992). *I make a difference* (pp. 66–77). Albany, NY: Delmar Publishers Inc.

Humphrey, C., & Milone-Nuzzo, P. (1996). Client teaching in the home. *Manual of home care nursing orientation* (pp. 7:2–7:20). Gaithersburg, MD: Aspen Publishers, Inc.

Kemp, J.E. (1985). *The instructional design process*. New York: Harper & Row Publishers.

Mager, R.F. (1984). *Preparing instructional objectives*. Belmont, CA: Lake Publishing Company.

Mason, J.E., & Hansen, J. F. (1991). How to teach patients. Teaching and learning: An overview. *Patient teaching loose-leaf library*. Springhouse, PA: Springhouse Corporation.

Pollock, D., & Altholz, J. (1993). *Caregivers handbook* (pp. 61–69). Tallahassee, FL: Health Trac Books.

Rice, R., et al. (1996). *Home health nursing practice concepts & application* (2nd ed., pp. 77–100). St. Louis, MO: Mosby-Year Book, Inc.

Sometimes a very simple intervention may lead to client learning.

Holt, J. (1995). Motivating Beth. *American Journal of Nursing*, 95(12), 60–61.

33

Motivating Beth

JEANIE HOLT

An innovative teaching strategy led to this special patient's success.

"Jeanie, guess what? I used my cards! I measured the spaghetti and the hamburger. Oh, and the peas, too!"

Beth was so excited that her words tumbled over each other, not quite keeping pace with her unbridled exuberance.

"That's great, Beth!" I replied. "Use a snack card tonight and we'll test your sugar in the morning." I, too, was excited at the prospect that my hard work had paid off and Beth's blood glucose levels were finally where they should be. And hard work it was.

I'd admitted Beth McCoy for home nursing services two months before. Beth, nearly 60, had non-insulin-dependent diabetes and was developmentally disabled. She couldn't read, and her ability to apply what she learned in one situation to another was limited. But despite these handicaps, she lived in an apartment, thanks in part to a local service that helped her with shopping, money management, and medical appointments.

Three months before, Beth's case manager at the disabilities services office had received a letter from her physician, who recommended an aggressive home care program to get her blood glucose levels and weight under control. Otherwise, he said, he'd be forced to recommend a more structured living environment, such as a group home. Beth had been receiving home care from another agency, but hadn't made adequate progress. So our agency was enlisted to provide diabetes care.

On my earliest visits, Beth wouldn't even look at me, answering my questions only with a reluctant word or two. I later learned that she missed the nurse who'd been coming to prefill her insulin syringes before our agency became involved in her case. Though Beth had been told about the switch, apparently she hadn't fully agreed to it. All I could do at that point was gently acknowledge her feelings of loss and helplessness.

Back at the office, I called the case manager, Cathy, for clarification. That's when I found out about the physician's letter—and the challenge ahead of me.

"The situation is urgent," Cathy said. "You've done so well with our other developmentally disabled patients that we figured you were our best shot."

Jeanie Holt is a staff nurse at Heritage Home Health and Hospice in Manchester, NH.

I suspected the agency thought I was a miracle worker, when, in fact, my patient would barely speak to me.

Over the next two weeks, I concentrated on identifying the cause of Beth's high blood glucose level and weight. I watched her inject her insulin, which she performed easily, and kept careful count of her syringes. She never missed a dose. I also observed her testing her blood glucose level using a glucometer. While her technique left room for improvement, the results were reasonably accurate. I tried to initiate an exercise program for Beth, but since she had severe arthritis in her knees, her mobility was limited. She also told me that both of her parents had been diabetic—and, she confessed, they "hid sweets and ate them when they thought no one was looking." I concluded that Beth's main problem was sticking to her diabetic diet.

We met with a dietitian, who took a detailed but rather inaccurate food history and designed a 1,500-calorie diabetic meal plan. All Beth got out of the meeting was that she could have a half cup of oatmeal for breakfast, which she mistook to mean a half cup *uncooked*, causing her to consume more than twice her allowance of breakfast calories.

I spent the next two visits teaching Beth to use the American Diabetes Association's booklet "Eating Healthy Foods," which the dietitian left for her. It quickly became clear that, though Beth recognized the pictures, the rest was far beyond her understanding. She couldn't even find the right page for a particular meal on her own. I pondered the problem several times that day while driving between patient visits. The solution finally came to me.

With renewed enthusiasm, I gathered supplies and headed for Beth's apartment. "Most women have a recipe box," I told her, "and you should too." She brightened a little at the idea of having something that most women have, and told me about the pretty recipe box her mother had. I explained to her that her box would have cards of four different colors with illustrated dividers, one for each meal of the day and one for snacks. I later added a clock face to each card with Beth's meal times drawn in.

With the box and divider cards ready, we began to make "recipes." For breakfast, Beth could have two starch exchanges, a piece of fruit, and a half cup of milk. We cut out pictures of foods from supermarket ads and made one card for each meal. "Look through the cards, pick the meal you want, shop for what you need, and then follow the card exactly," I explained.

During the next month, we made cards at every visit. But Beth's progress was slow. I could see that she was doing *something* with the cards between visits, but she admitted that she wasn't really using them. Her blood glucose levels, still well over 200, provided additional evidence. Still, she seemed to enjoy making the cards, and I'd heard she'd shown them off to her case manager and the local service staff.

When I arrived the next morning, Beth proudly showed me the card she had used to prepare breakfast and told me how she'd measured the oatmeal: "Three tablespoons *before* I cooked it!" Trying to sound casual, I asked for her glucose reading. "Two-sixteen," she said. I was a little disappointed, but I reminded myself that it was still one of the lowest readings we'd seen yet. Plus, Beth was bursting with life, interest, and enthusiasm.

Suddenly, I knew what I *had* accomplished. Using a simple tool—a recipe box—Beth had found the motivation to make the right decisions about what to eat. Realizing that we'd found common ground, as I too struggle with my diet, I began to enjoy my time with her as I would with any other woman. I'm not responsible for her blood glucose readings, only for understanding and encouraging her. Who knows, maybe one day I'll call her just to tell her that I've finally lost those five pounds I've needed to lose. I know now that, between us, we can work small miracles.

Case management is a term with many different meanings and therefore is not easily defined. This article presents one definition of case management and discusses the unique roles of the case manager.

What are the types of case management? What are the characteristics of each type of case management service? Discuss the current trends in case management.

Molloy, S. P. (1994). Defining case management. *Home Healthcare Nurse*, 12(3), 51–53.

Defining Case Management

SANDRA P. MOLLOY

Case management is a frequently used term in nursing; however, it is not easily defined. The discussion that follows examines the various meanings of case management and the roles of the case manager.

There is difficulty defining case management because it has many meanings. When some nurses hear the term, insurance company authorization comes to mind; others may envision the work done by county mental health programs, and still others may imagine nurses helping patients meet goals through standardized plans of care. These impressions are very different, yet they are all accurate, because case management can be categorized as a system, role, technology, process, and service.[1]

Even though case management has diverse applications, there are similar underlying component parts of all types of case management. These elements include assessment, coordination, integration of appropriate health and supportive care services over a length of time, and evaluation.[2]

Through these components of care, the system goals of cost-effectiveness, access of care, and quality of services are provided. As these goals become more difficult to achieve, yet mandated by consumers, a clearer understanding of case management and the roles of case managers is crucial to achieve these objectives.

● TYPES OF CASE MANAGEMENT

There are many models for case management. The American Nurses Association publication on case management describes 12 models.[2] The models can be categorized into three broad areas of case management. They include reimbursement-based, social welfare-based, and agency/institution-based case management systems (Table 34-1). All three have the same basic principles and goals. How these different systems meet the goals of case management will be discussed in the following sections.

Sandra P. Molloy, RN, MSN, CCM, is a case manager, Emanuel Hospital, Portland, OR.

TABLE 34-1 ● Comparison of Case Management Services

	Reimbursement Based	Social Welfare Based	Institution Based	Integrated System of Hospital and Home Care	Private Case Managers
Setting	Hospital, rehabilitation facility or home	Community agency offices or home	Hospital as inpatient; home healthcare agency	Across all settings	Usually across all settings
Length of service	Length of disease	Varies widely	Length of disease	Usually through health and illness	Usually through health and illness
Funding source	Funded by reimbursement based organization.	Usually government funding	Funded by the institution; some government funding	Funded by health system	Out of pocket
Type of case manager	Usually RN	Often social worker, may be RN	RN, often with advanced degree	Usually RN with advanced degree	RN or MSU
Roles & responsibilities of case manager	Insurance preauthorization; managing services provided to a trauma patient	Mental health case worker; Medicaid case worker, aging services case managers	Develop Critical Paths; assist in patient progress while admitted	Develop Critical Paths; assist in patient progress through health & illness	Develop life plan; manage finances, healthcare needs in home

Reimbursement Based

In the reimbursement-based case management system, assessment, coordination, integration, and evaluation are usually conducted by nurses. The title generally given to these care providers is case manager, many of whom have particular areas of specialty. Some of these case managers are based within an insurance company, and others are privately contracted to manage patients. The second group tends to be used to a greater extent in rural areas rather than urban settings.

The interactions of patients and case managers tend to focus on a particular health problem. For both groups of case managers, the assessments are often done by telephone. These may include calls for preauthorization of surgeries or home visits. However, out-of-office visits may be made if indicated.

The majority of the coordination and integration of appropriate services is also done by telephone. Additional roles of case managers are (1) monitoring the care provided; (2) exchanging healthcare benefits to pay for the care that better meets the patient's needs; and (3) evaluating the costs of care and benefits. The evaluation may be carried out in a variety of ways, such as through patient satisfaction surveys, through patient functioning tests, and by determining how many patients/clients change health plans.

Social Welfare Based

The social welfare-based care management organizations have been using the term case management for the longest period. It first appeared in the early 1970s.[2] These case management programs are often funded through the government. Social workers and nurses may fill the roles of case managers and case workers. The timeframe of social welfare-based case management varies widely. Client contact may last from one contact to several years. Interactions between the clients and case managers may be by telephone, at local offices, or in patients' homes.

The main functions are in assessment of need, connecting with resources, and coordination of care. On some levels, case managers may be responsible for rationing funds to provide greater access of services to a greater number of clients.

Another role that these case managers may perform is representative payee functioning, in which the case manager is given legal authority to manage and protect the assets of the client. By performing these various functions, the case managers work to meet the goals of quality of life and provide cost-effective services to the client.

● HOSPITAL/AGENCY BASED

Hospital Based

Since the institution of diagnosis-related groups (DRGs) in 1983, hospitals have made great strides in quantifying and standardizing care. This has led to the development of Critical Paths. Critical Paths are tools of case management that designate what care should be provided for a given healthcare problem within a specified timeframe. Care issues may include laboratory tests, assessments, teaching, procedures, diet, medications, and discharge planner needs. Usually, the increment of time used in a hospital setting is a day, but may be shorter in areas where care needs are intensive. This type of case management tool is usually focused on a particular health-related problem that requires hospitalization. Hospital-based case managers tend to be master's-prepared nurses. Their roles usually include developing, monitoring, and teaching Critical Paths. In addition, many case managers assist patients in obtaining patient-centered goals.

In developing the Critical Paths, case managers assess patients' needs on an aggregate level by disease. They coordinate care through the use of the Critical Paths. Integration of care is provided by use of the Critical Path throughout the patients' admissions to the hospital. The Critical Paths have been developed for a variety of patient care settings, such as the emergency room, intensive and nonintensive care units, and short-stay surgery.

Evaluation of care is performed by the case manager through analysis "variances" reports. Variances are occurrences that are not predicted by Critical Paths, such as extended hospital stays caused by surgical complications. Documented variances are reported by nursing staff. With this information, variance reports are generated by the coding and aggregation of data. These summaries can assist in problem identification and thus lead to resolutions.

Through the use of Critical Paths and assistance of case managers, case management is able to improve cost-effectiveness and quality of care. In addition, access to care is enhanced through the Critical Paths since they use staff to obtain the appropriate services.

Home Health Agency Based

With the shrinking reimbursement by insurance companies and with the Health Care Finance Administration planning the implementation of a DRG-type reimbursement in home care,[3] agencies have begun to look at case-managing home care patients.[4] The basic components of case management and the use of Critical Paths are easily transferred to home healthcare. Home care agencies are developing Critical Paths, which standardize care for health-related problems. The timeframes usually list the number of visits per admission for each diagnosis.[5]

In home healthcare agencies, the case managers' roles can be very similar to those of hospital-based case managers. In addition, primary field staff members may also be designated as case managers. For these field staff case managers, the assessments, coordination, integration, and evaluation tend to be on a patient-by-patient basis.

As in hospitals, home care case management achieves the goals of improved quality, reduced cost, and better access to healthcare through improved coordination of care, provision of expert knowledge, early problem solving, and close monitoring of services provided.

Case management is playing an essential role in several statewide geriatric programs, including those in New York and Connecticut. The New York State Health Department has implemented an innovative healthcare plan, called the Long Term Home Health Care program. This state-run system for healthcare is Medicaid wavered and is an option for state residence. Persons who choose this program are given free case management services as part of a benefits package. The case manager's role is to assist patients in meeting their long- and short-term health needs, while remaining in a safe home environment. Through the aid of the case managers, the patients are provided better-coordinated, less-expensive care.

● TRENDS IN CASE MANAGEMENT

Case management is evolving. Several trends can be identified. One recent development is the amalgamation of home- and hospital-based case management.[6] Through the integration of the case management systems of both, patient continuity and quality of care are greatly enhanced.

In addition to combining services, the timeframe of case management services is beginning to expand beyond a particular illness episode. For patients with chronic obstructive pulmonary disease (COPD), this new approach helps reduce hospital readmissions. Data have shown that this approach lowered hospital costs.[7]

Another innovative service in case management is provided by private case managers who assist individuals with life planning, economic, social, and medical care issues. In most instances, the services are an out-of-pocket cost paid by patients or family members.

A new development in case management is a certification for case managers. The process for certification was implemented this past year by the Commission on Insurance Rehabilitation Specialists. Those eligible for certification must hold a professional license or certificate in a healthcare field. Thus, registered nurses, medical social workers, occupational therapists, and physical therapists may apply for certification. In addition, candidates are required to have had previous case management experience, and pass an examination. In May 1993, approximately 4000 people completed the first test. A second test was offered in November of that year. This certification process ensures a common baseline of knowledge,[8] leading to higher quality of service.

As mentioned earlier, case managers are beginning to establish associations and publications. The National Association of Case Managers is open to case managers in all areas of practice. In addition, clinically focused case managers are beginning to organize associations by areas of expertise. One such group is the National Association of Geriatric Case Managers. To support case managers in their various roles, journals that focus on case management issues are being published. These include the *Journal of Case Management, The Case Manager, Definition,* and *Continuity of Care.*

● SUMMARY

The term case management is used in many different settings. However, the underlying principal functions are the same: assessment, coordination, integration, and evaluation. The goals are also the same: improved quality, reduced costs, and improved access to healthcare. The case manager plays the part of a "surrogate family member" to meet the goals of the identified patient and the society. Because of the importance of these goals, the use of case management principles and procedures certainly will grow in the future.[4]

● ACKNOWLEDGMENT

The author thanks the Emanuel Hospital case managers for assisting her in defining case management.

REFERENCES

1. Falk C. *Nursing Case Management: The Carondelet St. Mary's Model.* Presented at the Northwest Case Management Conference, Portland, Oregon, February 24, 1993.
2. Bower K. *Case Management by Nurses.* Washington, DC: American Nurses Publications, 1992.
3. Pasquale DK. A basis for prospective payment in home care. *Image* 1987; 19:186–191.
4. Sutton S. Experts see controlling utilization key to success in managed home care. *Home Health Line* 1993; April 14:158–161.
5. Zander K. Advertisement in *New Definition* 1993;8(4):IV.
6. Rogers M, Riordan J, Swindle, D. Community-based nursing case management pays off. *Nurs Management,* 1991; 22:30–35.
7. Haggerty MC, Stockdale-Woolley RS, Sreedhar, N. Respi-Care: An innovative home care program for the patient with chronic obstructive pulmonary disease. *Chest* 1991; 100:607–612.
8. Cline K. Certification update: Preparing for the first CM examination. *Case Management* 1993; 4:19–21.

Case management supports cost-effective, outcome-oriented care. Critically tied to the evolving system of reimbursing health care, it is not a static entity. This article describes how the role of the case manager has evolved.

How did the movement toward case management evolve? What are the similarities and differences between hospital-based case management and community-based case management? How can staff nurses become more involved in case management?

Cessna, T. G., & Falter, E. J. (1999). Case management: Its value for staff nurses. *American Journal of Nursing*, 99(1), 48–50.

Case Management: Its Value for Staff Nurses

TONI G. CESTA, ELIZABETH J. FALTER

As case management evolves, it functions are becoming more complex. And whether this intrigues or worries you, it will most likely affect you.

Case management, a nursing care delivery system that supports cost-effective, outcome-oriented care, has reinvented hospital and community health care—rather remarkable for a model that was first developed in the 1940s. Originally a public health tool used to manage catastrophic illness among various social populations, over the decades its use has shifted from the community setting toward the hospital and back again.

Many forces have driven the case management model forward: the escalating health care costs in the 1970s, the inception of the prospective payment system in the 1980s, and the managed care phenomenon in the 1990s. In the last decade, case management has had renewed appeal for providers in community settings, as they try to reduce costs and patient lengths of stay. Thus far, the model's flexibility has helped nurses to keep pace with a changing health care climate. And as leaders in the quest for high-quality, fiscally responsible patient care, registered nurses everywhere are uncovering new opportunities in this emerging discipline.

● THE HISTORY OF REIMBURSEMENT

In 1970, health care accounted for 8% of the gross national product. By 1993, this figure had risen to 14%, and according to a recent article in the *New York Times*, it's expected to reach 17% by 2007. This increase can be attributed, in part, to the lasting effects of legislation like the Hospital Survey and Construction Act of 1947 (also known as the Hill-Burton Act), which authorized federal grants to states to survey their hospitals and to plan

Toni G. Cesta is the director of Case Management at St. Vincent's Hospital and Medical Center in Manhattan, and director of the Case Management Program at the Lienhard School of Nursing, Pace University, in Pleasantville, NY.

Elizabeth J. Falter is the president of Falter & Associates, Inc., a health case consulting and financial planning firm in Croton-on-Hudson, NY.

and build additional public health facilities, thereby supporting the growth of specialist care and providing an incentive to fill those beds.

Also, people who received health insurance either through their employers or through the state (Medicaid) or federal (Medicare) government were relatively insulated from actual health care costs. Consumers wanted the most and best health care they could obtain; yet, because their care was paid for by third parties, they had little reason to consider—and in many cases, were completely unaware of—the associated costs. Medical technology has steadily grown more sophisticated and expensive, and, since the establishment of Medicare and Medicaid in the 1960s, more people have had access to it. The rising incidence of chronic illnesses in an aging patient population and increased litigation have also contributed to mounting health care costs.

To control Medicare expenditures, in 1983 the Health Care Finance Administration developed a prospective payment system using diagnosis-related groups (DRGs)—a move that helped establish the principle of paying for "average" rather than for actual costs. The system, which included 500 surgical and medical diagnostic categories, classified patients based on their resource consumption and length of stay, both indicators of cost of services. DRGs had a powerful effect on hospitals. With the dollar amount reimbursed by case classification now fixed, the prospective payment system fueled their need to reduce length of stay and resource consumption. In 1985, the New England Medical Center in Boston, Massachusetts, and Carondelet St. Mary's Hospital in Tucson, Arizona, were the first hospitals to look to case management for solutions, and others soon followed. Even today, hospitals continue to be reimbursed based on DRGs for certain patients. Appropriate case management for patients who may exceed the allotted resources for a particular DRG is crucial in order for a hospital to remain solvent.

DRGs focused on hospitals, and this system alone couldn't slow the continued growth of health care spending. During the late 1960s and early 1970s, health maintenance organizations (HMOs) began to proliferate, and health care purchasers, primarily employers, began switching to HMO-managed benefits, seeking to control costs by increasing the proportion of care provided in ambulatory or primary care settings.

Health maintenance organizations coordinate a patient's care by controlling access to other practitioners. Members choose a primary caregiver whom they consult for all their health care needs; in turn, this caregiver authorizes referrals to participating specialists and service providers. But HMOs can create higher caseloads and burdensome paperwork for clinicians who must work in partnership with other disciplines in order to shorten hospital stays when needed services and facilities might not be available. For example, an HMO may require a hospital's emergency department to refer a child in asthmatic crisis to an urgent care center without delay, yet there may be no 24-hour urgent care center in that community. Like the DRG system, then, managed care has heightened the need for case management.

Diverse insurance "products" are available to consumers today, ranging from high-cost premium plans with many choices to lower-cost premium plans with limited choices. The two most common plan types are the HMO and the point of service (POS). An HMO plan provides a comprehensive system of medical services to its members on a prepaid basis. A POS plan goes further; it combines the features of an HMO with an indemnity insurance option, allowing members to choose when, how, and from whom to seek needed services. If a member goes outside the HMO network, there are additional charges (higher copayments and deductibles) and paperwork (submission of claim forms).

Under capitation, another financial plan option being offered by managed care organizations, a provider organization accepts a uniform monthly or annual fee from the managed care company to provide services for all individuals (known as *covered lives*) who are covered by a plan. The dollar amount reimbursed per member per month does not deviate, whether the patient uses a lot of resources or never accesses the system. Case management is a way to make sure those fixed dollars are used optimally. Providers thus share in the financial as well as clinical risks associated with their decisions and care.

This model applies across all settings. Chronically ill patients, for instance, typically use many services, and one patient may be seen in several settings during the course of an illness. As providers have sought alternatives to hospitals for more cost-effective yet appropriate settings in which to deliver care, the hospital is now simply one venue for care delivery.

Ideally, a patient moves to the next care setting as soon as that's both appropriate and possible. A generation ago, a patient who underwent hip replacement surgery might have remained hospitalized for 10 days of postsurgical treatment and recuperation. Today, that patient moves to a rehabilitative or home care setting for physical therapy three or four days postsurgery.

● HOSPITAL-BASED CASE MANAGEMENT

When case management entered hospital settings in 1985, it was recognized that registered nurses were in an unparalleled position to manage patient length of stay and resource use. But although their responsibilities overlap somewhat, nurses and case managers have largely different roles. Case managers typically have three specific functions: clinical coordination and facilitation, utilization management, and discharge planning.

Coordination and facilitation are aimed at controlling costs and length of stay without compromising quality of care. As facilitator, the case manager expedites the patient's diagnostic tests, treatments, and consultations by ensuring that they take place promptly and in the proper sequence. The case manager also coordinates the patient's care plan with all involved disciplines, to make sure that needed services aren't overlooked and that service and resource redundancies are minimized. Case management plans are outcome oriented. That means that for each patient, as the case manager monitors the course of treatment in a given setting, the focus is on meeting a clinical outcome; when the patient moves on, the case manager looks for the setting that's the least costly yet appropriate to the patient. By providing care more efficiently, costs can be lowered without diminishing quality.

As *utilization manager*, the case manager advocates for patients and links them with physicians, institutions, and third-party payers. She reviews the services a patient receives to ensure that they're medically necessary and reasonable based on specific clinical guidelines; are provided in the most appropriate setting; and are at or above quality standards. Guidelines have been developed by organizations including the Agency for Health Care Policy and Research (AHCPR); medical specialty societies; disease-specific special interest groups; community coalitions like Healthy People 2000; and consulting firms. She also negotiates patient benefits with the third-party payer, which may mean seeking either an extension of current benefits or an allocation of benefits outside the patient's current benefits package.

Discharge planning involves assessment, planning, and implementation of the patient's health care needs following the current phase of illness. All team members contribute to the discharge plan. The case manager ensures that the plan is appropriate to the patient's clinical outlook and insurance benefits, and that necessary services are in place at the time of discharge.

● COMMUNITY-BASED CASE MANAGEMENT

Here, "community" refers to all settings outside the hospital where care is delivered—clinicians' offices, patients' homes, adult day care programs, subacute and acute care settings, and long-term care facilities. Case managers in the community have essentially the same functions as their hospital counterparts. One difference is that, in the community, the primary focus shifts from short- to long-term, and case managers and patients can potentially develop lifelong relationships.

Case managers use a number of care-planning tools to project expected outcomes. Critical pathways (also called clinical pathways), first introduced in hospitals in 1985, were designed to give short descriptions of appropriate interventions and the number of days allotted to the hospital stay. These tools were brief and organizationally specific. Current patterns of care usually determined their content, and their brevity meant that clinical care patterns didn't often change.

Since the first implementation of critical pathways, other, more comprehensive tools have been introduced, which are likely to be based on scientific principles, evidence, and literature. Algorithms, or decision trees—sequences of rules to be followed from beginning to end without deviation—are often used in critical care or emergency settings. Critical pathways today are still generally brief and based on site-specific recommendations that stem from current practice. They designate the time allotted for treatment, but because of their lack of specificity, they've been less than successful at changing clinical practice patterns, use of resources, and length of stay.

Multidisciplinary action plans (MAPs), the most detailed of all the tools, are developed collaboratively, representing all disciplines involved and incorporating all plans of care; outcomes are documented. For example, an orthopedic MAP would include medical, nursing, physical therapy, occupational therapy, and case management plans. Each discipline documents against its daily expected clinical outcomes for a patient.

Clinical practice guidelines are available from several sources and vary in format. Some are brief, while others are more sophisticated. Many health care organizations are developing their own internal guidelines, using the national guidelines as a standard.

● DESIGNING EXEMPLARS OF CARE

Case management models have been designed in a number of ways, and encompass variables including site, location, organization size, patient population, available resources, and case management goals and expected outcomes.

Patient populations for case management are identified by the health care organization and are selected based on criteria such as high patient volume and long length of stay. Targeting those diagnoses that most often require hospitalization—for example, congestive heart failure, acute myocardial infarction, hip fracture, stroke—makes sense. The larger the patient group, the greater the combined length-of-stay reductions will be for the hospital. The plan envisions state-of-the-art care by diagnosis.

Quality-of-care issues often arise for illnesses or conditions in which there are wide variations in physician practice and for which outcomes are inconsistent: for example, cardiac and orthopedic surgery and rehabilitation. Such concerns sometimes parallel an organization's desire to make itself a "center of excellence" in a specialty or around a product line. In addition, the organization may decide to target those diagnoses for which a more uniform treatment approach may benefit both patients and hospital.

Defining Target Populations for Case Management

Case management case types should be based on

• High volume
• Length of stay
• Quality of care issues
• Facility specialty
• Physician practice
• Homogeneous patient populations
• Continuum of care issues

The most common design is unit based. Case managers are assigned geographically within a facility to specific patient care units, or to a particular clinic or specialty area outside the hospital. With this approach, it's most effective to assign case managers to areas with relatively homogeneous populations, by unit (such as oncologic, cardiac, or pulmonary); the less the variation, the easier it is to implement practice guidelines and to monitor outcomes and variances.

Regardless of model design, it's important for case managers to focus on patient transition from one care setting to the next, in order to ensure a seamless flow process.

● CREATING THE ROLE OF CASE MANAGER

One of the first steps is choosing a design that uses available resources and meets the organization's goals. The case manager's functions must also be determined, but some organizations separate these functions among numerous case managers. However, maintaining several positions with similar functions may cause delays, or increase costs.

The case manager's position in the organization must also be designated. Will the case manager be a staff nurse or an equivalent, or should she be required to have an advanced practice degree? Although some organizations designate staff nurses as case managers as well as direct care providers, it has become evident that each job has its own discrete and complex functions, requiring specialized knowledge and skills. There are currently 20 case management masters degree programs and 30 certification programs across the country.

Successful case management cannot occur without the cooperation and support of virtually every department and discipline. The changes that case management initiates affect all parts of the organization. When change happens, it helps to understand why. Education about case management across all involved disciplines is essential for its successful implementation. Educational programs may be sponsored internally or offered at a national conference.

....
The AHCPR has developed hundreds of guidelines on clinical issues—including pain, incontinence, and specific diseases and surgical procedures—which are available free of charge. For information, contact the AHCPR Publications Clearinghouse at (800) 358-9295; it's also accessible online at http://www.ahcpr.gov/info.

● MEASURING SUCCESS

Most health care organizations evaluate the success of a case management program by measuring some common nonclinical outcomes, including patient and provider satisfaction, organizational efficiency, length of stay, and cost per case. The actual outcomes have less importance as measurements of the patient's clinical care than as measurements of the impact of case management on the organization itself.

To gauge patient and staff satisfaction, questionnaires are typically administered at intervals and examined for changes and trends. For example, a questionnaire might be administered every six months for a period of two years after implementation. And one way to evaluate organizational efficiency is to document and analyze turnaround times for tests, treatments, and procedures.

Cost-per-case measures, which assess the dollar amount spent in the care and treatment of a hospitalized patient, help an organization to determine whether or not it has reduced the use of unnecessary tests, treatments, or procedures. For community-based nursing, the term refers to dollars spent on outpatient visits to a physician or on home care services. If cost-per-case information isn't available, length-of-stay measures may be used. A dollar amount may be allotted for each day a patient's stay is shortened, and this amount can be counted as a cost savings for the hospital or health care system.

● BE PREPARED

You can become involved in case management in a number of ways, including:

- Variance reporting. Variance analysis allows health facilities to understand what improvements will ensure better outcomes. Since staff nurses work so closely with patients, they can communicate to them why an expected outcome wasn't achieved.
- Multidisciplinary action plans. Staff nurses who are experienced in a particular clinical area may be called on to serve on a MAP team.
- Education. As lengths of stay shorten, staff nurses may have limited time with patients, but they're in a prime position to educate patients on postdischarge care. The hospital nurse identifies patient needs as early as possible and notes them in the plan of care, and works closely with case managers, who will alert home care services of further educational needs.
- Discharge planning. The staff nurse can notify the case manager about patients who are at risk for not meeting a projected length of stay.
- Documentation. Staff nurse documentation substantiates the need for services being reimbursed at appropriate levels.
- Teamwork. Just as in sports, it's important to "pass the ball." For instance, staff nurses may be the first to identify high-risk patients, and can convey that information to the case manager so that she can appropriately intervene.

No matter how much management there is in an organization's managed care system, patient care remains the staff nurses' utmost responsibility. Understanding case management and learning how to advocate for better patient care can help prevent burnout. Information about case management is available in the following formats:

- In-house training. Short seminars provided by the health care organization that's implementing case management can be tailored to its needs.
- Formal training. Universities and other education venues sponsor seminars, courses,

and degree programs in case management—offered through continuing education programs, as course electives, and in some cases, as specialty tracks.

While much of the attention in health care today is focused on creating new care delivery systems and managed care and provider practice groups, the growing demands of patient care continue to be met primarily by staff nurses. Change can happen so quickly: regardless of setting and a patient's health status, chances are you'll be making more decisions on your own.

SELECTED REFERENCES

Altman, S.H., and Wallack, S.S. (eds.). Health care spending: Can the United States control it? In *Strategic Choices for a Changing Health Care System*. Chicago: Health Administration Press, 1996, p. 3.

Cesta, T.G., et al. *The Case Manager's Survival Guide: Winning Strategies for Clinical Practice*. St. Louis: Mosby, 1998.

Cohen, E.L., and Cesta, T.G. *Nursing Case Management: From Concept to Evaluation*. St. Louis: Mosby, 1997.

Doyle, R.L. *Healthcare Management Guidelines*. Albany, NY: Milliman & Robertson, 1997, vol. 1.

Halpern, R., et al. *Managed Care at a Glance*. Boston: Tufts Managed Care Institute, 1997.

Kongstvedt, P.R., [ed.]. *The Managed Health Care Handbook,* 3rd ed. Gaithersburg, MD: Aspen, 1996.

Pear, R. Sharp rise predicted in health-care spending in next decade. *New York Times,* Sept. 15, 1998, p. A21.

Tahan, H.A. The nurse case manager in the acute care setting: Job description and function. *J Nurs Adm 23*(10):53–61, 1993.

U. S. Agency for Health Care Policy and Research. *Clinical Practice Guidelines* (AHCPR Pub. No. 95-DP 10). Rockville, MD: U.S. Department of Health and Human Services, 1995.

Ethical decision-making in community-based settings considers factors that present challenges different from those found in acute care settings.

What challenges did Stan's situation pose to the home care nurse? What was the ethical dilemma in the case study? What ethical principles were represented by this dilemma? What decision resulted?

Erlen, J. A., Burger, A. M., & Tesone, L. (1990). Making an ethical decision in the home setting: The case of Stan. *Home Healthcare Nurse*, 8(6), 30–34.

36

Making an Ethical Decision in the Home Setting: The Case of Stan

JUDITH A. ERLEN, ALICE MAY BURGER, LAVONNE TESONE

Home health nurses are not immune to ethical dilemmas in their practices. In fact, the ethical dilemmas that are encountered in home health present a unique challenge to these nurses because of the relationship of the home care agency to the patient.

In today's society providing quality nursing care in the home is influenced by the increasing use of technology, the need to contain healthcare costs, the concern to respect the dignity of the patient, and the need to promote quality of life. Challenging questions and issues related to the nursing care of the patient frequently arise, and difficult decisions have to be made. There are the competing ethical principles, values, and interests of patients, families, and health professionals that need to be considered when making these choices.

Home health nurses are not immune to ethical dilemmas in their practice. In fact, the ethical dilemmas that are encountered in home health present a unique challenge to these nurses because of the relationship of the home care agency to the patient. The focus of an intermittent home care agency such as a Visiting Nurse Association (VNA) is to care for patients whose needs can be met by periodic visits that occur anywhere from twice a day to once a month. Although a VNA is not directly responsible for the 24-hour welfare of the patient, a VNA does focus on providing quality nursing care through either direct patient care or patient education. Thus, the resolution of ethical dilemmas in the home setting involves achieving a balance of ethical principles along with the patient's wishes, the standards of nursing care, the agency's philosophy and/or mission, the patient's health concerns, and the availability of resources. To achieve such a balance and determine the

Judith A. Erlen, PhD, RN, is an Assistant Professor, School of Nursing and an Associate, Center for Medical Ethics, University of Pittsburgh, Pittsburgh, PA.
Alice May Burger, MS, RNCS, is a Clinical Nurse Specialist with the Visiting Nurse Association of Allegheny County, Pittsburgh, PA.
Lavonne Tesone, BSN, RN, has been a staff nurse for 5½ years with the Visiting Nurse Association of Allegheny County, Pittsburgh, PA.

appropriate ethical choice can be both difficult and frustrating for home health nurses. Each situation requires that nurses be familiar with the process of ethical analysis and reasoning, as well as ethical theories and principles. This article describes the process of ethical decisionmaking and demonstrates the use of ethical inquiry in resolving ethical issues in a patient situation through a case presentation.

● ETHICAL DECISIONMAKING

The literature is replete with ethical decisionmaking models.[1-6] All of these models have certain basic features: delineating the ethical dilemma, identifying possible alternatives, choosing an alternative, and justifying the choice that is made. First, one must recognize that an actual ethical dilemma exists, that this is a situation in which one must make a choice from among various alternatives that are only partially satisfying. To identify the ethical dilemma requires that the individual gather all relevant information about the patient situation. This includes the medical/technical data, as well as the contextual data, values, and other nonmedical factors.[7] If there is an ethical dilemma, then examining this information will illuminate the ethical concerns present. For example, in reviewing the data related to the care of a confused patient, a nurse might note that there is a conflict among one's duty to promote the patient's welfare, the duty not to cause the patient harm, and the duty to respect the autonomy of the patient. These duties relate to the specific ethical principles of beneficence, nonmaleficence, and autonomy, respectively.

Briefly, autonomy refers to self-governance or self-determination.[8] Autonomous individuals are able to choose a plan and identify and carry out actions that fit with that plan. The choices made by autonomous individuals demonstrate that they are in charge of or in control of their lives. Beneficence centers on promoting the well-being of another.[8] Situations exist where it is necessary that others intervene in a positive way to prevent or to remove harm, as well as to contribute to another's welfare. These instances require either a provision of benefits or a balancing of benefits and harms.[8] Nonmaleficence, on the other hand, focuses on not doing harm including both actual harm and risk of harm.[8] This duty requires that one act with due care meaning that one is to act thoughtfully, prudently, and responsibly. Autonomy, beneficence, and nonmaleficence provide direction for the care of individuals. However, there are also those situations that require a consideration of the distribution of benefits and burdens within a broader context or the need to consider the principle of justice. This principle provides the basis for making allocation decisions within a society so that individuals will be treated in a fair way.[8] Thus, in order to discern the ethical dilemma clearly, a nurse needs information about the specific situation as well as an understanding of the relevant ethical principles.

Once the ethical situation becomes evident, one identifies possible alternatives and then chooses a particular course of action. DeWolf's research shows that nurses limit their options to two clearly opposing alternatives when asked to make a choice in an ethical dilemma.[9] Other models of ethical decisionmaking call for identifying and examining several possible options before choosing an alternative. The authors of this article suggest that whenever possible, home healthcare nurses need to specify several options. In fact, using a brain-storming technique is a helpful means for identifying alternatives because a person will be able to consider a broad range of options. An individual then reviews each possible alternative in terms of feasibility and congruence with ethical principles. This process provides the nurse with a rationale for the course of action that is selected. It is important and necessary that the justification for the decision be communicated along with the choice that is made. Knowing what one wants to do and why one wants to take that action helps a person to implement and later to evaluate the action. This knowledge also helps others to understand the basis for the particular alternative that was chosen.

As one engages in the process of ethical inquiry, one also needs to consider the time dimension.[5,6] Some decisions have to be made immediately, while others provide considerable time for effective deliberation. The acuity of the patient situation dictates whether or not a decision has to be made immediately. Many ethical decisions allow sufficient time to engage in deliberative decision-making and to explore various options. When one has time for data gathering, reflection, and deliberation, a more acceptable decision is likely.

Case

The following case is based on an actual patient situation. All names and other identifying information have been changed to provide anonymity and to maintain confidentiality.

Stan is a 69-year-old man who was diagnosed with amyotrophic lateral sclerosis (ALS) approximately 3 years ago. He has had rapid progression of the disease process and is currently bedridden. He can move his head and his eyes and has gross upper extremity movement. Stan is competent. He is alert and communicative but is unable to do anything for himself. For the past 18 months, Stan has had a tracheostomy, a gastrostomy tube, and a Foley catheter. Skin care and pulmonary toilet are major nursing concerns as are his elimination and nutrition. He is also an insulin-dependent diabetic. Stan lives in a high-rise building in a two-bedroom apartment. His caretaker is a female friend, Ruth, who has multiple physical limitations.

The staff nurse's initial contact with Stan began with his transfer from VNA rehabilitation services to VNA medical-surgical services for intermittent, skilled nursing assessments and Foley catheter changes. Although Stan was confined to his hospital bed and required constant care due to his disease process (ALS), he was in no acute distress and did not require any invasive treatments or procedures other than catheter insertions every 4 weeks. On the surface, his case was one of routine catheter maintenance in the home. Within 4 weeks, however, the patient's condition unexpectedly changed. He had a myocardial infarction and was hospitalized.

During this hospitalization Stan developed an aspiration pneumonia and dysphagia. He was eventually discharged to home care with a new gastrostomy tube, continuous feedings through a pump, a tracheostomy with continuous oxygen, and inhalation therapy treatments four times daily. Very little instruction was given to Ruth, the primary caretaker, while Stan was hospitalized regarding the gastrostomy tube and tracheostomy care in the home. Consequently, the staff nurse spent at least 3 hours on the initial visit frantically instructing Ruth and an aide on adequate and safe care of Stan in the home setting: maintaining a patent airway; providing tracheostomy care, oxygen, and continuous gastrostomy tube feedings; maintaining electrolyte balance; and managing his diabetes mellitus. The nurse left the home after this first visit totally frustrated and exhausted.

Subsequently, frequent and lengthy home care visits followed because of Ruth's knowledge deficits, the constant changing of aides in the home, and Stan's unstable condition. The primary nurse was overwhelmed by the multitude of clinical problems and the fact that she was physically alone when immediate decisions regarding appropriate clinical care had to be made. Her high expectations of providing excellent nursing care were offset by the reality of the home situation. She had to deal with the clinical problems and consider issues regarding the patient's autonomy and his quality of life. Thus, at this point, the staff nurse began to discuss the feasibility of VNA's involvement with Stan's care with the clinical nurse specialist.

(continued)

The primary nurse shared the data she had been gathering about Stan's situation and several concerns she had with the clinical nurse specialist. Stan's primary caretaker was willing to take full responsibility, but she herself was handicapped because of a below the knee amputation of her right leg, no lower extremity prosthesis, a visual deficit, and arthritis. She was confined to a wheelchair. As a result, the primary care-taker had difficulty standing at the patient's bedside to provide the necessary care. She also had difficulty maneuvering the wheelchair in the small, equipment-filled room. Al-though Stan had assistance from an aide from a government subsidized agency for 8 hours each day, the service was limited to noninvasive care. This essentially meant that the aide could not provide tracheostomy care and suctioning, dressing changes, and medication administration. The attending physician suggested that Stan be admitted to a skilled care facility to ensure the proper care necessitated by his multiple medical problems and frequent visits to the emergency department via the paramedic services. The local adult services agency questioned the liability surrounding the patient's care by their personnel. The administration of the home care agency also began to question patient safety and the agency's liability in this home situation.

Based on her assessment of the situation, Stan's primary nurse found herself asking the following questions: How could she facilitate the resolution of the above concerns? How could she deal with her own ideas of how to provide the best care? How would she be able to respect the rights and desires of the patient and his caretakers? How could she deliver care to Stan within the guidelines of the agency?

Stan's case also was of concern to the clinical nurse specialist since her role encom-passed offering support to the primary home care staff nurse by assisting with the de-cisionmaking process and the case management of the staff nurse's patients. The major concern was the visit pattern required to meet Stan's clinical needs and to do the necessary patient teaching to facilitate patient and caretaker independence. This exten-sive visit pattern was making tremendous demands on the staff nurse's schedule as VNA staff have a visit expectation. Both the primary nurse and the clinical nurse specialist were concerned about the patient's multiple nursing needs in regard to the tracheostomy, the gastrostomy, the Foley catheter, his insulin-dependent diabetes mellitus, and the caretaker's ability to attend to these needs between VNA visits. An-other concern was the limited and ever-changing community support available to the caretaker to assist with Stan's care. The turnover among the aides sent by the commu-nity agency to Stan's apartment necessitated repetitious teaching by the VNA nurse. Fi-nally, the clinical nurse specialist and the clinical supervisor were concerned because they were unable to offer the primary nurse an immediate solution to the situation that would decrease the demands this case made on her schedule, stamina, and commit-ment to the patient and still provide quality care according to home care standards.

Stan, too, realized that his constant care was indeed a challenge to the healthcare workers and Ruth; however, he refused placement to a nursing home, believing he would receive better care at home. He stated he would be transferred to such a facility "only when I am ready."

● ETHICAL ANALYSIS

Stan's case demonstrates how a staff nurse's concern for her patient's need for control was balanced against her concern for the patient's well-being. The dilemma that existed for the nurse was a conflict mainly between two ethical principles—respect for patient auton-omy and beneficence or promoting the patient's well-being. To identify this dilemma the primary nurse and the clinical nurse specialist gathered both medical/technical data and contextual data. The medical/technical data included Stan's requirements for care, his medical condition including both ALS and diabetes mellitus, his prognosis, and the type and amount of service that could be provided by the two agencies. The contextual data that was gathered included an understanding of Stan's values and value system, his desire for self-control, his level of competence, and the role of his caretaker. These data were collected over a period of several months. The primary nurse's ongoing assessment of Stan showed the same level of commitment by Stan to remain at home and to be in control. There was never any doubt about Stan's competence to make decisions. The repeated expression of Stan's values and the ongoing support of the caretaker further validated Stan's need to be autonomous. As a result, the primary nurse and the clinical nurse specialist realized that a way was needed to promote Stan's autonomy without further compromising his well-being or health status.

In searching for a resolution in Stan's case, several concerns were considered: the patient's autonomy, his competent decision to remain in his apartment, his prognosis, the caretaker's capabilities and willingness to provide care, and the VNA's responsibilities to meet Stan's needs. There were numerous multidisciplinary patient care conferences held among the VNA staff with the community agency's social worker to identify and discuss possible alternatives and to come to a decision about the case. During this time, VNA continued to service the patient two or three times each week with each visit being in excess of 1.5–2 hours. These visits provided additional opportunities to gather other contextual and medical/technical data necessary in seeking a resolution to the ethical dilemma that Stan's situation created.

The overall outcome of these conferences was a three-part resolution. First, the caretaker verbalized a willingness to continue her support, care, and participation in the treatment plan. Second, the government-subsidized agency promised to continue to provide an aide for 40 hours every week. In this case a hired caretaker was not an option due to Stan's financial constraints. Lastly, after all the patient teaching was completed, the VNA visit pattern would be once every 1–2 weeks with a limit of one extra visit per week if needed. This three-part resolution allowed Stan to stay in his apartment and to be in control of his situation, as well as VNA to service Stan in a manner more consistent with the agency's policy. The quality of care Stan would receive would be acceptable by home care standards. Stan understood the limits of VNA service and the risks of being maintained at home with limited support. If Stan could not be kept at home with this program, then he agreed to be placed.

The justification for this three-part resolution was based on the idea that it promoted Stan's autonomy despite his limited control over his body and yet protected his well-being. Potential harm to Stan was able to be kept to a minimum. In addition, the solution was within VNA guidelines enabling the primary nurse to continue to service Stan, yet care for her other patients.

This outcome has worked reasonably well. There were a few extra VNA visits and two hospitalizations in the last year. Ruth, the caretaker, became more independent in her ability to meet Stan's needs. However, a problem did remain because each VNA visit exceeded 1 hour.

● SUMMARY

This article has briefly described and demonstrated the process of ethical inquiry regarding caring for a patient in the home setting through an actual patient situation.

In this case the decisionmaking process occurred systematically and over time. As data were gathered, questions were asked and alternatives were considered that raised further questions or required the collection of additional data. Ethical principles and values were considered. The final resolution was not apparent when the ethical dilemma was first identified. Instead the resolution slowly emerged as all came to know and understand Stan's situation more completely. With the combined efforts of the VNA, the attending physician, the caretaker, and the government subsidized agency, Stan was able to remain in his apartment and to be cared for within the boundaries of Medicare and VNA requirements.

The discussion of Stan's case has shown that although the overall process of making ethical decisions in the home does not differ from an institutional setting, several important points relevant to the home setting need to be considered. These factors include: the time available for making decisions, the fact that the patient is being cared for in the home, the availability of a caretaker/support system, how to facilitate interdisciplinary communication, and the lack of an institutional ethics committee. A discussion of these considerations will be presented in a forthcoming article.

● ACKNOWLEDGMENT

The authors thank R. Helen Ference, PhD, RN, Manager of Training and Development, Visiting Nurse Association of Allegheny County, Pittsburgh, Pennsylvania, for her thoughtful comments on an earlier version of this manuscript.

REFERENCES

1. Thompson JE, Thompson HO: *Bioethical Decision Making for Nurses.* Norwalk, CT. Appleton-Century-Crofts, 1985.
2. Purtilo RB, Cassel CK: *Ethical Dimensions in the Health Professions.* Philadelphia, W.B. Saunders, 1981.
3. Brody H: *Ethical Decisions in Medicine,* ed 2. Boston, Little, Brown and Company, 1981.
4. Payton RJ: Pluralistic ethical decision making. In *Clinical and Scientific Sessions 1979.* Kansas City, MO, American Nurses' Association, 1979:9–16.
5. Aroskar M: Anatomy of an ethical dilemma: the theory. *Am J Nurs* 1980; 80:658–660.
6. Curtin L, Flaherty MJ: *Nursing Ethics: Theories and Pragmatics.* Bowie, MD, Robert J. Brady Company, 1982.
7. Benjamin M, Curtin J: *Ethics in Nursing,* ed 2. New York, Oxford, 1986.
8. Beauchamp TL, Childress JF: *Principles of Biomedical Ethics,* ed 3. New York, Oxford, 1989.
9. DeWolf MS: Ethical decision-making. *Sem Oncol Nurs* 1989; 5(2):77–81.

Community-based settings create different challenges to ethical decision making than in acute care settings. This article highlights some of these differences.

What factors influence ethical decision-making in the home? What can be done to assist nurses to manage ethical dilemmas more effectively? What resources can assist nurses to manage ethical dilemmas more effectively?

Burger, M. A., Erlen, J. A., Tesone, L. (1992). Factors influencing ethical decision making in the home setting. Home Healthcare Nurse, 10(2), 16–20.

37

Factors Influencing Ethical Decision Making in the Home Setting

ALICE MAY BURGER, JUDITH A. ERLEN, LAVONNE TESONE

Several factors influence ethical decision making in the home setting, including time to make decisions, the home setting itself, the patient's support system, interdisciplinary communication, and the lack of an institutional ethics committee.

Home healthcare nurses frequently are challenged by the ethical dilemmas confronting them as they provide care for their patients in the home. A previous article described the process of ethical inquiry through the use of an actual patient situation.[1] The salient features of that case are included in that report. Several important factors to consider when resolving ethical dilemmas in the home were identified. It is important at this time to read the original article in the November/December 1990 issue of *Home Healthcare Nurse* because the present article is based on and continues that earlier discussion.

The overall process of ethical decision making is not governed solely by the type of patient care setting. Instead, the nature of the relationship between the home care agency and the patient, in addition to the setting, requires that we focus on the way(s) in which particular factors may influence the resolution of ethical dilemmas.

Patients who are being cared for at home are in their own environment. Healthcare providers giving care in the home are guests and may be unaware of customary routines and family value systems. Thus, the home setting requires a reassessment of the patient–provider relationship.

Caring for the patient at home also differs because care is given on an intermittent basis. As a result, patients and their caretakers now assume more responsibility in the care-

Alice May Burger was a clinical nurse specialist with the Visiting Nurse Association of Allegheny County, Pittsburgh when this article was written. Judith A. Erlen, PhD, RN, is Assistant Professor, School of Nursing, and Associate, Center for Medical Ethics, University of Pittsburgh. Lavonne Tesone, BSN, RN, is a staff nurse with the Visiting Nurse Association of Allegheny County, Pittsburgh, PA.

> ### Case Report
>
> Stan, a 69-year-old insulin-dependent diabetic man, was diagnosed with amyotrophic lateral sclerosis 3 years ago. His disease progressed rapidly. Now he only can move his head and his eyes and he has gross upper extremity movement. Stan is competent, alert, and communicative but unable to care for himself. For the past 18 months, Stan has had a tracheostomy, a gastrostomy tube, and a Foley catheter. Stan lives in a high-rise building in a two-bedroom apartment. His primary caretaker, Ruth, is a friend with multiple physical limitations.
>
> Stan was transferred from Visiting Nurse Association (VNA) rehabilitation services to VNA medical-surgical services for intermittent, skilled nursing assessments and Foley catheter changes. His case appeared to be merely one of routine catheter maintenance in the home. However, 4 weeks later he had a myocardial infarction and was hospitalized.
>
> When discharged to home care, Stan had a new gastrostomy tube, continuous feeding via a pump, a tracheostomy with continuous oxygen, and inhalation therapy treatments four times each day. Very few instructions were given to Ruth by the hospital staff.
>
> Frequent and lengthy home care visits followed because of Ruth's knowledge deficits, the constant changing of aides in the home, and Stan's unstable condition. Despite these problems, Stan was adamant about remaining at home.

giving process. Surrogate caretakers may be needed to provide ongoing care. There are contracts established between the agency and the patients and their families which delineate the scope of responsibilities of all parties.

The purpose of this report is to discuss the following factors as they relate to ethical decision making in the home: the time available for making decisions, the fact that the patient is being cared for in the home, the availability of a caretaker and support system, facilitating interdisciplinary communication, and the lack of an institutional ethics committee. In addition, this article makes several recommendations that home healthcare agencies can implement to make home healthcare nurses' encounters with ethical dilemmas more manageable.

● THE FACTORS

Time

At first glance, it appears that more time is available to resolve ethical dilemmas in the home than in the hospital because visits frequently extend through a period of weeks. Yet, ironically, just the opposite is true. Home healthcare nurses visit the patient and caretaker on an intermittent basis and so have to assess quickly the total situation and determine what has value and meaning for that patient. These nurses are not with the patient and family 24 hours a day. In fact, once the initial assessment is made, nurses only spend, on the average, 40 to 60 minutes per visit with a patient three or four times a week. This is scarcely enough time to do the caretaking and teaching let alone to understand the complexity of the patient's situation. When a nurse visits a patient intermittently it is difficult to assess fully the patient's level of knowledge and understanding or that individual's capacity to make decisions.[2]

Administratively, the decision to provide service for the patient must be made immediately. The agency places considerable emphasis on establishing a plan of care within the first few visits. Without such a plan, the nurse and the patient and family will be confused about the goals for care. Stan's case was an example of the confusion and frustration that home healthcare nurses experience because of the potential for clashes between the overall goals of the agency and the ethical and professional responsibility nurses have to their patient. In his case, care continued to be given despite the fact that there was no way that his situation would improve, clinically or otherwise. There was no way to determine how long his support systems would remain in place. The nurse questioned how to provide service to others in her caseload when Stan was taking so much time. Stan's case demonstrated the importance of a thoughtful, deliberative evaluation of the caregiving situation with the patient and caretaker(s).

When the visitation pattern of a home healthcare nurse extends through a period of time, the nurse has more opportunity to assess the patient's and caretaker's wishes and values. The decision-making process is ongoing. As other treatments are introduced, long-term consequences can be reassessed. Discussing issues such as quality of life and the use of life-saving and life-extending technology may be easier because the nurse has developed a relationship that allows the patient and caretaker(s) to discuss these issues freely. In Stan's case, the nurse was able to identify areas of concern to him and his caretaker. There was time to engage in reflective thinking and to deliberate about available options. The nurse knew that Stan was adamant about not wanting to be placed in a nursing home. The long-term relationship and ongoing discussion of his condition clearly demonstrated that Stan wanted to continue to make decisions about his care and that he was competent to make those decisions. When the patient is competent, that person can exert control.

Involvement

In the home setting, patients and caretakers are often more intensely involved in the decision making that occurs regarding the plan of care. Patients and caretakers are active partners in their care. In addition, caretakers are intimately involved in direct patient care, which is an expectation of the agency. Caregiving cannot always be relinquished to others.[2] Patients and caretakers must assume responsibility for implementing the treatment(s) whenever nurses are not present.

In addition, instructing patients and caretakers to perform care activities in a particular way is more difficult when patients are cared for at home rather than in the hospital or a nursing home, which can raise ethical as well as professional concerns for nurses. For example, nurses often can make suggestions; however, they cannot always enforce restrictions on patients or make decisions for them. It is more difficult for a home healthcare nurse to treat a patient paternalistically, that is to treat the patient as if the nurse knows what is best for that other individual.[3] In the home, the patient has increased autonomy. In fact, as others have found, "the home setting can mute caregiver authority and encourage, even embolden, patient autonomy."[2]

This was the case with Stan. He demonstrated that he was a major participant in all decision making. Even though he was unable to care for himself physically, he could express those values that were important to him. Stan had established his definition of quality of life, which meant being at home and being cared for by someone special to him. He was able to continue to be involved in his care. His role in any decision making remained central. He was able to speak for himself. With Stan as a partner in his care, decisions that were made respected his dignity and considered what was in his best interest.

Stan's case demonstrates that even though he was unable to act physically on his decisions, others respected his autonomy. Collopy[4] notes that frequently whether a patient is able to act is confused with the patient's ability to decide. If this happens, patients can become increasingly dependent. In Stan's case, his ability to make choices was not confused with his inability to act alone on his decisions.

Support System

The accessibility, availability, and affordability of a caretaker is a third factor to consider when trying to resolve ethical dilemmas in home care. The type of caretaker, and how often and for how long the caretaker is available definitely affects available options. Patients being cared for at home may need caretakers. These caretakers need to be competent and reliable. Without an appropriate caretaker, alternatives for care in the home become fewer because of the potential risk of harm to patients. In other words, without an established caretaker, the nurse can be placed in an ethical dilemma: how to promote the patient's best interests and balance the risks and benefits of home care.[3]

This ethical dilemma is affected by the policies of the agency regarding eligibility. If a patient has adequate financial resources, it may be easier to find a caretaker and to acquire the necessary support system. Without sufficient funds, the patient is limited by the availability of community services (e.g., Area Agency on Aging). Affordability and accessibility are linked. In addition, patient age is frequently another criterion used to determine eligibility for services.

Another concern regarding available support services is that they may not be able to provide the type of care that the patient requires. For example support services may be available to provide part-time but not full-time services. Or there may be caretakers who are available to feed and bathe patients but who are not able to give medications, do suction, or to do catheter care.

An additional problem is that caretakers have only a limited amount of time to spend with patients because of other commitments and responsibilities. Similarly, not every willing individual can be a caregiver. Personal limitations, such as physical or mental deficits, affect such a decision. A patient's ability to withstand intensive caretaking over time is also a consideration.[6] Caretakers begin with the best of intentions. There is genuine concern for the well-being of the patient. Realistically, however, it may be impossible to implement the original care plan, thus creating an ethical dilemma for the patient and caretaker(s).

Stan had a friend who was willing to be his caretaker. However, due to her physical limitations and Stan's extensive needs, she was unable to be his only provider. Instead, a service system was created to try to meet Stan's needs and wishes.

Interdisciplinary Communication

A fourth consideration influencing ethical decision making is a professional practice concern: how to promote effective communication between and among the healthcare team members. Home care complicates interdisciplinary communication because a nurse does not always have an established relationship with a patient's physician.[5] Home care nurses and doctors do not interact with each other on a regular basis; face-to-face conversation is missing. Frequently the only way these health professionals communicate is *via* the telephone. Returning telephone calls takes time and telephone messages can get lost. Therefore, home care impoverishes communication between the nurse and the physician.

Home care presents limited opportunities for direct communication among the different health-care professionals involved in the care of a particular patient. Better resolutions to ethical situations occur whenever health professionals and, if possible, the patient can come together and discuss the situation. Such discussions provide a forum to share information and an opportunity to identify other perspectives and alternatives. Yet, a problem exists in that it is difficult to get all individuals involved in the care of a particular patient in one place at one time.[5,6] Schedules are difficult to coordinate because individuals may come from different service agencies. This is somewhat easier when all the healthcare professionals involved in the care of a patient are from a VNA. Frequently, though, that is not the case. Yet, unless the healthcare professionals can meet to discuss a particular case, communication difficulties continue and the ethical dilemmas related to patient care may remain unresolved.

Without the commitment of all the agencies and the physician involved in Stan's care, the three-part resolution was not possible.[1] On-going communication enabled the physician and the agencies to be apprised of Stan's wishes and to work toward a compromise to allow Stan's needs to be met at home.

Ethics Committee

A final concern when ethical decisions are made in the home setting is that usually there is no ethics committee or an ethicist available to consult with the nurse and/or the patient and family when a situation seems unresolvable.[2] Hospitals are establishing ethics committees and are beginning to hire clinical ethicists. To date this has not been the case in the home healthcare setting. Therefore nurses and patients and families feel alone when ethical dilemmas arise. Similarly, no mechanism exists for patients and families to use when they seek help to resolve a difficult issue.

There is the concern and fear that unless the ethical dilemma is resolved within a reasonable period of time the patient's welfare will be jeopardized. All participants in the care of the patient need to know what resources are available to assist them in resolving the ethical dilemma. Patient care conferences provide one means to examine these issues. In instances in which there are particularly difficult situations, the option exists to invite an ethics expert to attend these conferences to offer insight into the case. The use of such outside resources depends on the availability and the arrangements that have been to provide consultation services.

Stan's case prompted issues related to an on-going need for care; yet no one knew how long this need would exist. Although a case conference was initiated, there was no mechanism readily available to invite an ethicist to assist with the discussions. The management of Stan's case demonstrated the need for home healthcare nurses to be knowledgeable about ethical decision making and ethical principles to analyze and resolve ethical dilemmas systematically in their practice because outside resources may be unavailable.

● RECOMMENDATIONS

Collopy and colleagues[2] call for fuller exploration of the ethical issues in home healthcare. Ethical dilemmas will continue to confront nurses. What can be done to assist nurses to manage the dilemmas more effectively and to avoid becoming overwhelmed by them?

One recommendation is to educate the home healthcare staff in ethical decision making. This can be done through one-day seminars, although ongoing staff development programs are probably more effective. These programs need to focus on the moral foundation of nursing and then discuss ethical issues as they are presented within the context of the nurse–patient relationship in the home setting. Forums for discussion of nursing ethics need to be initiated. A nurse can present a particular patient situation and follow that with a discussion of the ethical problems in the case. Journal clubs can be started. Staff nurses can come together on a regular basis to discuss an article that focuses on a particular ethical dilemma in nursing. Through on-going educational programs, staff nurses can increase their awareness of ethical issues in their practice, as well as their knowledge of the nursing role and professional responsibilities when trying to resolve ethical dilemmas.

Home care agencies need to consider employing a personnel counselor or a chaplain to assist nurses with managing the stress of ethical dilemmas, as well as other patient care problems. These counselors do not have to be full-time employees, although that is certainly advantageous. If they are employed full-time, nursing staff will have better access to them. The counselors can conduct stress management workshops or can work with nurses on a one-to-one basis.

Counselors can help to develop nurse support groups within the agency. Support groups can be an effective means whereby individuals with common problems and concerns can come together and share their experiences. Others in the group can offer suggestions regarding ways to manage particular patient-related issues. Support groups have been used with groups of nurses in hospital settings and have been found to be an effective resource to help nurses cope with professional concerns.[7,8]

Another way that a counselor or a chaplain can help home healthcare nurses is by serving as a consultant. Patients and families may experience problems that nurses feel ill equipped to manage. The chaplain or counselor can be asked to visit and to assess a patient and family in relation to their ability to cope with the situation. Then this individual and the nurse can meet and discuss the situation. These discussions can help to clarify the ethical dilemmas in managing a patient's care.

A third recommendation is to have an ethicist available to nurses in the agency with whom they can consult. The ethicist needs to be an individual with whom nurses can consult directly on particular cases. Therefore accessibility is necessary. Patients and/or families also need to know that this service is available so that they can make self-referrals when troubling situations arise and no answers seem available.

Finally, agencies need to establish ethics committees composed of individuals from throughout the agency. The committee needs to have members from the various healthcare disciplines, as well as a lawyer, ethicist, and a lay person. These committees can serve several functions, *i.e.*, educational, consultative, policy making.[9] Ethics committees in home healthcare agencies are an idea whose time has come because ethical dilemmas in home care will only increase. There needs to be a forum within the agency through which these ethical dilemmas can be discussed and possible resolutions/policies can be considered.

● SUMMARY

The process of ethical decision making does not differ according to the patient care setting. However, various factors in home care affect the way in which decisions are made. The factors to consider are the amount of time needed to make a decision, the involvement of the patient and family, the need for support systems, the difficulties with interdisciplinary communication, and the lack of an ethics committee. Recognizing the ways in which these variables affect the decision making can help home healthcare nurses resolve the ethical dilemmas they face. In addition, staff education programs, the use of consultants, and the development of ethics committees are possible strategies to facilitate ethical decision making.

REFERENCES

1. Erlen JA, Burger AM, Tesone L: Ethical decision making in the home setting: The case of Stan. *Home Healthcare Nurse* 1990;8(6):30–34.
2. Collopy B, Dubler N, Zuckerman C: The ethics of home care: Autonomy and accommodation. *Hastings Center Report* 1990;20(2):1–16(Suppl).
3. Beauchamp TL, Childress JF: *Principles of Biomedical Ethics, Third edition.* New York, Oxford, 1989.
4. Collopy, BJ: Autonomy in long term care: Some crucial distinctions. *Gerontologist* 1988;28 (Suppl):10–17.
5. Cary AH: Home health care. In: Lambert CE, Lambert VA, eds. *Perspectives in Nursing: The Impacts on the Nurse, the Consumer, and Society.* East Norwalk, CT: Appleton's Lange, 1989, pp 379–402.
6. Barkauskas VH: Home health care: Responding in need, growth, and cost containment. In: Chaska NI, of *The Nursing Profession: Turning Points.* St. Louis: CA Mosby, 1990, pp 394–404.
7. Ceslowitz SB: Burnout and coping strategies among hospital staff nurses. *J Adv Nurs* 1989;14:553–557.
8. Weiner MF, Caldwell T: The process and impact of an ICU nurse support group. *Int J Psychiatry Med* 1983–1984;13:47–55.
9. Gibson JM, Kushner TK: Will the "conscience of an institution" become society's servant? *Hastings Center Report* 1986;16(3):9–11.

Occasionally the nurse may not feel safe entering a client's home or neighbourhood. No nurse should ever disregard personal safety in an effort to visit a client. The following article provides practical steps and precautions needed to predict violent incidents and suggestions for implementing simple self-protection techniques.

What were the goals of this violence prevention program? Identify some predictors of violence. What is the role of the environmental assessment? What can you do if you sense an assault?

Durkin, N., & Wilson, C. (1999). Simple steps to keep yourself safe. *Home Healthcare Nurse*, 17(7), 430–435.

Simple Steps to Keep Yourself Safe

NANCY DURKIN, CYNTHIA WILSON

With increasing incidences of violence in the patient's environment, home healthcare staff are at risk in and out of the client's home. This article addresses the practical steps and precautions needed to predict violent incidents and provides suggestions for implementing simple self-protection techniques when encountering situations in which violence is escalating.

Healthcare journals stress the need for safety awareness and training programs (Cohn, 1996; Hunter, 1997; Page, 1996) and OSHA (OSHA 96-53; OSHA 3148) along with accrediting agencies that want to see agency policies in place that address this issue. It is well documented in the healthcare industry journals (Hunter, 1997; Simonowitz, 1994; Vandergaer, 1997) that there is an increasing incidence of violence in the patient's environment, placing visiting staff at greater risk while providing home care. Many studies conducted on workplace violence give quantitative data to support the need for violence prevention training.

We are managers in a home healthcare agency in central Massachusetts covering 20 rural and suburban towns with 140 professional and 90 paraprofessional staff who make an average of over 700 home visits each day. In 1997 we created a workplace violence prevention program that included a lecture on general safety precautions along with demonstrations of basic nonviolent self-defense techniques. We set two program goals:

1. to increase staff awareness of potentially violent situations; and
2. to empower employees with the skills necessary to respond to verbal and physical assaultive behaviors in a manner that promoted staff and patient safety.

Nancy Durkin, MSSW, LICSW, is a Social Services Clinical Manager, VNA of the Greater Milford-Northbridge Area, Mendon, MA, where Cynthia Wilson, BSN, RN, is VNA Education Manager.

An outcome study of the staff reactions to and utility of the program was published in *Home Healthcare Nurse Manager* (Durkin & Wilson, 1998).

As the program's creators, we strongly believe in the need to implement a violence prevention program in order for staff to understand the appropriateness of establishing and maintaining safety boundaries that can be used both professionally and personally. This article provides helpful information and tips to increase your safety awareness as well as preventative moves you can use during an escalating dangerous situation.

● PREDICTORS OF VIOLENCE

It's important to understand that violence comes in many forms. There are no conclusive studies on race or ethnicity as an indicator or predictor of violent tendencies.

For example, a visiting staff person lost a tooth when a patient with dementia assaulted her. Although no one blames the patient, that kind of experience fits the definition of a violent encounter. Often people become violent when they feel they have no other options available. All patients and families need to be evaluated based on the predictors that follow:

- Studies show that people with a history of using violence will do so again as will people who are members of a subculture (e.g., a gang).
- Stressful environments can also trigger violent responses (e.g., an overwhelmed caregiver who becomes rough with the patient).
- Men have a higher frequency of using violence than women, however, women do become violent (Beck, 1987).
- Often, the unpredictability of what might happen creates a stressful environment that can affect the staff member's job performance in the patient's home and for the rest of the day. For example, no one knows what an abuser of substances will do when high or drunk—this can be a very dangerous situation for a staff member.
- Younger people tend to use physical violence and elderly people tend to use verbal violence.

Other high-risk predictors (such as low socioeconomic status, i.e., living at or below the poverty level) or history of head trauma or cognitive impairments can lead to violent behavior. These concepts are based on the theory that people become violent when they feel they have no options (Beck, 1987; Pastor, 1995).

Definitions

Abuse. To physically or verbally attack or injure.

Anger. A feeling of displeasure resulting from injury, mistreatment, opposition, etc., and usually showing itself in a desire to fight back at the supposed cause of this feeling.

Assault. A violent attack, either physical or verbal.

Frustration. A feeling that results from an interference with one's ability to attain a desired goal or satisfaction.

Rage. Violent anger; fury, enthusiasm; rapture (raging, raged). To be furious with anger, to be violently agitated.

Violate. To injure; to outrage; to desecrate; to profane; to transgress.

Violence. Moving, acting, or characterized by physical force, especially by extreme and sudden or unjust or improper force.

Source: Anderson, 1994, Gifis, 1996, *Webster's Dictionary*, 1984.

A verbal assault is as devastating as a physical assault. Battered women in support groups often talk about how it is "easier" to be hit than to experience verbal violence. Verbal violence is also more accessible because it can occur on the phone. Supervisors and office staff often experience this type of assault; it needs to be responded to just as quickly and seriously as the physical confrontation.

● ROLE OF ENVIRONMENTAL ASSESSMENTS

Home care providers must at all times remain aware of the environment in which they work. There is a story of a visiting staff person who arrived for a visit and found that the house was surrounded by police. She still tried to go inside to see the patient. Attention must be paid to the big clues as well as the little ones.

Our agency policy states that the staff person is to leave immediately if a gun is out in the open and the patient or family refuses to put it away (VNAGMNA, 1995). If people in the home are physically or verbally assaulting each other or staff, it is important that staff leave the site. We tell the visiting staff that once they are out of the situation and personally safe, they are to call the agency immediately to report the circumstance. However, if they feel that there is someone in the house who is still at risk, they are to call the police before calling the agency (VNAGMNA, 1995). Every staff member who visits patients in the community must review the agency's policies and procedures regarding safety precautions and incidence reporting requirements on a regular basis.

● YOUR PHYSICAL ENVIRONMENT

Part of the environment is your own physical being. Our bodies are wonderful communicators if we just listen to them. When a person is in a dangerous situation, the body undergoes physical reactions (e.g., the feeling that the hairs on the back of your neck are standing; your stomach churning; and your heart pounding rapidly). Those are big clues something is not right and you might need to flee the situation. Be sure to listen to your own body and your intuition.

As you go on your first visit to a home it's important to invest some time for your own safety by:

- driving around the block (this may take more time but you learn a lot about potential cues to violence);
- checking out the specific environmental clues of the neighborhood;
- being careful not to walk through crowds or staying on an elevator with the other passengers if you feel uncomfortable; and
- looking for potentially dangerous weapons as well as guns and knives, animals, and objects that can be thrown or made into assault weapons.

Body Language and Rage

Visiting staff need to pay attention to the body language of *anyone* in the home, not just the patient. You also should be aware of your own body language and how others might interpret it. Although anger is a normal reaction and feeling, rage goes beyond that and encompasses everything. For example, if you arrive late for a visit, the enraged client may not only be angry that you are late, but may also harbor long repressed feelings, hostilities, and thoughts that can affect your interaction.

Signs of Rage

You can tell if a person is becoming enraged (which is beyond angry), for they will show the following signs:

- their face and/or neck are flushed and red;
- the veins on their neck or forehead are "popping out";
- their hands can be clenched, or they can be clenching and unclenching their hands;
- if sitting, their knees could start bouncing up and down, or;
- their feelings become more out of control as they start to pace.

If You're About to Become Assaulted

When a person is about to verbally or physically assault you, rationalizing is no longer an option. This is not the time to talk to the person about why they are being unreasonable. They will not be able to listen or appropriately respond to anything you say or try to do.

If You Are Assaulted: The Aftermath

It is important to realize that whether the assault is verbal or physical you need to spend some time talking to your supervisor and others whose support you might find helpful. Talking about what happened and how you feel about it can prevent emotional, physical, or cognitive problems that are all related to the stress of the incident, called *critical stress reaction*. Some of the signs and symptoms of critical stress reaction to be aware of include:

- inability to concentrate on your work;
- loss of appetite;
- fatigue;
- fear of going on home visits;
- memory loss;
- stomach upset;
- insomnia;
- severe startle reaction;
- emotional extremes; and
- apathy, depression (Lewis)

Remember to Care for Yourself

Caregiving for yourself is vital in order to minimize the symptoms. Tips such as maintaining a healthy diet and regular sleep schedule, use of quiet time for relaxation, and other stress management techniques are recommended. However, if you find that these symptoms are affecting your work performance or your personal life, contact your Employee Assistance Program or seek a referral for a counselor skilled in critical stress management.

Tips to Consider Regarding Equipment, Dress, and Accessories

Lock Up Equipment. Personal belongings need to remain locked in the car, preferably in the trunk. We had a case of a patient's daughter who would go out "to check the rabbits" when staff arrived. People would leave wallets and purses in the car but not lock it because they felt it was "the country," "a nice neighborhood," and "a nice family." After one

What to Do If You Sense an Assault

Know the location of the door. Always stay closest to the door, and don't let anything block your way. You may end up stuck behind the table with your back to the wall and someone blocking the exit if you don't pay attention to all the clues.

Pay attention to your own body language. We suggest staff stay at the same eye level but not to make ongoing eye contact with a person in a rage. Direct eye contact can be very threatening and could escalate a situation. However, staying at eye level communicates a respectful attention. Therefore, if the person stands up, you stand. When they sit, you sit.

Distance yourself at least three to four arm lengths away from the person. If the person starts waving their arms (even without the intention of hitting you), you have enough of a buffer zone to avoid blows.

Do *not* cross your arms or shove your hands in your pockets. This stance may convey a message of hostility or not caring. Keeping arms relaxed and loose at your sides or adopting a stance with one arm crossed with the other resting on it, holding your chin in your hand conveys attention and keeps your hands available to deflect blows or thrown objects.

Be aware of the inflection and tone of your voice. Your voice should become clear and almost monotone. Shouting will only make your throat sore and can escalate the situation.

Convey respect. This is not the time to make a joke or to minimize the situation. Even though you want to yell or scream, for your own protection adopt a respectful and calm demeanor.

Assume a body stance. As the potential victim, you need to stand with your feet spread hip width apart and at a slight angle to the enraged person. Point your front foot at the other person and your back foot perpendicular to your front foot. This will help you maintain your balance if you are hit or shoved.

Once you have left the house do *not* return to retrieve bags or other items left behind. Walking back into the house skyrockets the person's potential for becoming even angrier. At that point you are *the* least welcomed person in that house. Nothing is more valuable than your life and well-being. Even if you left your purse—which should never have been taken into the house—and you really need it, request the police to retrieve it for you.

Remember: The adrenaline rush that both you and the enraged person will have is going to last at least 1 hour. The enraged person may appear to have calmed down after 15 minutes of yelling, but because of all the adrenaline coursing through the body he or she could easily flare up again. Once out of the situation and in your car, your adrenaline rush will last for 1 hour and it can affect how you drive, therefore, find a spot to calm down before deciding on your next step.

home health aide lost all her holiday shopping money, we finally tallied all the money "missing" for the various different staff (nurses, therapists, social workers, and aides) assigned to that case and found it was over $200—not counting other noncash items.

Plan Your Dress. Even if your staff doesn't wear uniforms, spend time thinking about how you are going to dress for the job. Here are some good rules to remember:

• Sensible shoes, like our mothers always told us, are the best. Twisting an ankle due to high heels or falling out of a clog prevents a person from making a safe and a quick exit.

- Long necklaces and neck ties can choke; long earrings can be ripped out.
- Pins of a political or religious nature can offend and potentially escalate someone's rage.
- Clothing that is binding or restricts movement is not the best option when making home visits.

Other Safety Accessories. Other accessories that promote your safety are:

- a working cellular phone;
- a flashlight (especially if conducting evening visits);
- your vehicle—regular maintenance and a full tank of gas are minimal recommendations (Myers, 1998)

Some suggest mace or pepper spray. However, organizations such as the National Police Association caution that users of these sprays often end up spraying themselves.

Make Your Whereabouts Known. If you are entering a potentially dangerous house—one that has been identified as a concern—let office staff know the time of the visit and ask that they page you approximately 15 minutes into the visit. This will give you a reason to call out of the house and through "yes" and "no" answers can let the office know if the situation is safe. If unsafe, you have an easy excuse to leave by saying, "that's my supervisor and she wants me to come into the office right away." Everyone is advised to leave their schedules with the office and at some agencies it may even be standard policy.

What You Can Do to Prevent Violence

If your agency does not have a violence prevention training program, encourage them to develop one. Know your agency's policies and procedures if you encounter a violent situation. If an incident occurs, document it—even if you would prefer to forget about it. Your agency may not even realize the frequency of incidents that are occurring if staff fail to take the time to document them. There are several main points to remember to help yourself and your patients:

- **Get to know the community, especially the differences between neighborhoods.** Local radio and newspapers are a great source of information, as are our patients. The local police department should have a community liaison officer who can also provide information.
- **Get to know your patient.** Find out all you can about the patient and his or her household before your first visit. Does the referral source know of any violent history associated with the patient or the people living in the household? (Hunter, 1997)
- **Know your agency policies and procedures and follow them.** You may want to advocate for some changes but you first need to know the current guidelines.
- **Keep your supervisor informed of any potentially violent situations with your caseload.** Case conferences are not only clinically necessary but keep the multidisciplinary team unified and cognizant of any safety plans.
- **Take the opportunity to attend courses and lectures on safety and self-defense.** Our staff found the program valuable in their personal lives as well as on the job. Assaults, unfortunately, do happen in our homes, when shopping in the mall, on vacation, etc. Personal protection is an issue for everyone 24-hours a day.

Remember, it is important that you respect yourself, your patient, and the people caring for the patient at all times. A respectful approach to someone who is extremely angry can possibly calm them. Respect for those working with a patient, whether in a professional or personal role, helps you to understand the emotional impact of a verbal or physical assault and the need to get support after a violent encounter. Respect for yourself establishes the internal self-protection mechanism that says "this is getting dangerous, it's time to leave!"

REFERENCES

Anderson, K. (Ed.). (1994). *Mosby's Medical, Nursing, and Allied Health Dictionary.* St. Louis: Mosby.

Beck, J. (1987). The potentially violent patient: Legal duties, clinical practice, and risk management. *Psychiatric Annals, 17*(10), 695–699.

Cohn, S. (1996). Safety Policies and procedures at your workplace. *Social Work Focus, NASW,* Boston *23*(11).

Durkin, N. & Wilson, C. (1998). The Value and Impact of Violence Prevention Training in a Home Healthcare Setting. *Home Healthcare Nurse Manager, 2*(6), 22–28.

Gifis, S. (1996). *Law Dictionary.* Hauppauge, New York: Barron's Educational Series.

Hunter, E. (1997). Violence prevention in the home health setting. *Home Health Nurse, 15*(6), 403–409.

Lewis, G. (1998). *Introduction to Critical Incident Stress (CIS).* Unpublished manuscript, COMPASS, Framingham, MA.

Myers, H. (1998). Street Smarts: Guidelines to Safety for Home Care Aides. *Caring, xvii*(4), 10–14.

Page, L. (1996). First federal guidelines issued on workplace violence. *American Medical News, 39*(14), 8.

Pastor, L. (1995). Initial assessment and intervention strategies to reduce workplace violence. *American Family Physician, 52*(4), 1169–1174.

Simonowitz, J. (1994). Violence in the work place: You're entitled to protection. *RN, 57*(11), 61–64.

U.S. Department of Labor. (1996). Protecting community workers against violence. *OSHA 96-53.* Washington, DC: OSHA Publications office.

U.S. Department of Labor. (1996). Guidelines for preventing workplace violence for health care and social service workers. *OSHA 3148.* Washington, DC: OSHA Publications office.

Vandergaer, F. & Sud, S. (1997). Your thoughts: Decrease violence—Increase safety. *Home Health Focus, 3.*

Visiting Nurse Association of the Greater Milford-Northbridge Area (VNAGMNA). (1995). Staff Security: Management of Environment. *Policy and Procedures Manual.*

Webster's Dictionary. (1984). New York. Modern Publishing.

Webster's New World Dictionary, 2nd Ed. (1980). New York: Simon and Schuster.

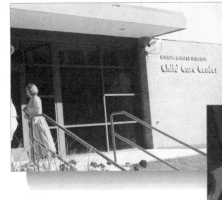

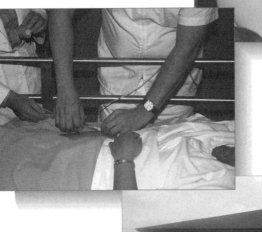

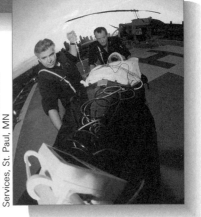

Discovering Your Niche in Community-Based Nursing

Lifelink III Mobile Intensive Care Services, St. Paul, MN

Multiple opportunities for employment exist in community-based settings. Your first challenge will be to take charge of your own professional career and do some serious planning. Discovering your niche requires exploring options and possibilities that perhaps you weren't even aware existed. Reviewing these articles, which describe the myriad of programs and roles, will expand your outlook regarding the possibilities available in community-based settings. As specialties emerge in nursing practice, develop your own niche based on your gifts, talents, interests, competencies, personal and professional expertise, and the needs of the population you desire to serve.

Taking charge of your career is imperative as the role of the nurse continues to evolve in the changing health care environment.

Why do corporations seek nurses? Identify your own priorities and skills. Complete a SWOT analysis as provided in the article. How might you fit your expertise and special interests into the changing marketplace? What are steps to follow to plan your career plan? What are your next steps as you plot your career plan?

Hoffs, B. B. (1998). Taking charge of your career. *American Journal of Nursing*, 98(1), 36–40.

39

Taking Charge of Your Career

BARBARA BETZ HOBBS

Here's how to prevent the waves of change in health care from carrying you in the wrong direction.

With the changes in this country's health care system, many nurses face uncertain futures, confronted with organizational restructuring or job loss. As downsizing continues and managed care moves patients from acute care settings to outpatient facilities, you're probably seeing some nursing units close, never to reopen. And, as each door closes, feelings of insecurity increase. You wonder if your unit will be next.

Though it may sound trite, when one door closes, another usually opens. The changes in health care are creating new and exciting career opportunities in hospitals, community settings, businesses, and health care organizations. Instead of looking back regretfully at the closed door, you need to envision the many roles you might play in the future—in all the possible new settings.

In this article, I'll provide an overview of the career-planning process. I'll suggest strategies to help you make decisions and discuss possible opportunities and career choices.

● ASSESS THE TRENDS

The current trend toward managed care has resulted in reduced hospital reimbursement rates, shorter hospital stays, and more outpatient services. All that translates into an income reduction at the institutional level that forces hospitals to lower costs, restructure, and reduce staff.

To adhere to budgetary constraints, hospital administrators often reduce the number of RN positions, or limit the hours RNs work, while increasing the numbers of lower-paid, unlicensed staff. While these changes may cause you to feel uneasy, you can take control of your professional future by acting now.

Barbara Betz Hobbs is an instructor and student services coordinator in the department of nursing at South Dakota University, Rapid City, SD.

● INVESTIGATE THE MARKET

In many ways, health care is changing for the better. When an acute care facility eliminates a nursing service, it's often because outpatient nursing services have proved so effective. This affords a wide array of opportunities to the experienced clinician. It's important that you investigate new areas and explore options that didn't exist in the past.

Consider the case of Joan, an RN working in an acute care pediatric unit. The number of infectious disease cases in her unit decreased steadily, while the number of outpatient surgeries increased. The net result was a drop in the total number of hospital beds reserved for pediatric patients and the number of pediatric nurses employed in Joan's facility. Joan responded to these changes by exploring opportunities for the experienced pediatric nurse outside the acute care setting. She took stock of her clinical expertise and broadened her scope, considering positions in different settings—such as a clinic, surgical center, or school. Joan even considered roles that focused on employee and family health in an industrial setting.

As you investigate the market, try to imagine how you might apply your expertise in new settings. While you may not be able to envision the perfect setting for your next career move, you need to identify where nurses will be needed in the future. In doing so, you may be able to create an opportunity where none currently exists—where the need for a nurse has yet to be identified.

Depending on the situation—and the needs of your new clients—your scope of practice may change. Take the time to research current openings, network with other nurses, and market your ideas to managers and executives.

The results will benefit you and your career, even if you don't change your current position. It's your education, experience, and expertise that will allow you to successfully venture into new arenas.

● WHY CORPORATIONS SEEK NURSES

Your assessment and problem-solving skills make you an asset to many disciplines. Several professions outside health care value the same traits that make you an excellent nurse. You have the ability to care for and about others, and a willingness to work as part of a team. You're responsible, accountable, and credible. That's why so many positions in pharmaceutical research, biomedical services or data collection, financial case management, biomedical informatics, and media consultation are being filled by nurses.

Many nurse managers are responsible for large numbers of employees and administer million-dollar budgets. Non-health care corporations recognize the value of this experience, and it's reflected in their hiring practices: They hire nurses. And the spectrum of corporations seeking nurses as employees grows ever wider. Recently, for example, a nurse researcher working in a university setting was approached by the Honda Corporation. The corporate leadership felt that her unique combination of education and experience could enhance their operations. They offered her a position as a vice president of medical health services. She acknowledged their vote of confidence and accepted the position.

Though most nurses still work in acute care settings, over 30% of nurses in the United States don't work in hospitals. And the number of non-hospital-based nurses is expected to increase as more of us complete nurse practitioner programs and move into clinics, rural health care, and private practice.

● EVALUATE YOUR PRIORITIES AND SKILLS

In exploring career opportunities, evaluate your own interests and expertise. If staying in the acute care setting is important to you, consider what forces drive changes in hospitals and which clinical areas are expanding. For example, if you're an experienced ICU nurse with strong computer skills, consider a position developing information systems for ICU nursing care. As a coronary care nurse, you may want to consider using your skills in an inpatient or outpatient cardiac rehabilitation facility. And, because hospital reimbursement plans continue to change, the need for care managers and financial case managers continues to grow.

Alternative, high-touch, high-tech clinical opportunities are more abundant than ever. As the focus of health care moves from treatment to prevention, clinical positions in community and public health are increasing. In the next eight years, the number of grade school students is expected to increase to 54.4 million, creating more opportunities for school nurses. Recognizing that spiritual health must be supported by physical and emotional health, some religious denominations (including Lutheran and Methodist congregations) now seek nurses to work within their health ministries. As paid employees of the health ministries, they provide physical, emotional, and spiritual nursing care to congregation members.

The number of home health care agencies is increasing rapidly, providing the experienced clinician with a wonderful setting in which to apply broad-based expertise. Investigate opportunities in nurse-managed clinics. You can transfer skills gained in geriatric acute care to an Alzheimer's day care center or a hospice. Regardless of the role or setting, your nursing experience and problem-solving skills will prove useful.

● POTENTIAL IN ADVANCED PRACTICE

While investigating career options, explore opportunities in advanced practice nursing. To work as a clinical specialist, midwife, educator, administrator, or nurse anesthetist, you may need to invest in further education. The investment, however, will yield additional career choices. If you choose to become a nurse practitioner, you'll be able to focus on a specialty area such as family practice, neonatal care, women's health, geriatrics, or mental health. New areas of practice are defined each year.

All types of advanced practice nurses are forging ahead in the field of health care delivery as entrepreneurs—as practitioners providing services for fees. As entrepreneurs, these nurses are responsible for starting and running businesses, including nursing clinics, home health agencies, health care supply firms, and education companies.

But entrepreneurial opportunities aren't limited to those in advanced practice. You can use your skills and expertise to develop a consulting business. Consultants are employed by organizations to fulfill specific needs or complete special projects. For example, legal nurse consultants review malpractice cases or testify as expert witnesses.

Many corporations in other fields, seeking to minimize down-time caused by sick employees, have developed an interest in wellness programs. Use your interest in health maintenance and wellness care as an opportunity to develop and market this type of program.

Explore the possibility of sharing your nursing expertise with publishers or television or video producers in the capacity of media consultant. Consider collecting patient data for pharmaceutical companies conducting research studies on new products.

You don't even necessarily have to leave your job setting to express your entrepreneurial spirit constructively. As an "intrapreneur," you identify a need *within* the institution where you currently work. You then use your entrepreneurial instinct to develop a strategy that meets the need. For example, if you're a pediatric nurse, consider developing a system for providing sick-child care for employees at your institution. You can find new opportunities while providing a service at the institution.

● DEVELOP A CAREER PLAN

After you've explored various opportunities, you're ready to develop your career plan. Such a plan helps direct your search for employment, while allowing you to expand your professional knowledge and maximize your earning potential.

You begin by defining your needs. Do you want a job or a career? Generally, a job has limited opportunities for advancement. It may be short-term or even dead-end: It's a way to pay the bills. A career, on the other hand, is a dynamic, life-long process. It changes and grows with your experience and education.

When you became a nurse you chose a career; embrace it as such. Nurture the health of your career with the same intensity that you care for your patients. Instead of reacting to outside forces such as downsizing, become proactive (see *Career Planning Tips and Strategies*).

Plot your course systematically, following these six steps:

- Step one: Envision your future as you'd like it to be.
- Step two: Assess yourself and factors influencing your decision-making process.
- Step three: Identify career options.
- Step four: Set both long-term and short-term goals, and assign target dates for meeting those goals.
- Step five: Develop strategies that allow you to meet your goals.
- Step six: Evaluate and revise your plan regularly; career growth is dynamic and changes in response to new situations.

● SELF-KNOWLEDGE IS KEY

Having a vision is the first step in the process. Try to imagine what would make you feel fulfilled and accomplished within your career. Reflect on the reasons you wanted to be a nurse. Write down ideas about different jobs that sound interesting or exciting, using recruiting ads in nursing journals as a reference. This will help you envision possible opportunities. Don't eliminate any choice until you have a clear understanding about the type of career move you want to make.

Regardless of your age, your level of experience, or satisfaction with your current position, you need to plan for your future. And because there are no guaranteed positions in today's health care market, it's essential to try to be flexible and to develop a contingency plan.

The second step may be the most difficult: You must honestly assess yourself. Start by examining your motivation—the factors driving your decision to consider new career choices. Is your primary motivation fear of losing your current job, a personal need to grow, or a desire for a more influential position? Identify your personal, professional, and family interests, including relocation, the need to work around children's schedules, finances, and desirable length of shifts. Are you close to retirement or planning to continue your education? In developing a career plan, you must consider timing.

Career Planning Tips and Strategies

- Keep a positive attitude.
- Focus on your future.
- Build on past accomplishments and work experience.
- Do your homework—research and learn about career options.
- Network with colleagues, nursing leaders, and other health care professionals.
- Complete your self-assessment and SWOT analysis.
- Target opportunities that match your best characteristics and traits.
- Develop a proactive, systematic career plan based on your self-assessment.
- Plan your future in one, five, and 10-year goals.
- Devise a system for periodic evaluation of your progress.
- Attend workshops and local professional meetings.
- Go to the career planning seminars provided by the college of nursing in your area.
- Develop expertise in two or three nursing areas as a contingency plan.
- Join professional organizations.
- Read nursing journals in the specialty areas in which you're interested.
- Review, edit, and update your résumé for each area of nursing you are considering.
- Tailor your résumé to each position, highlighting the talents that make you a viable candidate.
- Contact college career personnel.
- Attend job fairs.
- Submit articles for publication in your area of expertise.
- Explore the Internet for career opportunities (search for the term "careers"). Two of the larger, general employment lists are America's Job Bank (<http://www.ajb.dni.us>) and Career Path (<http://www.careerpath.com>).

For nursing career opportunities, browse the following resources:

- <http://www.nursingcenter.com/career>
- <http://galaxy.tradewave.com/Galaxy/Medicine/Health-Occupations/Nursing.html>
- <http://www.healthcareers-online.com>
- <http://www.travcorps.com> or <http://www.aacn.org> (An alliance between the American Association of Critical Care Nurses and TravCorps, a health care placement service, has fostered the creation of Career Development Services [CDS]. CDS offers members of the AACN direct access to career counseling and a range of career-enhancing resources.)

Self-assessment also involves using a decision-making tool known as a SWOT analysis, which helps you identify and examine strengths (S), weaknesses (W), opportunities (O), and threats (T) as they apply to achieving your goals. The SWOT analysis enables you to recognize your strengths and special qualities as well as factors that might interfere with your success (see *Performing a SWOT Analysis*).

The final component of self-assessment is a detailed examination of the alternatives and opportunities you've identified. Focus on areas of nursing that interest you. Review the applicable literature, noting the current trends and anticipating future needs in the desired fields. Are the nursing specialties you're interested in new and expected to grow, as are nursing informatics and geriatrics, or are they all but being eliminated by technology and new health care methodologies? For example, if your interest is in pediatrics, recall that immunizations have nearly eliminated pediatric hospitalization for childhood diseases.

Performing a SWOT Analysis

A SWOT analysis is used to formulate a plan of action. It allows you to systematically analyze a large amount of complex information in order to arrive at a balanced decision. Think of the SWOT analysis as a large box and each of its four components (your strengths, weaknesses, opportunities, and threats) as building blocks within the box.

STRENGTHS

Since it's difficult to evaluate your strengths objectively, ask a colleague you respect to help you identify your skills and accomplishments. These might include:

- expertise in a nursing specialty;
- years of experience;
- job performance;
- special talents in caring for clients and their families, and
- education, including certifications and special training.

WEAKNESSES

Keep in mind that weaknesses include limitations as well as deficiencies. Limiting factors may make it difficult for you to take the necessary risk involved with changing jobs. Some limitations are related to family or personal needs (for example, for medical or vacation benefits), geographic factors (such as family immobility), or financial constraints. These might include:

- the need for more education or training;
- limited experience in the specialties you find interesting;
- insufficient knowledge about opportunities;
- lack of self-confidence;
- comfort in your present position, which may make it difficult for you to risk changing jobs;
- a reluctance to take risks;
- poor communication style; and
- a lack of persistence (while an initial rejection can be off-putting, persistence may open new doors).

By identifying possible weaknesses, you give yourself an opportunity to change them into strengths. For example, although you may not have the formal training required for a position, your expertise and experience can be validated by references.

OPPORTUNITIES

Take note of any situation, personal or professional, that supports your future direction. These might include:

- the chance to work with an expert or a mentor in your chosen field;
- the ability to network with peers and nursing leaders;
- references and referrals from colleagues;
- membership in local or national nursing organizations;
- attendance at local business and educational meetings related to your desired field;
- work on political action committees or advanced education programs; and
- involvement in developing new programs in your hospital.

(continued)

Performing a SWOT Analysis (*Continued*)

THREATS

First list those factors you consider threats to your current situation, including:

* shift reduction;
* salary cuts; and
* elimination of the position.

Next list those factors that may threaten a career move; including

* competition for a specific position and
* inability to meet the entry level requirements.

● FINDING A GOOD MATCH

Once you've performed your self-assessment, you're ready to move to step three. Identify the various career options that might match your self-assessment. If the specialty you're interested in requires relocation, consider the local and regional competition for clients. If a city of 50,000 has three dialysis programs, for instance, is that financially viable? The chamber of commerce in the area you're considering should have information and statistics about local and regional health care facilities. In addition, local newspapers may carry information about recent mergers, acquisitions or contract agreements.

Because the health care market is in a state of flux, it's essential that your career plan include more than one option. Evaluate and select two or three options that you may be interested in pursuing.

In step four of your career development plan, you set long- and short-term goals. Your goals are based on your self-assessment and should include target dates for completion. It will be helpful to target goal achievement with one-, five-, and 10-year plans. Remember, since your career plan is dynamic, your goals and timelines may need to be adjusted.

Having developed goals with specific career options in mind, you can move on to step five. Develop strategies to meet your goals. Gather detailed information about the two or three career options you've selected. Identify the relevant journals, and read literature written by experts in the selected fields. Contact clinical and professional organizations about job postings. Speak with the nursing services coordinator at a college or university. Review the latest career guides for more information. Attend specialty meetings in your selected specialties and speak with nurses currently practicing in these areas to get their views of the field. If possible, contact the experts in your area of interest and ask them to help you identify future trends. If possible, "shadow" a nurse in the position or field you desire.

Examine the current local, regional, and national employment opportunities by scanning career advertisements and job postings, discussing placement with staffing agencies, and searching the Internet. The World Wide Web provides nurses with access to information about all types of job openings. Note the number of openings and types of positions advertised in any given locality, as well as opportunities in the surrounding area. If there is only one major hospital in the desired locale, consider opportunities in neighboring clinics, home health care agencies, and industry. Don't forget to investigate factors affecting the area's economics, such as recent hospital mergers or announcements of managed care contracts, as well as local salaries.

At this point, you're ready to take action. Review and revise your résumé. Use the goals you've set to define and describe your objective. Focus your résumé on your strengths-your nursing education, experience, and special skills. Capitalize on your professional commitment to nursing, caring attitude, and flexibility. Describe your best characteristics, such as efficiency or accuracy. List advanced or continuing education programs completed, all nursing certifications, and special awards. Although a certification may not be directly applicable to your new position, it's evidence of your initiative and ability.

● MARKETING YOURSELF

Once your plan is in place, and you're prepared to explore new opportunities, it's important to market yourself. Network with your colleagues. Go public by writing and publishing articles in your local newspaper, a nursing organization newsletter, or a nursing journal. Volunteer as a board member for an agency, local charity, or nonprofit organization affiliated with your desired specialty. Observe—and use—the strategies adopted by other successful nurses.

Having a career plan enables you to be flexible and prepared for change. It's your map, providing you with direction, allowing you to change course without getting lost. As your life and your nursing career grow and change, the sixth step of career planning, reevaluation and revision, comes into play. When new opportunities arise, use your unique plan, built on the strengths of your professional and personal life, to accept the challenge and to expand your nursing expertise.

The changes in the delivery of health care are cause for concern. Despite downsizing, however, there are new and exciting choices for nurses. Explore these opportunities and envision the roles you might play in the future.

SELECTED REFERENCES

American Association of Colleges of Nursing. *Media Backgrounder.* Washington, DC, The Association, 1996.

Chitty, K.K., ed. *Professional Nursing: Concepts and Challenges,* 2nd ed. Philadelphia, Saunders, 1997.

Cooper, M.C. *Pathway Evaluation Program for Nursing Professionals.* Research Triangle Park, NC, Glaxo Wellcome, 1995.

Mundinger, M.O., ed. *The Pfizer Guide: Nursing Career Opportunities.* Old Saybrook, CT, Merritt Communications, 1994.

Nunnery, R.K. *Advancing Your Career: Concepts of Professional Nursing.* Philadelphia, Davis, 1997.

Wise, P. S. Y. *Leading and Managing in Nursing.* St. Louis, Mosby, 1995.

A primary role of the nurse in community-based care is providing specialized nursing. This specialized care often involves use of technology and development of expert clinical skills. One of the most common types of high-technology care is medication administration using home IV therapy.

What types of IV treatment do clients receive in home settings? Which clients are appropriate choices for home IV therapy? What special education do these clients need? What are some of the Medicare reimbursement guidelines for home infusion therapy?

Masoorli, S. (1996). Home IV therapy comes of age. RN, 59 (10), 22–25.

40

Home IV Therapy Comes of Age

SUE MASOORLI

Here's an update on the growing area of home infusion—including types of treatment, patient selection, and nursing considerations.

Just in case you had any doubt about the rise of home health care, consider the statistics: There are more than 15,000 home health agencies in this country and they deliver care to more than seven million patients. Experts predict both these numbers will increase by 10% in each of the next five years.[1]

One of the most rapidly growing segments in this market is home infusion therapy—now a $4 billion a year industry.[2]

Not surprisingly, an increasing number of home health agencies are offering home infusion services in an effort to compete for patient referrals. And health care facilities are eager to supply them, since home IV therapy fits right in with their cost-cutting strategies. A 30-day IV antibiotic regimen of one common cephalosporin, for example, costs about $5,000 when given in the hospital; it's just $1,600 at home.[3]

That being the case, it's likely that sooner or later, whether you work in a hospital, an outpatient setting, or in home care itself, you'll be caring for patients who are either candidates for home infusions or are currently receiving them. To bring you up to date on this area of practice, we'll start with a look at which IV therapies are now being used in the privacy—and hopefully comfort—of the patient's own home.

● WHAT TYPES OF TREATMENT ARE PATIENTS GETTING?

Antibiotics, hydration, and total parenteral nutrition (TPN) are three of the most common forms of home IV therapy, and they're often started at home without any prior hospital admission. Other, less frequently used, therapies include pain medication, chemotherapy, and dobutamine (Dobutrex) administration.

Sue Masoorli is president of Perivascular Nurse Consultants, Inc., a Philadelphia-based company that provides infusion nurse specialists to home health agencies, hospitals, and nursing homes.

IV antibiotics may be ordered to treat osteomyelitis, Lyme disease, pneumonia, and subacute bacterial endocarditis. The length of therapy can range from a few days to a few months. Short-term antibiotics are usually administered through conventional peripheral IV catheters; long-term therapy may be given through a central line.

IV hydration is frequently prescribed for patients with AIDS, pregnancy-induced hyperemesis, or cancer—before or after chemotherapy. Usually it is ordered for a few days to a few weeks through a peripheral IV line. Keep in mind, however, that venous access is often difficult in dehydrated patients, so fluids may have to be given through a central line.

Total parenteral nutrition may be ordered for patients who can't absorb nutrients through the GI tract. Candidates include those with short bowel syndrome, radiation enteritis, severe Crohn's disease, and ulcerative colitis.

Usually, TPN is prescribed for a minimum of three months—but sometimes for life—and is infused through a central line. When given in the home, the total infusion is delivered over eight to 16 hours, preferably overnight.

IV pain medications may be prescribed for either chronic or acute pain. Among the most likely candidates are oncology patients and patients discharged after same-day surgery. The home is often the ideal setting in which to deliver IV pain meds because many patients receiving them are terminally ill and in extreme pain, and transporting them to a hospital may worsen their condition. The drugs are usually administered through a central line—including a peripherally inserted central catheter (PICC)—or by means of a continuous subcutaneous infusion.

Chemotherapy is still administered primarily at a physician's office or outpatient clinic. However, some patients do now receive the drugs at home, the most common one being fluorouracil (5-FU, Adrucil). Some drugs, like cisplatin (Platinol), take up to five hours to infuse and a nurse must be present for the entire infusion. That's because the drugs are so toxic that an RN must be on hand to administer IV antiemetics during the infusion. As you might expect, both Medicare and private health insurers may balk at reimbursing for some of these regimens.

Dobutamine infusions, once only administered in the ICU, are now used as palliative therapy for home care patients with severe refractory congestive heart failure and for those awaiting a heart transplant. The drug is infused through a central line to maintain a constant blood level and to minimize the risk of IV infiltration. As with home chemotherapy, reimbursement from Medicare and private insurers for these home infusions is also limited.

● WHO'S A GOOD CHOICE FOR HOME IV THERAPY?

Since few patients can afford to pay for infusion therapy out-of-pocket, one of the most important factors in determining who receives it at home instead of in a hospital or clinic is insurance coverage. Medicare, and many private insurers, will reimburse part of the expense for home infusions, but only if certain criteria are met.

In the case of Medicare, the patient must be homebound, which means if he's able to leave his home to go to a drugstore or to shop for food, he doesn't qualify. In the case of TPN, the government also stipulates that the treatment must last at least 90 days to be eligible for reimbursement. Other criteria are outlined in Fig. 40-1.

Of course, candidates for home IV therapy need to be stable enough to receive treatment at home rather than in a hospital setting. With proper training, many of these patients are capable of administering and monitoring their own infusions. Others can have someone else in the family do this for them.

Medicare reimbursement guidelines for home infusion

The following federal guidelines apply to home care patients seeking insurance coverage under Medicare Part-B Durable Medical Equipment Benefit.

Total Parenteral Nutrition

►Therapy duration must be at least 90 days; and
►TPN must be the patient's only source of nutrition, and documentation must demonstrate that the patient is unable to absorb nutrition from the gut.

Antibiotics

►Must require an infusion pump for safe delivery;
►May not be delivered by a disposable infusion device, such as an elastomeric pump; and
►Must be one of the following four drugs: acyclovir, amphotericin-B, fosarnet, and ganciclovir.

Dobutamine

►The patient must have documentation of a significant physiologic response to dobutamine therapy, including evidence of clinical deterioration when the drug is discontinued even with

the addition of ACE inhibitors, digoxin, and a diuretic; and
►The patient must be on an active cardiac transplant list, or receive a Medicare waiver.

Chemotherapy

►Must be administered via an external infusion pump;
►Must be administered over a 24-hour period or longer; and
►Must be one of the following drugs: doxorubicin, bleomycin, cytarabine, fluorouracil, vinblastine, or vincristine.

Pain Management

►Must have a diagnosis of intractable pain due to cancer;
►It must be documented that the pain is unrelieved by PO, PR, or topical narcotics;
►The drug must be administered via an external infusion pump; and
►Must be one of the following drugs: morphine, hydromorphone, meperidine, or fentanyl.

SOURCE: Herbert, J. R., (1996). Medicare reimbursement for home infusion therapy. *J. Intraven. Nurs.*, *19*(2), 99. © Intravenous Nurses Society. Used with permission of Lipponcott-Raven Publishers.

FIGURE 40-1. Medicare reimbursement guidelines for home infusion.

● WHAT KIND OF EDUCATION DO THESE PATIENTS NEED?

Once a patient is discharged on IV therapy, the home care nurse will evaluate the ability of the patient and his family to handle the rigors of home infusion therapy, especially if they have not been fully trained before the patient is discharged. Many patients are taught in the hospital how to administer their IV therapy using equipment that they may not use at home. For instance, hospitals tend to use IV pumps for a great majority of infusions but in home care, it's easier for the nurse to teach patients how to administer gravity infusions.

Similarly, if a pump is required for infusion therapy in the home, many home infusion companies select user-friendly units, rather than the more complex models that are used in the hospital, because they're easier to prime and troubleshoot.

Regardless of the type of equipment the patient will be using, he and his family will have to be taught as much as possible about the medication regimen. Depending on the type of regimen and the patient's abilities, he may also be taught how to infuse the medication himself.

To identify individual teaching needs—and ensure effective nursing care—the home care nurse needs to obtain an intake form listing basic information on the patient's IV protocol from the referring facility when accepting patients. With that in mind, hospital nurses should be prepared to provide the detailed clinical information needed to ensure continuity of care.

As an example, the intake form for patients with PICC lines should provide the date the line was inserted, the brand and gauge of the PICC, the total length of the catheter, as well as the number of inches inserted and exposed. The form should also list the exact anatomical location of the catheter tip, the name of the accessed vein, and any complications that have developed to date.

All home infusion patients need to be taught the basic principles behind the therapy and how the vascular access device works. Most patients receive the bulk of this training during the first visit from the home care nurse, but they may require one or two follow-up visits depending on the complexity of the treatment. The home care nurse will demonstrate each technique—priming the tubing, connecting and disconnecting the IV tubing, and so on—and then may ask the patient or caregiver for return demonstrations.

Having step-by-step written instructions or videos makes the learning process easier, too. So does a patient teaching checklist, which should contain a list of patient education outcomes, teaching methods, and the date and time each item is taught. Among the topics to be covered:

- Infection control principles and procedures,
- Drip rate calculation,
- Catheter flushing,
- Dressing changes,
- Signs and symptoms of an allergic reaction and infiltration,
- Needle disposal, and
- Emergency response to catheter ruptures.[4]

For most home infusion patients, the list of things to learn also includes how to set up the pump, troubleshoot the alarm system and—if they are getting TPN—how to add medications to the solution. Many patients must also get in the routine of monitoring and recording their weight, fluid intake and output, and body temperature. TPN patients need to be able to recognize the signs and symptoms of metabolic complications such as hypoglycemia and know what emergency measures to take if these complications occur.

● WHAT SKILLS AND SAVVY DO NURSES NEED?

Once the patient has mastered IV therapy, he'll still need follow-up assessment. The home care nurse has to anticipate all sorts of patient problems and, in emergencies, take charge of the situation and inform the physician later. That requires expert assessment and IV skills, which is why home care accrediting agencies look for records of inservice training and other documentation to demonstrate competency.

Thorough documentation is also key—and the best type of legal protection in the event of a malpractice suit. All patient education should be documented, including the fact that he's been instructed on emergency procedures in the event that the catheter inadvertently falls out or develops a leak.

In the case of a PICC line, that would involve immediately occluding the exit site to prevent air from entering the system, and calling 911 when appropriate. If the line falls out, its length should also be measured, documented, and compared to the length of catheter previously inserted. If there's a discrepancy, it probably means that part of the line is still in the patient. If that's the case, he will have to apply a tourniquet until help arrives.

The fact that the patient has been given written instructions should be documented and the teaching checklist should be signed by both the nurse and patient.

Although there are no definitive guidelines on the need for home care nurses to get informed consent, I would strongly advise that they do so before any treatment or hands-on training begins. That applies whether the patient has a peripheral IV catheter or a PICC line, or needs a port accessed.

Nurses who are on call for a home health agency that provides 24-hour coverage must also have 24-hour access to the agency's policies and procedures. That means the supervisor on call should have a copy of the procedures manual available when the field nurse calls in or each nurse should have her own copy.

The growing field of home health will no doubt provide employment opportunities for many nurses in the years ahead. But along with the new opportunities comes the obligation to stay current with this ever-changing field. Keeping up to date will make your professional life more fulfilling and ensure your patients the best possible care.

REFERENCES

1. National Association for Home Care (1995). Basic statistics about home care. Available from the NAHC Internet site: http://www.nahc.org.
2. Geniusz, G. (1995). Future trends affecting the home infusion therapy industry. *Caring,* *14*(5), 58.
3. Milkovich, G. (1993). Outpatient parenteral antibiotic therapy: Costs and benefits. *Hospital Practice,* 28(Suppl. 1), 39.
4. Graves, D. (1995). Home infusion therapy: Meeting a need. *Nurs. Manag., 26*(8), 32J.

One of the most important roles of the nurse in community-based care is the role of educator. If you enjoy teaching in the acute care setting, you will find abundant teaching opportunities in community settings. Currently there is a shortage of nurse educators with graduate degrees so if you know that teaching is for you, this article may provide some ideas for opportunities in the educational arena.

What are some opportunities for teaching? What are some of the benefits of teaching? What are some challenges of teaching?

Burke, S. (1996). Take your skills to the classroom. RN, 59(11), 43–37.

Take Your Skills to the Classroom

SHELLY BURKE

I'd been a staff nurse for a year when my family and I moved back to our small hometown of Genoa, Nebraska. There's just one hospital within commuting distance. They had no vacancies, so I had no luck getting another staff position. Like many nurses today, I worried that I'd have to leave the profession.

To my relief, and surprise, I found that I could continue to practice—just not in the traditional way. Rather, I could capitalize on a skill I'd used as a staff nurse: teaching.

I didn't realize just how many opportunities there were—from teaching clinical concepts and techniques to students and colleagues, to teaching everything from childbirth preparation to cardiopulmonary resuscitation to the general public. Here is a look at a few of the teaching jobs I have explored that may work for you, too. Keep in mind that the earnings cited for each of these opportunities reflects the going rates in my hometown; compensation varies considerably across the country.

● WHO BETTER TO EDUCATE UP-AND-COMING NURSES?

There are about 1,500 basic RN programs, more than 1,000 programs for LPNs,[1] and many, many training programs for certified nursing assistants and care staff members—nursing assistants with additional training that allows them to pass meds. As a result, qualified instructors will always be needed.

Experience and knowledge in the area you plan to teach are key job requirements. Most nursing school faculty are also required to have, or be working towards, an advanced degree. While many faculty members are at least master's-prepared—50% have PhDs[2]—there are openings for BSN-prepared instructors as well.

Teaching options include lecturing in a specialty like med/surg or oncology, supervising student nurses on clinical rotations, or being a skills lab instructor. As a part-time instructor in a program for LPNs, I got to try my hand at two of the three.

I taught an OB class, lecturing about 25 students a semester in six, four-hour sessions.

The author is an independent education consultant for Genoa Community Hospital in Genoa, NE.

The college provided me with textbooks and some old tests, but I had to develop a class—with objectives, handouts, and the like—on my own.

Sometimes, I'd be asked to assist with the med/surg clinical rotation whenever there were too many students for one instructor to supervise. Teaching clinical is a good way to stay involved in hands-on nursing, but it's a big responsibility since you're accountable for your students' actions. I had to be very attuned to their skills and abilities before assigning them to patients.

Since I worked part-time, I was paid $14 an hour for my efforts in the classroom and on rotation. I was also reimbursed at the same rate for the time I spent preparing at home—daily class planning, correcting tests, and so on. I spent almost as much time preparing for classes as I did teaching them.

If you're interested in joining the faculty of a nursing program, consider getting a taste of the work by starting out on a part-time basis. Contact the program's personnel office or the dean of the nursing department to discuss your qualifications and their needs.

● FULL-FLEDGED NURSES REQUIRE INSTRUCTION, TOO

Health care facilities need nurses to teach nurses, too. I offer monthly inservices at a local nursing home, meeting with the staff several weeks before the presentation to discuss educational needs. If there's been an increase in falls, for instance, I'll do an inservice that reviews how to prevent them.

Each inservice usually lasts an hour, and I present it several times a day over a period of two or three days. I'm paid $13 an hour, both for the inservices themselves and the time I spend preparing them.

Although no special training is required to teach inservices, you are expected to have up-to-date knowledge on the topic you're teaching and the skills to teach. You might consider attending workshops offered by your community college or hospital to improve your teaching abilities. It's also a good idea to read up on teaching strategies—such as how to establish objectives or organize your discussions—in the nursing literature.

Contact health care facilities in your area to see if they need inservice providers. If you're a staff nurse, your workplace may already encourage you to present inservices as part of your performance evaluation.[3] This may be the perfect opportunity to explore this realm of teaching.

● USE YOUR SKILLS WITH EXPECTANT PARENTS

Nurses are experienced at teaching patients. Teaching members of the public—like parents-to-be about childbirth—is a natural extension of that role.

Childbirth instructors can be trained in a variety of techniques, such as Lamaze or the Bradley Method. They work for hospitals and physician groups or market their services independently. Opportunities are also available through colleges and universities.

As a certified Lamaze instructor, I've found this work rewarding. For 2½ hours a week over six weeks, I teach eager parents-to-be about such topics as the anatomy and physiology of a pregnant woman, the stages of labor, and strategies for coping with labor and delivery. The connection I make with my students endures even after the series of classes end: Parents I have taught proudly show off their children whenever they see me.

The pay isn't bad, either. At the local community college where I teach, pay for childbirth instructors starts at $11.50 an hour. It then increases 50 cents an hour for every five series of classes taught.

To become a childbirth instructor, you need training and credentials—although requirements will vary depending on the technique you plan to teach. A prospective Lamaze instructor, for example, must participate in a program that takes six to 12 months. You will be required to complete a home-study component and attend a three to four day hands-on seminar. Then you will have to take a certification examination.[4]

For information on how to become a childbirth instructor, contact your local hospital or one of these organizations:

- ASPO/Lamaze, American Society for Psychoprophylaxis in Obstetrics, Inc., 1200 19th Street, NW, Suite 300, Washington, DC 20036; (800) 368-4404.
- The Bradley Method of Natural Childbirth, American Association of Husband-Coached Childbirth, P.O. Box 5224, Sherman Oaks, CA 91413-5224; (800) 4A-BIRTH.
- International Childbirth Education Association, P.O. Box 20048, Minneapolis, MN 55420; (612) 854-8660.

● NURSES, THE PUBLIC: BOTH NEED CPR TRAINING

More than five million people receive CPR training each year[5]—including members of the lay public and nurses who must stay current in CPR as part of their licensure requirements.

Because of this demand, CPR instructors are needed by hospitals, employer-sponsored wellness or health promotion programs, colleges, and community centers. In Genoa, I earn around $12 an hour teaching at the community college.

Course content isn't strictly limited to CPR. Classes generally also cover the anatomy and physiology of the cardiovascular and respiratory systems, healthy living strategies such as diet and exercise, and safety.

Like childbirth instructors, a CPR instructor needs training and credentials. I had to pass an advanced course in CPR and then enroll in and pass an instructors' course. To continue as a CPR instructor, I am required to teach at least one CPR class a year and attend a review class every two years.

While teaching requirements vary by location, ultimately you'll need to pass an instructors' course approved by either the American Heart Association or American Red Cross. For information on courses, contact a local chapter. For the one nearest you, call the AHA at (800) 242-8721 or the Red Cross at (703) 206-7090.

● THE OPPORTUNITIES ARE ENDLESS

If CPR or childbirth education isn't for you, consider checking into your high school or college community education program to see if they need nurse instructors to teach health promotion classes.

You can also explore more specialized teaching opportunities at health care facilities. See if they need a diabetes educator, a cardiac rehab nurse, an enterostomal therapy nurse, or a lactation consultant if you have knowledge in these areas. Ask if instructors are needed to teach classes for children who will be having surgery, for instance, or who have chronically ill siblings. Or, ask if they need a nurse to provide continuing education classes or staff development programs.

To get an idea of the facility's needs, talk to the DON or the education department. Don't be shy about presenting some of your own ideas for classes, too.

● THE PROS AND CONS OF TEACHING

Teaching is a wonderful way to make use of your nursing education while having the flexibility that most traditional nursing jobs don't offer. Many teaching opportunities are part-time. And classes are usually held during the day or evening, with few weekend or holiday commitments.

Another benefit is the variety—both in the kinds of students you instruct and what you teach. One day you may be teaching CPR to a group of people with no health care background; the next, you might be updating fellow nurses on a new standard of care. For each group you'll need to be proficient at altering your teaching style to address the varying needs of your students.

Yet teaching does have its challenges. Your students may not be motivated to learn. Some might say, "I'm taking this CPR class as a job requirement" or "My wife made me come to Lamaze class." It takes persistence and experience to motivate reluctant learners and to give constructive criticism to students who need to improve.

Class size can be another problem. If not enough students sign up, the class may be canceled—frequently with very short notice. Or, if there are too many students, the instructor may have trouble getting her lesson across to each student.

Add up the pluses and minuses, though, and I've found that nurse instructors come out ahead. My advice? Try teaching a class or two: It may open up a whole new career.

REFERENCES

1. National League for Nursing. (1995). *Nursing data review:* 1995 (Pub. No. 19-2686). New York: National League for Nursing Press.
2. Berlin, L.E., Bednash, G.D., & Scott, D.I. (1996). 1995-1996 *Faculty salaries in baccalaureate and graduate programs in nursing.* Washington, DC: American Association of Colleges of Nursing.
3. Inglis, A.D. (1992). Ten commonsense teaching strategies for effective inservice presentation by staff nurses. *Journal of Continuing Education in Nursing, 23*(6), 263.
4. American Society for Psychoprophylaxis in Obstetrics, Inc. (1996). *Excel in your profession.* . . . Washington, DC: Author.
5. American Heart Association. (1996). *Cardiopulmonary Resuscitation (CPR).* Washington, DC: Author.

Never has there been a time when the demand for quality day care has been greater. Increasingly, it is the nurse who is responsible for the health and safety of children in this setting. Day care consulting is a tremendous opportunity for the RN who enjoys working with children in the community setting.

What are some disease prevention and health promotion activities appropriate for day care settings? How does documentation support disease prevention and health promotion activities coordinated by nurses in the day care setting?

Schneider, B. (1996). Day care consulting: It isn't kids' stuff. RN, 59(3), 53–55.

Day Care Consulting: It Isn't Kids' Stuff

BARBARA SCHNEIDER

Never has the demand for quality day care been as great as it is today. More than 60% of women with children under the age of 5 have kids in day care; and that number is expected to increase to 75% by the year 2000.[1,2] The demand could increase still further if states pay for job training and child care to help wean single parents off of welfare.

And if you are an RN, here's one more thing to keep in mind: These societal changes, combined with declining hospital inpatient census, have set the stage for a new and exciting career—day care nurse consulting.

I began my career as a nurse consultant in 1975, just at the point when day care centers began realizing the benefits of hiring RNs to help keep children healthy and safe. Today, some states, including my home state of Washington, actually *require* day care facilities caring for four or more infants under age 1 to employ nursing consultants.

Even though the work may not have the sense of urgency that acute care nursing does, it can literally save lives. Three years ago in Seattle, for example, an *Escherichia coli* epidemic landed more than 100 youngsters in the hospital. Four of the children, including one toddler who died, were in day care at the time they became ill. But because nurse consultants had helped ensure that the day care centers adhered to infection control policies, the spread of the virus was contained and a potential calamity was averted.

If you are a licensed RN and have experience in pediatric or community nursing, or simply have experience raising your own children, you may already be qualified to become a day care nurse consultant. And there's no need to leave—or take—a full-time job to do it: No more than one on-site visit to the day care center is required each month, though depending on what services you contract for, you can spend much more time. (RNs typically charge between $40 and $50 per visit.) You can contract to work one hour a month for one day care center, or more hours with several centers. It's truly a "career" you can shape yourself.

The author is a certified pediatric nurse practitioner in private practice in Bellevue, WA. She has 20 years of experience providing nursing and health services to day care centers.

● PREVENTING DISEASE THROUGH EDUCATION

The first thing I do when I begin consulting for a center is ask to see its health and safety policy. Every center must have a detailed policy covering the admission and exclusion of children, and how such things as illness, infant care, hand washing, diaper changing, cleaning, employee health, care of pets such as gerbils and hamsters, medical emergencies, and first aid are to be handled. I review the policy on a quarterly basis, making adjustments as necessary.

During my monthly visits to the center, I assess and monitor four main areas: child health and safety, staff health, family health, and the health practices of the center itself. If any area isn't up to snuff, I provide the remedial instruction needed to get it there.

I zero in on infection control practices with particular vigor, since without them, disease can run rampant. I teach staff members the basics—why and how to routinely wash their hands and arms after wiping children's noses and changing diapers, the need to clean changing areas, tables, highchairs, and beds with a chlorine solution after each use, and the importance of disinfecting toys in the infant and toddler rooms on a daily basis.

Even with the best of training, however, some children are going to become sick, as will teachers and other staff members on occasion. Working parents who have little or no time off have no other option but to bring their sick children to day care. As a result, influenza, herpes simplex virus, and gastrointestinal diseases—conditions that can become more virulent in adults—are common in this setting.

To keep diseases from spreading, I train staff members in how to assess various symptoms, and which of them warrant a phone call to a parent to remove the child from the center. To make sure staff members aren't the ones spreading disease, I review communicable disease prevention measures, make sure they've been tested for TB, and monitor their personal health. I also make sure that staff members have been certified in first aid and CPR by the American Red Cross or the American Heart Association, so they're prepared for emergencies.

Since disease and accident prevention is important in the home, as well, I educate parents, and respond to any concerns they have. And they have plenty: I field questions on everything from nutrition and growth and development to behavior and seasonal health concerns—this is where the expertise in child rearing or pediatrics really pays off. Some consulting nurses address parents' most common questions and concerns by assembling timely information—such as common illnesses and disease prevention tips—on a monthly bulletin board at the center or in a health newsletter.

● KID-FRIENDLY TEACHING, KID-SPECIFIC CARE

Health education isn't for adults only. A large part of a day care nurse consultant's job is teaching kids—even the very young ones—about physical fitness, personal safety, and hygiene. To help make learning fun, I suggest or acquire materials for educational activities and guest speakers.

Along with teaching the children, I monitor their growth and development, watch how they interact with staff and other kids, and keep track of their immunization status. And because health and nutrition go hand in hand, I make sure they're eating right. I review menus with the day care staff and ensure that meals and snacks include items from the five food groups. I also observe the meals being served to make sure that the portions aren't too big or small.

Knowing *when* to serve meals and snacks is just as important as knowing what to serve.

For example, children who spend three to four hours in day care shouldn't be given a snack less than two hours before the next scheduled meal. A child who attends day care for nine hours or more needs two meals and two snacks. Children who are still at the center after 5 p.m. should receive a third, small snack.

Along with giving health and nutritional advice, some consulting nurses offer "hands-on" health services for an additional fee, such as TB testing for employees, hearing and vision screening of preschool children, and developmental screening.

Still other consulting nurses provide primary care such as well-child exams, school physicals, immunizations, and assessment and treatment of common childhood illnesses. Such "easy access" care is especially welcomed by low-income families and those who have no health insurance or regular health provider. Nurses who perform these services, however, ought to be advanced practice nurses.

● KEEPING TABS ON COMPLIANCE

All day care nurse consultants must document their work in a monthly report that's filed at the center and made available to state health department licensers and inspectors during their periodic or yearly visits. You note each area that you've assessed or monitored, any teaching, suggested policy revisions, or other interventions.

The report is a valuable tool: By calling attention to problem areas, it helps both the nurse and state regulators assess how well a center is complying with its own policies and state health and safety regulations.

One report I filed alerted officials to the fact that at one day care center more than 20 children had been left without adult supervision. That's both unsafe and illegal. (I ended up staying at the center until the situation was corrected.) When a lawsuit was later brought against the center, my report was used as evidence.

● JOBS IN DAY CARE: A LOOK AT THE FUTURE

Although many states now require day care centers to contract with consulting nurses, regulatory control over the centers themselves is weak. In 1992, for example, half of all states had regulations for the licensure of day care centers that did not meet the health and safety standards for out-of-home care set by the American Public Health Association and the American Academy of Pediatrics.[2]

Nurses have a role to play in promoting the health and safety of kids in day care as well as working in the field themselves. RNs have a personal stake in both, considering their commitment to keeping people healthy and the dwindling number of acute care jobs. Here are some steps you can take:

- Work with parents, social and health advocates, and physicians to pass more comprehensive health and safety regulations. Standards should mandate that teachers and center directors meet educational requirements in early childhood education and undergo background checks and fingerprinting by the police.
- Encourage employers to offer day care for their employees' children or to give subsidies to workers to help pay for quality care.
- Lobby city and county governments to subsidize day care centers for low income parents, particularly for single mothers.
- Educate parents on child health and safety by writing articles for newspapers and magazines and public service announcements for radio and television. Volunteer to talk to school and church groups and on local talk shows.

If you love children, want a flexible schedule, and are looking for a chance to apply your clinical knowledge in a community setting, day care nursing may be the ideal career choice. After 20 years in the field, I still enjoy the challenges and rewards it brings, both large and small. Helping others help themselves isn't just a saying—it's a consulting nurse's way of life.

REFERENCES

1. Chira, S. (1992, October 13). Motherhood: It's not like Mrs. Cleaver now. *The (Bellevue, WA) Journal American,* pp. C7.
2. Thacker, S.B., Addiss, D.G., et al. (1992). Infectious diseases and injuries in child day care. *JAMA, 268*(13), 1720.

EXPLORING YOUR OPTIONS

Parish nurses work in conjunction with a congregation and community health providers to deliver holistic nursing care.

What are the roles of the parish nurse? What are the requirements of the position? Where are the employment opportunities? Is parish nursing a good fit for you?

Dunkle, R. M. (1996). Parish nurses help patients—body *and* soul. RN, 59(5), 55–57.

43

Parish Nurses Help Patients—Body *and* Soul

ROSENE M. DUNKLE

How to make health care more accessible? It's a tremendous challenge, and one that nurses and doctors alike have spent a great deal of time wrestling with in recent years.

One solution that has slowly emerged over the past few years is parish nursing, where RNs work in conjunction with a congregation and community health providers to deliver holistic nursing care. Parish nursing is a logical way to provide accessible care when you consider that more than 65% of Americans have a formal membership in a church or synagogue, and about 40% attend some sort of weekly service.[1]

This career path, however, is still the one less traveled. In 1994, there were only 2,500 parish nurses in various churches—and synagogues—across the country.[2] But the concept is relatively new, created just 12 years ago by a Lutheran minister who felt that congregations could play a larger role in health promotion and disease prevention.[3]

And that's just what parish nurses do. They provide information on healthy life-styles and ways to prevent illness. But they also focus on meeting patients' psychosocial and spiritual needs. Schedules are flexible, with most parish nurses working between 16 and 20 hours a week and making themselves available to congregation members between and after services.[3] They also keep regular office hours at the church and make hospital, home, and nursing home visits when necessary.

Contrary to what you might think, however, parish nurses aren't always employed by the church. Some work for a hospital and contract their work out to local congregations, while others work for both a hospital and a church that have come together in a collaborative effort.

Pay arrangements vary. Approximately 60% of parish nurses work as volunteers and receive money for gas, continuing education, and medical supplies.[4] The remaining 40% earn, on average, $30,000–$35,000 a year if they're employed by a hospital, $22,000–$25,000 if they're employed by a religious congregation.[5]

The author is an on-call, part-time resident nurse at the Willow Valley Lakes Manor nursing home in Willow Street, PA. This article is based on her extensive research in the field of parish nursing.

● HOW A PARISH NURSE PROVIDES HOLISTIC CARE

Parishioners, who have either met the parish nurse at church functions, or heard about her through the church bulletin, seek out the parish nurse to discuss a broad spectrum of issues—everything from the side effects of a new medication to coping with growing old.

Helping these parishioners requires the nurse to assume a variety of roles, including that of educator, referral agent, volunteer coordinator, and overall troubleshooter.

Educator. The majority of a parish nurse's time is spent teaching her patients. She may, for example, review discharge instructions with a patient recently released from a hospital, explain the potential side effects of a medication, or describe what's involved in a particular diagnostic test. She may also teach—one-on-one or in a class—preventive care, such as how to protect against skin cancer or reduce the risks of heart disease.

If enough patients ask questions about such health issues as their blood pressure or cholesterol, a parish nurse may organize a health fair—to cover a variety of health issues.

Referral Agent. The parish nurse offers parishioners health care options they may not have known existed. For example, one nurse learned of a parishioner who was driving an hour to a health care facility for physical therapy sessions. The nurse gave her the name and phone number of a physical therapist who was just 15 minutes away.

The parish nurse makes other referrals as well, to shelters in cases of domestic violence and to support groups, like Overeaters and Alcoholics Anonymous. And, when a needed resource doesn't exist, a parish nurse is likely to establish one.

After hearing several parishioners complain about the effects of old age, for example, one of my colleagues started a support group specifically for senior citizens. This group meets periodically to talk about common health problems, such as hip replacements and cataracts, and to share effective coping strategies.

In other cases the need for support is of a spiritual nature. To help parishioners deal with chronic illnesses, for example, some parish nurses coordinate "healing services" where parishioners can attain spiritual peace by praying in a group.

Volunteer Coordinator. To augment her efforts, the parish nurse frequently organizes volunteers to provide parishioners with things like transportation, meals, baby-sitting services, and respite care. Some volunteers even help fellow parishioners fill out Medicare and insurance forms.

To get volunteers out into the community, the nurse selects willing and qualified community members and trains them. She also acts as their clinical resource when questions arise.

Volunteers can make a tremendous difference, as one colleague of mine found. This nurse was concerned about an elderly woman who lived alone and had been sent home for two weeks of rest after triple coronary bypass graft surgery. The nurse rounded up some volunteers to do the elderly woman's housework and cooking and to pick up her medications from the pharmacy. The work of these volunteers made a full recovery possible.

Troubleshooter. In this role, the parish nurse helps prevent patients from "falling through the cracks." At the most basic level, this means loaning out (and teaching the proper use of) things like crutches and wheelchairs to patients who, for financial or other reasons, might not otherwise obtain them. Many parish nurses keep such supplies in their offices.

Sometimes, the troubleshooting is a bit trickier, requiring the parish nurse to take on the role of patient advocate. I remember one instance in particular when a parishioner sought help from a local health care facility for severe abdominal pain. She was told it would be more than a week before she could get a CT scan—and a diagnosis. When she told me of her predicament, I recommended another facility and helped her get an appointment there the next day. (It was a good thing, too, since the scan revealed she needed immediate surgery.)

At still other times, troubleshooting requires the parish nurse to play detective. One nurse was called to the home of an elderly widow who was complaining that her pain medications weren't working as well as they used to. After spending some time talking with her, the nurse examined the medications and found many of them outdated. She disposed of them, helped set up a doctor's appointment, and arranged for the new drugs to be delivered to the patient's home.

Whatever the role she's filling at the moment, the parish nurse is careful to document the care she provides and the referrals she makes, just like a nurse in a traditional setting would do. But, unlike those in more traditional settings, the parish nurse brings to each of her roles the freedom to read from the Bible and pray with her patients.

● HOW TO QUALIFY FOR THE JOB

To become a parish nurse, a candidate must be licensed in the state, have at least two years of nursing experience, and have liability insurance. Coverage is a must because, even though parish nurses don't do invasive procedures, they do give advice and suggest interventions.

Also a must: knowledge of holistic health philosophy and the congregation's health ministry statement, which outlines the parameters in which the parish nurse can provide care to parishioners. She must also be familiar with community resources, including shelters, support groups, and hot lines.

Though it isn't necessary for employment, nurses committed to parish work may want to expand their background in the holistic and spiritual aspects of the job through seminars or courses for credit from local colleges, universities, and seminaries. Marquette University in Wisconsin, for example, offers an eight-day program worth 5.4 continuing education units on parish nursing, while Loyola University in Illinois offers a dual nursing/divinity masters degree program. Some hospitals also offer parish nurse programs.

● JOB OPPORTUNITIES: THEY'RE UP TO YOU

While some institutions and churches publicly advertise for parish nurse positions, the majority are created by individuals who approach a congregation or health care facility with a proposal outlining the need for such a program and how it can be implemented.

But whether a nurse gets the job through an ad, or through the proposal process, she'll need at least a brief training period with the spiritual leaders of the church or synagogue where she'll be working. If the nurse is filling an existing position, the nurse who's leaving will probably show her the ropes. However, if it's a new position, the nurse will need to work with the pastor or rabbi to establish the program.

Once she's on her own, the parish nurse meets on a weekly or monthly basis with the leader of the congregation to keep him abreast of her activities and to talk about concerns and new ideas. This holds true for all parish nurses—whether they're employed by a congregation, hospital, or both. Those with ties to a hospital, however, must also report regularly to their nursing supervisor.

Resources for Parish Nurses

The National Parish Nurse Resource Center
205 West Touhy Avenue
Suite 104
Park Ridge, IL 60068
(800) 556-5368
This group offers documentation and assessment tools, videos and a curriculum for parish nurse education. (Prices are listed in the center's *Catalog of Resources*.)
The Health Ministries Association
P.O. Box 7853
Huntington Beach, CA 92646
(800) 852-5613
(714) 965-0085
Nearly 30 chapters across the country provide information—including how to start a new program—and networking opportunities. Membership in the association is on an individual congregational or institutional basis.
The International Network for Interfaith Health Practices
Saint Francis Hospital
355 Ridge Avenue
Evanston, IL 60202
(708) 316-4040
E-mail: Interaccess.com/ihpnet
This electronic forum lists job openings and provides networking and training opportunities. The network is accessible through an E-mail gateway to the internet that's available through several on-line services. If you don't have internet access, phone or write to Dennis Fey, manager of congregational relations at the number above.

For additional support, the parish nurse can also turn to such groups as the National Parish Nurse Resource Center, the Health Ministries Association, and the International Network for Interfaith Health Practices [see display].

Clearly, parish nursing is still an emerging career option, but it's one alternative that's already proven to be both professionally and personally rewarding. It's also one that makes accessible health care a reality—a boon to patients trying to navigate today's complex health care system.

REFERENCES

1. Moore, D.W. (1995). Most Americans say religion is important to them. *Gallup Poll Monthly, 353,* 16.
2. Solari-Twadell, A., McDermott, M.A., et al. (Eds.). (1994). *Assuring viability for the future: Guideline development for parish nurse education programs.* Park Ridge, IL: The National Parish Nurse Resource Center.
3. Schank, M.J., Weis, D., & Matheus, R. (1996). Parish nursing: Ministry of healing. *Geriatric Nursing, 17*(1), 11.
4. Lloyd, R.C., & Solari-Twadell, A. (1994). Organizational framework, functions and educational preparation of parish nurses: A comparison of national survey results. In *Proceedings of the Eighth Annual Westberg symposium* (pp. 107–115). Park Ridge, IL: The National Parish Nurse Resource Center.
5. Djupe, A.M., Lantz, J.C., et al. (1994). *Reaching out: Parish nursing services—An institutional/ congregational partnership.* Park Ridge, IL: National Parish Nurse Resource Center.

An infinite number of volunteer opportunities are available to nursing students. Most are in community settings caring for the underserved. These opportunities often provide valuable clinical experiences for students.

What are some of the benefits of volunteering? What are some volunteer opportunities in your community? What volunteer opportunities would allow you to explore areas of nursing that are unfamiliar to you? Which volunteer opportunities would expand your clinical expertise?

Savage, N., Ryan, M. T., & Hieber, K. (1996). Nursing on your own time. RN, 59 (7), 47–50.

Nursing on Your Own Time

NANCY SAVAGE, MARJORIE THIEL RYAN, KATHERINE HIEBER

Joe is a regular visitor to the Southwestern Ohio Nurses Association (SONA) Nurses Clinic in inner-city Cincinnati. The 43-year-old has hypertension. He's come in today to get his blood pressure checked and to talk to a nurse about how he's been feeling. When it's his turn, he sits down, pulls out a card containing his weekly BP record for the past month, and proudly hands it to the nurse.

Joe's condition in and of itself is not noteworthy. Nor is the treatment prescribed by his doctor: An antihypertensive and a low-salt diet. What is significant is that he comes to the clinic for follow-up care on a regular basis.

You see, Joe is homeless. And if it weren't for the clinic, which occupies a small room in The Drop-Inn Center homeless shelter where he stays intermittently, Joe probably wouldn't be so conscientious.

For Joe, and the handful of other homeless people who visit the clinic every Wednesday, basic health care is just a short walk down the hall to a place where being homeless is nothing to be embarrassed about and where the nurses take the time to get to know their patients.

Patients like Joe are lucky. They're not the only ones: The nurses who care for them—all volunteers—feel lucky too.

Many feel a tremendous sense of satisfaction knowing that they can provide direct patient care to those who sorely need it. It's a refreshing change for many hospital nurses who spend countless hours away from the bedside coordinating fragmented patient care. For others—educators like us—the work provides a chance to step outside of academia, roll up our sleeves, and get to the business of helping people directly.

All of us, however, share a single satisfaction in knowing that we're meeting a community need, one that, until a year-and-a-half ago, was going largely unmet.

Nancy Savage is an associate professor at the College of Nursing and Health, University of Cincinnati. Marjorie Thiel Ryan and Katherine Hieber are, respectively, associate and assistant professor, in the department of nursing at Miami University, in Oxford, OH. All are volunteers at the SONA Nurses Clinic.

● A SPECIAL POPULATION IN NEED OF HELP

Cincinnati, like most major cities across the country, has a large homeless community—more than 200,000 people, by some estimates.[1] Sadly, a large number of these people don't get any health care, either because they're ashamed to admit that they're homeless, or because they fear they'll be treated with a lack of respect and dignity.[2]

It was to fill this need that a VA nurse who worked with homeless veterans at The Drop-Inn Center contacted SONA three years ago. She suggested that the association establish a clinic there. The idea was that SONA nurses would provide basic supportive and preventive care.

The SONA Human Rights Committee picked up the ball and ran with it. The shelter administrators eagerly embraced the concept and the committee. The committee established three initial goals: Obtain space at the shelter for the clinic, acquire the necessary funds and supplies, and recruit volunteer nurses.

The shelter provided a small room with a sink in a remodeled area of the building for the clinic to operate from. It afforded privacy for patients and hand-washing facilities for volunteers.

The committee obtained funding and supplies through several sources. SONA contributed start-up funds to purchase supplies ranging from stethoscopes and latex gloves to loose-leaf binders. The association also provided a storage cabinet and sweat shirts and T-shirts with the SONA logo and the slogan "Nurses Care."

Individual SONA members donated more supplies and the Procter & Gamble Fund responded to a committee request with a check for $1,000. Though efforts to obtain funding are ongoing, SONA provides for any shortfall in the nursing clinic's small budget.

The committee enlisted volunteers through SONA's newsletter and at membership meetings. When all was said and done, 12 of us volunteered. The committee turned over the rest of the organizational tasks to us volunteers—stipulating only that we each had to have our own liability insurance that covered our volunteer work, and that the nursing tasks we would perform had to fall within the scope of the Ohio Nurse Practice Act. That's especially important since the nursing clinic has no direct physician involvement.

● ORGANIZING RESOURCES WITH SECURITY IN MIND

The clinic is located in a high crime area where drug deals and shootings are common occurrences. So safety was a major factor in many of our decisions.

For one, we decided it was best not to dispense over-the-counter drugs at the clinic. Not only were we concerned about liability, but we didn't want the clinic to be perceived as a place to get drugs—OTC or otherwise. As an added measure, we decided to make a point of telling patients that there were no drugs in the clinic.

Other security measures we took include keeping supplies in a locked cabinet and holding office hours only during the daylight—every Wednesday from 4 p.m. to 6 p.m.—when there's more activity on the streets. Working on the safety-in-numbers theory, we decided to have two nurses at the clinic at any given time.

● THE SONA NURSES CLINIC OPENS ITS DOORS

We opened for business on November 9, 1994 to serve the homeless men and women who stay at the shelter. The male residents of a non-medical, substance abuse treatment program housed at the shelter were also welcome at the clinic.

Since the beginning, the clinic has served a steady stream of patients. We typically see between two and 17 people each week with a wide range of health problems—we get everything from headaches and toothaches to diabetes, hypertension, and psychiatric disorders.

The care we give is by no means high-tech. The bulk of our time is spent on nursing basics: taking histories, conducting physical exams, teaching about diet and medications, providing psychosocial support, making referrals to area clinics and hospitals, and documenting care.

Still, the work is immensely rewarding—especially considering how many of these people might fall through the cracks of the health care system without our help.

Take Katie. She was young and four months pregnant when she visited the clinic and described the trouble she was having getting prenatal care. Because she was on Medicaid, she needed a medical card to see a physician. But she couldn't get a card without seeing a physician first. To get her foot in the door, the nurse referred Katie to the public health clinic where she could finally see a physician and get the care she needed.

Not all of our patients are like Katie. A rare few already have health care providers, but they visit our clinic anyway. Some come by to see whether the symptoms they're experiencing warrant a trip to their physician. Others see us between doctor appointments to keep an eye on health problems that are worrisome to them.

That was the case with Pete, who was already on antihypertensive medication when he came in for a blood pressure check. It was a good thing he did—his BP was 160/110. The nurse told him that he couldn't wait the five days until his scheduled appointment with his physician. She urged him to call the doctor and report the reading immediately. Her sense of urgency impressed him; Pete saw his physician that day and got a new prescription.

Finally, there are the patients who just want someone to talk to. Mary, an outgoing, middle-aged woman who has bipolar disorder, frequently stops by the clinic to talk with the nurses. She tells us that she'd rather talk to us than to the other residents of the shelter because she trusts us. Talking with us, she says, makes her feel calm.

● WORK AT THE CLINIC HAS ITS SHARE OF DILEMMAS

Just because we provide basic care doesn't mean we don't face problems. Take the frustrating case of Tammy, who'd had a seizure in the shelter. When the nurse got to her, she found her fairly alert with elevated vital signs. Tammy told the nurse that she'd been discharged from the hospital recently where they'd started her on anticonvulsant medication.

The nurse told Tammy that she needed to return to the hospital right away for re-evaluation, but Tammy refused. The nurse tried again to convince her to get help, emphasizing her health risks, but to no avail. Tammy refused to seek further medical attention and left the shelter.

Though that nurse did all she could, the situation was a good reminder to us all of how important it is to explain to our patients the risks of not seeking treatment, to accept the fact that they have a right to refuse care, and to document this refusal.

Jim, a man in his 70s, presented a different kind of dilemma. He came into the clinic on a cold winter day, shoeless and limping. After determining that Jim was not ill—just very cold—a nurse gave Jim a pair of new socks and asked his shoe size. Discovering that Jim wore the same size as he did, the nurse asked if Jim would accept a pair of shoes that he no longer needed. Jim agreed, the nurse made a trip home and soon returned with the pair of shoes. That patient left with warm feet.

Did the nurse's actions foster codependency in the patient? The nurse doesn't think so: Jim's feet were freezing; there was no other practical way for him to get shoes that day; giving Jim the shoes was simply the humane thing to do.

● OUR EFFORTS CONTINUE; SHOULD YOURS BEGIN?

Clearly, the Jims of the world have a tremendous impact on us: They bring out our very best and renew our faith that the care we provide makes a difference.

Our experience at the clinic has been so rewarding—and well received by our patients and the shelter administration—that we're planning to expand it. At the request of the female residents of the shelter, we're developing a women's health program. We may also offer additional services to the residents of the substance abuse treatment program.

If our efforts remind you of why you got into nursing in the first place—or of how long it's been since you felt the satisfaction we've described—why not consider volunteer work yourself. Call your local nurses association and ask whether they run a nursing clinic. If they don't, contact a shelter in your area to see if they need a volunteer nurse. You could also volunteer at an HIV-clinic or a local school.

Volunteer work needn't eat up too much of your time. (Each of us works once a month.) In return, you'll rediscover the passion you once felt for nursing. Our experience has given us immense fulfillment, which we bring to our daily jobs and carry in our hearts.

REFERENCES

1. Greater Cincinnati Coalition for the Homeless. (1993). *Homelessness in Greater Cincinnati in 1993: A summary of the report.* Cincinnati: Author.
2. Plumb, J.D., McManus, P., & Carson, L. (1996, March). A collaborative community approach to homeless care. In R.L. Perkel and R.C. Wender (Eds.), *Primary care: Models of ambulatory care* (pp. 17–30). Philadelphia: W. B. Saunders Company.

EXPLORING YOUR OPTIONS
....

Do you enjoy the intensity and immediacy of nursing care depicted in the popular medical emergency television series? If so, flight nursing may be for you.

What are the requirements of flight nurse positions? What are the primary roles of the nurse in flight nursing? What clinical skills are essential?

Semonin-Holleran, R. (1996). These nurses take flight. RN, 59 (9), 57–60.

45

These Nurses Take Flight

RENE SEMONIN-HOLLERAN

"Air Care One, respond to the scene of a truck rollover with multiple victims."

Hearing that page, the flight nurse runs to the ED, grabs two units of O-negative blood, a bag of Mannitol, and several bags of warm IV fluids, then proceeds to the helipad. The BK117 is already running. Once the flight team is secured on board, the helicopter lifts off the rooftop and heads to the site of the accident.

Sound like a scene out of M*A*S*H? Well, in a way it is. Except in this case the injured aren't soldiers but civilians. And the setting isn't a war zone but a busy state highway, a rugged mountainside, or an open field miles away from any hospital.

Nurses have been flying to the aid of patients for more than 60 years. Flight nursing began with the inception of the Emergency Flight Corps in 1933, but it really gained acceptance during the Korean and Vietnam Wars when the care and transport of wounded soldiers in aircraft became more common.

The use of air ambulances for civilians began in 1972, when the first hospital-based helicopter program was created in Denver to increase access to the surrounding mountainous areas.[1,2] Today there are approximately 225 hospital-based flight programs throughout the United States.[3] Most of them have made nurses an integral part of their operation.[4]

● A VIRTUAL HOSPITAL IN THE SKY

The medical personnel on the flight crew varies from program to program, but the majority of teams are comprised of a nurse and a paramedic.[4] Other combinations include two nurses, a nurse and a physician, or a nurse and a respiratory therapist.

Flight teams attend to patients in airplanes when traveling long distances, but more commonly they ride in helicopters, which can access difficult-to-reach areas. Each aircraft

The author is chief flight nurse with University Air Care at the University of Cincinnati Hospital in Cincinnati, and president of the Emergency Nurses Association.

is outfitted with battery-operated, light-weight equipment, including infusion pumps, defibrillators, intra-aortic balloon pumps, cardiac monitors, and ventilators. Such portable equipment makes it possible to transport any patient over short and long distances.

Some of the patients are relatively stable; they're flown from referring hospitals to distant facilities that are better equipped to treat them. But most airlifted patients are severely ill or injured. They need to get to the hospital the quickest way possible—and they need skilled health care professionals to keep them alive until they do.

● CAREGIVER, SAFETY GUARD, COMFORTER, TEACHER

When the aircraft arrives on the scene, the flight nurse assists EMS personnel with hands-on care or triage if necessary. Depending on the situation and the nurse's skills and training, this may require some unconventional techniques—say, rappelling down a mountainside.

Once the patient is stable enough to be evacuated, it's up to the nurse to ensure his safety on board—that means securing him appropriately in the cabin. A sick or injured child, for example, would be placed in a car bed or a car seat.

Once in flight, the nurse continuously assesses the patient, monitoring his airway, breathing, and circulation with a pulse oximeter, cardiac monitor, or end-tidal CO_2 monitor if he's intubated. As a matter of course, she checks that all the equipment is functioning properly. And, as needed, she performs a range of interventions, such as cricothyroidotomy, administering medication and blood transfusions, or applying devices such as external pacemakers.

The ability to anticipate problems is key. Depending on the length of the flight and the severity of the patient's condition, the nurse may elect to intubate the patient if he's having trouble breathing. Or she may choose to use physical or chemical restraints on a patient who's becoming agitated.

She also tries to keep the patient comfortable—using blankets and warm IV fluids when he's cold, for instance, and providing protection for his ears from the noise of the aircraft.

Once at the hospital, the flight nurse turns the patient over to the receiving health care team. Then it's usually back to the base to prepare for another flight.

When she's not on call, the flight nurse spends a great deal of her time educating. She teaches EMS providers and personnel from affiliated facilities how to safely approach an aircraft, signal the aircraft, or set up a landing area. Sometimes she teaches continuing education courses on topics such as how to treat a stroke patient.

The flight nurse also preaches prevention to community groups. For instance, our program conducts "Prom Drills" at local high schools in collaboration with area fire departments. We simulate a car crash and then demonstrate how rescue and care efforts would be undertaken. We also speak with the students about the importance of always wearing their seat belts, and of not driving under the influence of drugs or alcohol.

● THE DIFFICULTIES OF NURSING IN THE AIR

Just as in other fields of nursing, there are some unique challenges to the practice of flight nursing. Noise, vibrations, and lack of light hinder your ability to assess and monitor the patient. To compensate, you must rely more heavily on your observation skills, on palpation, and on the equipment on board.

Being in flight also exposes you to high levels of physical stress, including hypoxia, fatigue, and dehydration.[5] The team may also experience some emotional strain, especially when a patient dies during transport.[6]

To cope, you must be able to recognize the signs and symptoms of stress, and know how to relieve it. Supplying extra oxygen at high altitudes to relieve hypoxia, or doing deep breathing exercises to ease tension are just a few of the remedies. But there's still no escaping the fact that these flights are high-pressure situations.

● ARE YOU QUALIFIED FOR THE JOB?

There are no national standards for becoming a flight nurse, and those established by individual programs vary. However, there are some general requirements; one of the most important is experience. Flight nurses must be able to make rapid comprehensive assessments, reach quick conclusions, and initiate critical interventions—all of which come with experience.

Exactly how *much* experience is necessary varies. But one study of 80 flight programs gives some idea of the kind of preparation needed: A third of the flight nurses had 10 to 15 years experience as an RN.[4]

Flight nurses generally have training in advanced cardiac life support (ACLS) and pediatric advanced life support (PALS). Some states also require that they take an emergency medical technician or a prehospital nursing course.

Certification in a nursing specialty, such as emergency or critical care nursing, is desirable too. Most flight nurses are CCRNs or CENs with salaries that are commensurate with these specialties. (At my hospital, flight nurses generally earn about $40,000–$45,000.) Some are also certified flight registered nurses (CFRNs). But the majority take this exam only after they've been nursing in the air for a while.

Flight nurses must also have demonstrated clinical skills in a variety of areas—basic and advanced airway management, vascular access, and cardiac monitoring, to name a few. And they need to be familiar with the nurse practice act in the states in which they practice or fly across so that they know whether they have the authority to perform certain procedures. In some states, for example, nurses aren't allowed to insert chest tubes or perform surgical cricothyrotomies.

In addition to having the necessary patient care skills, many flight programs have weight and physical requirements that ensure that the flight nurse can handle the physical demands of the job (the box lists some of these). The geographic location of the program, the size of the aircraft, and the types of patients transported determine what sorts of physical requirements are in place.

● GETTING YOUR WINGS AS A FLIGHT NURSE

If the idea of providing care in the air appeals to you and you have the necessary skills and training, see if there's a program in your area. While the vast majority are hospital-based, some services operate under the auspices of the military, local municipalities, or police departments.

You will probably be required to go through some additional training to meet the specific requirements of the flight program. So, do some further reading. I've written and edited two books on the subject: *Flight Nursing Principles and Practice* and *Prehospital Nursing: A Collaborative Approach* (St. Louis: Mosby Year Book).

Also, take courses that apply directly to flight nursing. Such courses are offered by the

How Flight Nurses Shape up

Researchers who surveyed 134 hospital-based flight programs found a number of uniform physical requirements. In most cases, flight nurses were required to:

- Meet provisions of the FAA Class III physical exam, which includes the ability to hear a whispered voice at three feet, a visual acuity of 20/30, and no history of psychiatric disease, epilepsy, cardiovascular disease, hypoglycemia, or other ailments that could interfere with the nurse's performance of her duties.
- Report to work in a mentally alert state and be able to cope with the stress of working outside the walls of the hospital.
- Have an annual audiogram.
- Be able, with one partner to carry a stretcher loaded with 100 pounds.
- Perform chest compressions for five minutes in the aircraft.
- Wear the seat belts installed in the aircraft.
- If pregnant, obtain written medical clearance to perform as a member of the crew.

Source: Wraa, C., & O'Malley, B. (1992). Flight nurse physical requirements. *Journal of Air Medical Transport, 11*(10), 17.

U.S. Department of Transportation, the National Flight Nurses Association, and the Emergency Nurses Association.

As a flight nurse, don't expect all of your shifts to be filled with nonstop action. Some days you'll have back-to-back flights, but on other days you'll sit around waiting for your pager to sound. Overall, though, flight nursing is one of the most demanding jobs a nurse can have, and one of the most exhilarating. It gives you the opportunity to soar—in more ways than one.

REFERENCES

1. Lee, G. (1987). History of flight nursing. *J. Emerg. Nurs., 13*(4), 212.
2. Sheehy, S.B. (1995). Flight nursing update: The evolution of air medical transport. *J. Emerg. Nurs., 21*(2), 146.
3. *Association of Air Medical Services.* (1995). Pasadena, CA: Association of Air Medical Services.
4. Bader, G.B., Terhorst, M., et al. (1995). Characteristics of flight nursing practice. *Air Medical Journal, 14*(4), 214.
5. Brown, L., Bodenstedt, R., et al. (1987). The nine stresses of flight. *J. Emerg. Nurs., 13*(4), 232.
6. Andersen, C.A. (1987). Preparing patients for aeromedical transport. *J. Emerg. Nurs., 13*(4), 229.

Index

Page numbers followed by *f* indicate figures; *t* following a page number indicates tabular material.